Health Care
fraud *and*
abuse

A Physician's Guide to Compliance

Second Edition

Hoyt Torras

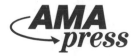

Health Care Fraud and Abuse

A Physician's Guide to Compliance, Second Edition

© 2003 by the American Medical Association
All rights reserved.
Printed in the United States of America.

Internet address: www.ama-assn.org

Additional copies of this book may be ordered by calling 800 621-8335.
Mention product number OP083503.

ISBN 1-57947-353-9

Library of Congress Cataloging-in-Publication Data

Torras, Hoyt W.
   Health care fraud and abuse : a physician's guide to com-
pliance / Hoyt Torras. — 2nd ed.
      p. ; cm.
   Includes bibliographical references and index.
   ISBN 1-57947-353-9
   1. Insurance, Health—Law and legislation—United States—
Criminal provisions. 2. Medical care—Corrupt practices—United
States. I. Title.
   [DNLM: 1. Delivery of Health Care—legislation & jurisprudence
—United States. 2. Ethics, Medical—United States. 3. Fraud
—United States. 4. Insurance, Health—legislation &
jurisprudence—United States. W 32.5 AA1 T688h 2003]
   KF3605.T67 2003
   345.73'0263—dc21

2002015294

BP41:02-P-048:12/02

Preface

The first edition of *Health Care Fraud and Abuse* was published in early 2001. That edition was written shortly after release of the Office of Inspector General's Compliance Program Guidance for Individual and Small Group Physician Practices on September 25, 2000. Since that time, the government has released new information that medical practices need to ensure compliance; and, the authors have developed new insights and tools to help readers improve their compliance efforts.

The authors have also become more convinced that a properly designed compliance program will help improve the results of the coding, billing, and accounts receivable management processes in most physicians' offices. Compliance does not have to be another administrative impediment to achieving a smooth running medical practice focused on patient care.

We continue to believe that the vast majority of physicians are making an honest attempt to comply with very complex laws and guidelines while they attend to patients' medical needs. The examples of fraudulent billing activities that make media headlines are usually so blatant that most physicians cannot envision themselves being involved in such obviously illegal schemes. However, the reimbursement system is so complex that billing errors can occur, even in well-managed and well-intentioned practices. Thus, physicians should understand what actions need to be taken to keep compliance risks low. There are many relatively easy steps physicians can take to reduce and manage their compliance risks.

Obvious fraudulent schemes are clearly illegal and are not the focus of this book. Rather, this book is written to help physicians identify and avoid situations where compliance implications are not as obvious and where errors could occur. There are many misconceptions that can increase compliance risks or cause unnecessary worry, expense, and even loss of income.

Health Care Fraud and Abuse is written to help physicians:

1 Understand the implications of the fraud and abuse laws in their day-to-day practice.

2 Identify areas where violations could occur in their practice.

3 Determine what steps they should consider and take to minimize exposure and ensure compliance.

Every physician should know: Who is making sure the information checked on internal billing forms is transferred properly to insurance claims filed with Medicare and other payers? Who makes sure the practice's computer is processing information correctly? Who is keeping up and ensuring compliance with changes in reimbursement and coding guidelines impacting one's practice? What are the practice's real compliance risks and how are the risks best managed?

Health Care Fraud and Abuse covers effective compliance actions that even the smallest practice can afford to implement as well as those concerns that the largest groups must address. This book provides numerous examples of potentially illegal activities, permissible arrangements, and where to go for information (including Internet sites) that will help physicians and their staff effectively manage their compliance risks.

Chapters 1 and 2 include an introduction to fraud and abuse; definitions of and the distinction between fraud and abuse; examples of recent government fraud and abuse initiatives; statistics; and examples of potentially improper billing activities and possible government targets for the future.

Chapters 3 through 5 provide a summary of federal laws commonly used to prosecute alleged instances of fraud in criminal proceedings, levy civil monetary penalties, or exclude physicians and others from participation in government health care programs. These chapters also emphasize the risks under antikickback laws and Stark I and II.

Chapters 6 through 8 discuss the role of Medicare carriers, state Medicaid Agencies, and various federal law enforcement agencies; prepayment computer edits; prepayment and post-payment audits; how physicians are targeted for an audit; tips for surviving an audit; physicians' appeal rights to adverse audit findings and claim denials; medical services denied for lack of medical necessity; non-covered vs denials for lack of "medical necessity"; Advance Beneficiary Notification waiver forms; documentation that demonstrates medical necessity; reviews; and hearings.

Chapter 9 includes ways to minimize chances of an audit, including self-auditing to detect any problems early enough to take corrective action.

Chapters 10 and 11 discuss the CPT® and ICD-9 coding systems from the perspective of compliance; where coding problems are most likely to occur; techniques for avoiding errors; bundling edits; The Medicare Correct Coding Policy Manual; common situations where Medicare coding and reimbursement rules differ from those of private payers; and how best to "describe" the patient encounter accurately by using code (from a billing perspective).

Chapters 12 through 14 are devoted to compliance programs; what is required by law; the essential elements of a compliance program; developing an effective compliance program; how to respond if an error or impropriety is identified; coding and billing reviews; legal analyses; items that should be included in a written compliance plan; tips for handling compliance efforts in smaller medical practices; kicking off a compliance program and keeping it going; and the recently released Office of Inspector General Compliance Program Guidance for Individual and Small Group Physician Practices.

Appendix A provides more examples of governmental actions against physicians and other health care professionals.

Appendix B discusses how (and when) to request an advisory opinion from the government on planned activities that could represent a compliance issue.

Appendix C is the *OIG Compliance Program Guidance for Individual and Small Group Physician Practices* released September 25, 2000.

Acknowledgments

Health Care Fraud and Abuse was written with the assistance of MAG Mutual HealthCare Consultants, Inc (MMHCI). MAG Mutual Healthcare Consultants, Inc is a subsidiary of MAG Mutual Insurance Company, a company headquartered in Georgia and owned by its physician policyholders.

MMHCI is a full-service medical practice management consulting firm with specialized expertise in health care fraud and abuse. Its staff includes attorneys experienced in fraud and abuse, former Medicare hearing officers, auditors, and instructors in educational programs on coding, billing, and compliance. MMHCI consultants assist physicians, their legal counsel, and others to prepare for audits, develop appeals, implement cost-effective compliance programs that prevent improper billing, and meet mandated compliance requirements imposed by government enforcement agencies as part of fraud or abuse settlements.

MMHCI acknowledges its appreciation to the staff of the American Medical Association who assisted in this project including Marsha Mildred, Shelley Benson, Katharine Dvorak, Rosalyn Carlton, Ronnie Summers, and Boon Ai Tan.

MMHCI also expresses its appreciation to the MAG Mutual Board of Directors, including those who are AMA Delegates: William C. Collins, MD; Alva L. Mayes, Jr., MD; Jack F. Menendez, MD; and Roy W. Vandiver, MD (Chairman of MAG Mutual Board). The MAG Mutual Board and Tom Gose, President and Chief Operating Officer, encouraged MMHCI during the original project and this revision to "do whatever is necessary to provide physicians the information they need to manage their compliance risks."

James R. Lyle, President
Rodney Benefield, Publications Manager
MAG Mutual HealthCare Consultants, Inc.

Contents

Introduction: Health Care Fraud and Abuse

In recent years, the federal government and many state governments have become very aggressive in identifying and prosecuting health care professionals and entities suspected of what is commonly referred to as fraud and abuse. During this period, the government has increased funding and personnel devoted to fraud and abuse detection and prosecution. Recent legislation—most notably the Health Insurance Portability and Accountability Act of 1996 (HIPAA) and various state efforts—has expanded fraud and abuse statutes, even to nongovernmental health care programs. The government is also performing more random audits to detect improper payments and inappropriate activity, rather than simply targeting so-called outliers.

It is easy for the public to get the impression that many physicians are billing inappropriately: some media publicity makes it sound like most health care professionals are billing fraudulently; some private attorneys openly solicit—and offer to pay "bounties" to—patients and employees for reporting possible fraudulent activities; and the government issues fraud alerts that could be misinterpreted by the elderly and others.

No one is quarreling with the need to identify and prosecute those who bill fraudulently, because it hurts everyone. However, the vast majority of physicians are making an honest attempt to comply with very complex laws and guidelines while they attend to patients' medical needs. Honest mistakes by physicians are no more indicative of fraudulent billing than a carrier's failure to issue a correct payment in response to a clean health insurance claim form is indicative of fraud on the government's part.

In an environment of increasing public concern over health care fraud and expanded enforcement efforts, many medical practices are establishing formal compliance programs to prevent, detect, and correct possible deficiencies. In fact, the government has indicated that the presence of an effective compliance program that is designed to prevent inappropriate billing practices might mitigate ultimate fines and penalties in the event of a fraud or abuse action. Mandatory compliance programs, called corporate integrity agreements, typically are part of fraud and abuse settlements.

Although most physicians and other health care professionals are making an honest attempt to bill appropriately, it certainly makes sense for them to assess their situation and adopt reasonable compliance efforts to keep risks low.

The goal of this book is to help physicians assess their situation with respect to fraud and abuse, identify areas where violations could occur, and determine what steps they should consider to minimize exposure. There are many relatively easy steps physicians can take to reduce and manage their compliance risks.

More Than Just Medicare

Private insurers are becoming more active in pursuing overbillings. The relatively new HIPAA includes provisions that make it easier for commercial insurers to recoup payments and pursue other legal actions. HIPAA also includes provisions aimed at ensuring privacy and security of patient information. Those aspects of HIPAA are not addressed in this book.

Are You Sure That Your Billing Activities Are Appropriate?

The authors of this book encountered a situation that clearly indicates the risks physicians take if they do not make sure their medical practice implements effective fraud and abuse safeguards. While engaged to evaluate a seemingly desirable medical practice for a potential purchaser, billing consultants assessed the practice's equipment, patient base, payer mix, gross billings, receipts, overhead, and other factors. Because receipts seemed greater than average for the physician's specialty, a sample of records was reviewed to determine the accuracy of billing.

The additional revenue was traced to a well-meaning billing clerk who routinely upcoded evaluation and management codes above what the physician marked on encounter forms because she "found that this would get the practice reimbursement closer to what they wanted." This physician was putting his practice in jeopardy with Medicare and managed care plans because his billing profiles indicated a much higher percentage of CPT® code 99214 than peers did.

While Medicare and other payers had not audited the physician, the risk associated with the improper billing practices squelched the deal and left the physician quite concerned about his audit exposure.

The above example is not an isolated case. Sometimes billing staff change ICD-9 codes and other codes or modifiers because they find doing so bypasses certain payer computer edits or screens. Sometimes, the patient's condition or the payer's billing rules justify the changes. In other cases, the medical practice might be increasing audit risks if medical record documentation or coding conventions do not support the change.

These are good examples of what a compliance program would help prevent. Periodic monitoring would have identified such problems very early. If physicians implement a compliance program correctly, it should help identify deficiencies in their billing and collection operations and it might actually increase revenue. Again, the Department of Health and Human Services Office of Inspector General (OIG) indicated that a compliance program that is really designed to prevent abusive billing practices might mitigate ultimate penalties in the event of a fraud and abuse action.

Admittedly, a full-blown, formal compliance plan may be difficult for a small practice to implement cost-effectively. However, there are a number of compliance checks that even the smallest practice can implement to help identify improper billing activities.

The examples of fraudulent billing activities that make media headlines are often so blatant that the vast majority of physicians and other health care professionals cannot see themselves ever being charged with involvement in such obvious schemes. However, improper billing activities that do not rise to the level of fraud may still lead to recoupment of funds Medicare carriers paid in excess of the "correct" amount.

Thus, one may avoid the exorbitant penalties imposed on fraudulent activities and potential criminal sanctions but still have to repay substantial funds (plus some hefty interest charges). In fact, many more health care professionals will be involved in recoupment efforts that do not carry criminal sanctions or civil monetary penalties than will ever be involved in fraud investigations.

Stripped to basics, Medicare carriers pursuing recoupment efforts will commonly audit a small number of medical records and determine an overpayment percentage.

The carrier may then extrapolate the overpayment percentage over several years' worth of payments to determine the amount it will seek. Although several levels of appeal may allow physicians to reduce the overpayment request, this may become a costly, stressful, and time-consuming process. Again, effective compliance programs will help physicians avoid such recoupment efforts.

The point should be clear—it is prudent to take reasonable efforts to ensure compliance.

Fraud vs Abuse—What Is the Difference?

The distinction between fraud and abuse can be very important in determining the potential fines and penalties that might apply. In terms of the possible penalties and sanctions, abuse is not as serious as fraud.

Unfortunately, the distinction between abuse and fraud is not always clear. The degree of intent by the individual or entity under investigation is often the determining factor.[1] What might start as a limited audit by a Medicare carrier—because it has identified a potentially abusive billing pattern—could become a fraud case turned over to the OIG and/or the Justice Department for criminal prosecution if new information, additional billing irregularities, or an intent to defraud is discovered.

It is unfortunate that the phrase *fraud and abuse* has become so widely used to describe alleged instances of noncompliance with billing requirements. A more appropriate phrase would emphasize the distinction between unintentional billing errors and fraudulent schemes. In either event, physicians may still be responsible for repaying funds collected in error, but additional penalties beyond interest payments do not apply where criminal or fraudulent intent is not present. As we will see in a moment, the government can allege fraudulent intent in some cases when one should have known, or one acted in deliberate ignorance or reckless disregard of the truth.

The instances of fraud reported in the media often involve deliberate schemes to bill repeatedly for services never performed, services that are clearly not medically necessary for the patient's symptoms or condition, services induced by payment of kickbacks or fees to referral sources, and the like. These types of schemes may carry criminal sanctions and/or involve civil monetary penalties (in addition to the actual refunding of amounts collected through fraudulent activities).

Obvious fraudulent schemes are clearly illegal and are not the focus of this book. Rather, this book is written to help physicians identify and avoid situations where compliance implications are not as obvious and where errors could occur.

Cigna Healthcare—the Medicare carrier for North Carolina, Tennessee, and Idaho—provides these simplified definitions of fraud and abuse on their Web site (www.cignamedicare.com/afraud/index.html):

> *Fraud,* as defined by the Centers for Medicare and Medicaid Services (CMS), is an intentional deception or misrepresentation that someone makes, knowing it is false, that could result in the payment of unauthorized benefits.
>
> A scheme does not have to be successful to be considered fraudulent.
>
> *Abuse* involves actions that are inconsistent with sound medical, business, or fiscal practices.
>
> Abuse directly or indirectly results in higher costs to the Medicare program through improper payments that are not medically necessary.
>
> The primary difference between fraud and abuse is a person's intent. That is, did they know they were committing a crime?

Definition of Abuse

Abuse may, directly or indirectly, result in unnecessary costs to a program such as Medicare or Medicaid, improper payment, or payment for services that fail to meet professionally recognized standards of care or that are medically unnecessary. Abuse may also involve payment for items or services for which there is no legal entitlement to payment. Typically, however, the physician or other health care professional has not knowingly and willfully misrepresented facts to obtain payment.

Some of the more common examples of abuse are as follows:

- Performance of services considered by the carrier to be medically unnecessary
- Failure to document medical records adequately (in the payer's view)
- Unintentional, inappropriate billing practices such as misuse of modifiers
- Medicare limiting charge violations
- Failure to comply with a participation agreement

The key words in the definition of abuse are "not knowingly or willfully." One's intent is the most significant factor in determining whether noncompliance is considered abuse, rather than a fraudulent practice.

Although abuse may be less serious than fraud, it is not without consequence. In many cases, abusive billing practices may carry economic consequences almost as serious as those of fraudulent activities. Again, one who should have known, or who acted in deliberate ignorance or reckless disregard of the truth, may have his or her case referred to law enforcement agencies for further investigation and potential criminal penalties.

Definition of Fraud

Fraud relates to intentional deception or misrepresentation to obtain some benefit, such as payment for medical services. Thus, intent is an essential element in fraudulent billing. However, this does not mean that physicians can necessarily protect themselves from charges of fraudulent billing by "closing their eyes to the facts."[2]

In defining persons who have filed a false claim, federal legislation includes the following language:

> . . . including any person who engages in a pattern or practice of presenting or causing to be presented a claim for an item or service that is based on a [CPT®] code that the person *knows or should know* will result in a greater payment to the person than the code the person knows or should know is applicable to the item or service actually provided.[3]

The HIPAA specifically states:

> . . . the term *should know* means that a person . . . (A) acts in deliberate ignorance of the truth or falsity of the information; or (B) acts in reckless disregard of the truth or falsity of the information, and no proof of specific intent to defraud is required.

Medicare Carrier's Manual for Fraud Unit Procedures, Section 14011. Coordination With Carrier MR (Medical Review) Unit

The MR unit's [the carrier's Medical Review unit's] responsibilities include looking for questionable billing patterns and practices, i.e., program abuse. The term "abuse" describes incidents or practices of providers that are inconsistent with accepted sound medical practice. Abuse may, directly or indirectly, result in unnecessary costs to the program, improper payment, or payment for services that fail to meet professionally recognized standards of care, or that are medically unnecessary. Abuse involves payment for items or services when there is no legal entitlement to that payment and the provider has not knowingly and intentionally misrepresented facts to obtain payment.

If the MR unit finds, or suspects, such practices, it should consult with the fraud unit to determine whether the case should be referred to the fraud unit for further action.

Medicare is most vulnerable to overutilization of medical and health care services. Abuse takes such forms as, but is not limited to, claims for services not medically necessary, or not medically necessary to the extent furnished (e.g., a battery of diagnostic tests is given when, based on diagnosis, only a few are needed).

Although these types of practices may be considered abusive, under certain circumstances, they may constitute or evolve into fraud. If a provider appears to have knowingly and intentionally furnished medically unnecessary services or filed claims for services not furnished as stated on the claim form, or made any false statement on the claim form to receive payment, the case is discussed with the fraud unit. If the fraud unit agrees that there is potential fraud, the MR unit then refers the case to the fraud unit. When reviewing such situations, do not assume that the abuse is the result of an error or misunderstanding of program requirements. At a minimum, ascertain whether there have been similar complaints or warnings, and whether the provider has been the subject of MR previously.

The fraud unit often receives complaints alleging fraud that are determined to be abusive rather than fraudulent. When this occurs, the fraud unit will decide if it is more cost and time effective to complete the case or refer it to the MR unit.

In all situations where abuse has been identified, the unit completing the case must notify the provider that the particular practice or behavior is abusive and must cease.

If the situation does not appear to involve fraud (and the fraud unit concurs), the MR unit notifies providers that particular practices or behaviors are abusive and must cease. Refer cases involving providers who fail to correct their practices or behavior following the educational contact and warning to the fraud unit.

In the notice to a provider regarding abusive practice or overpayment situations resulting from unnecessary services or excessive charges, the MR unit must include a sentence informing the provider that continuation of the abuse or repeated unnecessary care problems could result in his/her being excluded from the Medicare program in accordance with 1128 of the Act.

If the MR unit detects what clearly appears to be fraudulent practices, it should refer them to the fraud unit immediately.

If there are repeat violations by a provider, forward the case to the fraud unit for development and, if appropriate, the fraud unit refers the case to OIFO (i.e., the OIG's Office of Investigations, Field Office).

Serious Implications of Both Abuse and Fraud

Where fraudulent intent is established, the government may pursue criminal prosecution, civil monetary penalties, or exclusion from participation in federal health care programs. These sanctions do not apply to abusive billing practices that are handled at the carrier level rather than being referred to law enforcement agencies.

When a Medicare carrier identifies what is ultimately deemed an improper billing practice, the physician will be required to repay any monies received inappropriately plus interest. Depending on the carrier's discretion, it may simply ask for a return of monies for a relatively small number of services. However, a Medicare carrier can use the overpayment percentage calculated from a small sample of patient encounters to determine amounts to be recouped for payments received over several years for similar services.

As a simplification of this sampling process, assume a Medicare carrier audited documentation for 15 patient encounters and determined that a physician upcoded five of the claims, resulting in an overpayment of $125 (or $25 per claim). The carrier could ask for repayment of $125 plus interest for the five encounters reviewed and write a letter to "educate" the physician regarding proper billing requirements. Increasingly, Medicare carriers will ask for repayment of $25 each on 33.3% of similar services paid by the carrier over the past 3 or 4 years. This could be quite a large repayment request.[4] (This example is a simplification, and audit extrapolations will be discussed in detail later.)

Most overpayment requests will include interest assessments for the period of time involved. The interest rates are high—in the 12.5% to 14% range during the past few years. Additionally, carriers may require physicians to submit documentation such as office notes with all future claims for a period of time.

Potentially, carriers can also refer the case to the Department of Justice or the OIG for further investigation. The OIG could exclude the health care professional from participation in Medicare and all other federal health care programs without a criminal conviction (of course, there are appeal rights). Exclusion could then lead to loss of hospital privileges and denial of participation in some managed care plans. Finally, law enforcement agencies could allege fraudulent intent, as discussed previously.

The point to this lengthy discussion is that there is not always a clear distinction between abusive and fraudulent activities. Clearly, there are serious implications for either abusive or fraudulent actions.

What may begin as a seemingly routine audit of a small number of medical records could expand into a large overpayment request or even a criminal investigation. What may clearly be the result of billing errors could result in a large overpayment request if the error occurred often enough. Finally, fraudulent intent could be alleged for billing irregularities where the health care professional should have known, or for which he or she acted in deliberate ignorance or reckless disregard of the truth.

To avoid awkward discussions in many remaining sections of this book, the term noncompliance will be used where the distinction between fraud and abuse is not particularly relevant.

Enforcement Agencies and Statutes

A number of enforcement agencies could be involved in fraud and abuse actions: the Department of Justice, including the FBI, the Centers for Medicare and Medicaid Services (CMS), the OIG, the Drug Enforcement Agency, Medicare carriers, state licensing boards, Medicaid fraud units, state attorneys general, the Internal Revenue Service, and postal inspectors. There is evidence of increased cooperation among the various federal and state agencies in recent years. Several states have even established special task forces to combat fraud and abuse. We will discuss the enforcement agencies in greater detail.

A number of statutes—including mail and wire fraud statutes, the False Claims Act, provisions of HIPAA, and the Social Security Act—may be used to prosecute violators and/or impose sanctions or penalties (administrative remedies, criminal prosecution, and/or civil actions). We will discuss many of these statutes in more detail later.

It is critical that any fraud or abuse settlement include all potential sanctioning bodies and causes of action.[5] There are cases where a fraud action is settled through one agency, but another agency later applies sanctions for the same offense. For example, one might settle a fraud investigation with the Department of Justice and then face action by the OIG. Similarly, investigations of alleged Medicare fraud could be investigated by state authorities when Medicaid is also involved.

Some Recent Government Fraud and Abuse Initiatives

In May 2002, the government released the following fact sheet that is available at the Web site www.hhs.gov/news/press/2002pres/fraud.html:

(Fact Sheet)
May 7, 2002
Contact: HHS Press Office (202) 690-6343

Reducing Payment Errors and Stopping Fraud in Medicare

Overview: The Department of Health and Human Services (HHS) plays a critical role in ensuring that beneficiaries and taxpayers get their money's worth from the Medicare program. Each year Medicare spends more than $240 billion on health care benefits for nearly 40 million senior citizens and other Americans with disabilities. As steward of the Medicare program, the Center for Medicare & Medicaid Services (CMS) is responsible for ensuring Medicare pays correctly for covered services. CMS implements the coverage and reimbursement policies that Congress establishes in the law.

To achieve this goal, HHS has expanded efforts to help doctors and health care providers understand and follow Medicare law and regulations. CMS also is working to simplify requirements to further reduce payment errors. These efforts are showing significant results. Medicare's estimated error rate has fallen by more than half, from 14 percent in fiscal year 1996 to 6.3 percent in fiscal year 2001, according to annual independent reviews conducted by the HHS Office of Inspector General (OIG). The error rate measures payments made by Medicare which are not properly supported by health care providers' documentation or which otherwise do not meet Medicare reimbursement requirements. The error rate does not measure fraud or abuse in the Medicare program.

In cases where evidence may suggest fraudulent billing practices, HHS works closely with its OIG, other law enforcement agencies and CMS to investigate and enforce the laws in order to protect beneficiaries and taxpayers. Health care providers are not subject to civil or

criminal penalties for innocent errors, as the laws only cover offenses involving actual knowledge, reckless disregard or deliberate ignorance of the falsity of claims. In fiscal year 2001, the federal government recovered more than $1.3 billion in judgments, settlements, and administrative impositions in health care fraud cases and proceedings—including more than $1 billion returned to the Medicare Trust Fund.

Background

HHS' strategy to reduce Medicare payment errors includes efforts focusing both on helping providers to file Medicare claims correctly so that Medicare pays it right the first time and on vigilant oversight of claims payments to stem fraud, waste and abuse. Specific efforts include:

- Increasing the focus of CMS and its claims processing contractors on provider education as a means to decrease errors.

- Clarifying Medicare's reimbursement and coverage requirements to make it easier and simpler for physicians, providers and suppliers to bill for the services they perform.

- Addressing program vulnerabilities by promoting voluntary compliance while focusing anti-fraud resources on the small fraction of providers trying to defraud the program.

- Strengthening oversight of Medicare contractors and enhancing Medicare's financial accountability.

These efforts have helped reduce Medicare's estimated payment error rate in half, from 14 percent in fiscal year 1996 to 6.3 percent in fiscal year 2001. Although Medicare pays virtually all claims correctly based on the information submitted, payments are considered "improper" if they lack sufficient documentation, if the service provided is found to have been unnecessary, or if the service is coded improperly by a physician or other health care providers. Medicare's "improper payment" estimate is not a measure of fraud, though it may include fraud.

Improving Provider, Supplier and Physician Education

CMS is enhancing its education activities and improving carriers' and fiscal intermediaries' communications with physicians and providers. The Medicare program primarily relies on these private sector contractors to process and pay Medicare claims, to educate physicians and providers, and to communicate policy changes and other helpful information to them. CMS is taking a number of steps to ensure Medicare contractors provide consistent, unambiguous, timely, and accurate information to physicians and other providers.

Centralized Education Efforts. CMS has centralized educational efforts in the Division of Provider Education and Training, whose primary purpose is to educate and train both the contractors and the physician and provider community about Medicare policies. CMS is providing contractors with in-person instruction and a standardized training manual for them to use in educating physicians and other providers. These programs help ensure that the contractors speak with one voice on national issues.

Improved Customer Service. CMS is working to improve the quality of the Medicare contractors' customer service to physicians and other health care providers. In 2001, the carriers and fiscal intermediaries answered 24 million telephone calls from physicians and providers. CMS has developed performance standards, quality call-monitoring procedures, and contractor guidelines to make the Agency's expectations clear and to ensure that contractors are reaching those expectations.

Customer Service Training Plan. To improve responsiveness to the millions of phone calls the provider call centers handle each year, CMS is collecting detailed information on call center operations, including frequently asked physician questions, the call centers' use of technology, and the centers' training needs. CMS will analyze this information to further improve the quality of customer service to health care providers. CMS has also

developed a new Customer Service Training Plan to bring uniformity to contractor training and improve the accuracy and consistency of the information that contractor service representatives deliver over the phone.

Internet Options. CMS has implemented new website architecture and is tailoring it to be intuitive to physicians to help meet their office and billing needs. Once this new website is successfully implemented, CMS will organize similar web navigation tools for other Medicare providers. The Frequently Asked Questions section has been improved, making it more intuitive and easier to search.

Expanding the Medicare Learning Network. The Medicare Learning Network homepage (http://www.hcfa.gov/medlearn) provides timely, accurate, and relevant information about Medicare coverage and payment policies, and serves as an efficient, convenient physician education tool. In the Fall of 2001, the MedLearn website averaged more than 250,000 hits per month, with the Reference Guides, Frequently Asked Questions, and Computer-Based Training pages having the greatest activity. Physicians and other providers can email their feedback directly to the MedLearn mailbox on the site.

Providing Free Computer and Web-Based Training Courses. Interested physicians, providers, practice staff, and others can access a growing number of web-based training courses designed to improve their understanding of Medicare. Some courses focus on important administrative and coding issues, such as how to check in new Medicare patients or correctly complete Medicare claims forms, while others explain Medicare's coverage for home health care, women's health services, and other benefits.

Installing a Satellite Learning Channel. CMS recently completed the installation of a network of satellite dishes at all contractor call centers to improve training efforts with contractor customer service representatives to improve their customer service skills and expand their knowledge of the Medicare program.

Clarifying Medicare Requirements

Clarifying and streamlining Medicare rules represents another significant way to further reduce Medicare payment errors. HHS is committed to taking steps to make Medicare more understandable and user-friendly to help physicians and other providers avoid unintended errors.

HHS Regulatory Reform Committee. Secretary Thompson has formed a regulatory reform group to identify ineffective regulations that prevent physicians, hospitals, and other health care providers from providing quality care to their patients. The panel will make recommendations about how to change or revise regulations that interfere with providers' ability to provide quality care to patients. The committee is now conducting hearings across the country to gather suggestions from patients and providers for specific changes in regulations.

The Physicians' Regulatory Issues Team (PRIT). In 1998, CMS created the PRIT to improve the agency's responsiveness to the daily concerns of practicing physicians as the agency reviews and creates Medicare requirements. The team, which includes physicians working throughout CMS, seeks to make Medicare simpler and more supportive of the doctor-patient relationship. PRIT members work within the Agency to serve as catalysts and advisors to policy staff as changes and decisions are discussed. Team members have assisted in:

- Streamlining Medicare forms, including the physician enrollment form;

- Improving operational policies;

- Working to improve current channels of input from practicing physicians;

- Clarifying oversight policies; and

- Identifying and changing excessively burdensome requirements.

The Practicing Physicians Advisory Council (PPAC). The council, established by Congress in 1990, advises CMS on proposed changes in Medicare regulations and manual instructions related to physician services. A CMS physician leads the PPAC, and all 15 members are practicing physicians who bill Medicare and represent a wide variety of specialties and both urban and rural areas. More information about PPAC is available at http://www.hcfa.gov/medicare/ppacpage.htm.

Open Door Policy Forums. In 2001, CMS Administrator Tom Scully established 13 Open Door Policy Forums to interact directly with physicians, hospitals, nursing homes, health plans and other health care providers and suppliers, as well as beneficiary groups, to strengthen communication and information sharing between these stakeholders and CMS. The Open Door Policy Forums facilitate information sharing and enhance communication between CMS and its partners and beneficiaries.

CMS Expert Panel. Chaired by a practicing emergency room physician, this panel of CMS staff is being challenged to suggest meaningful changes and develop ways that we can reduce burden, eliminate complexity, and make Medicare more "user-friendly" for everyone.

Clinical Preceptorships. CMS is participating in and co-sponsoring "preceptorships" with local county medical societies, where policy staff "shadow" physicians, watching them provide care, listening to lectures, and even observing operating room procedures. This program provides CMS staff with a first-hand observation of clinicians' daily work life and the challenges they face in providing care to Medicare beneficiaries.

Targeting Program Vulnerabilities

Full Implementation of Program Safeguard Contractor Strategy. Since 1999, CMS has used special contractors with program integrity experience to target problem areas, such as reviewing claims for therapy services and developing data analysis centers to identify and stop payment errors and possible fraud. This year CMS is significantly expanding this program by separating out the fraud and abuse prevention and detection activities from all fiscal intermediaries and carriers and competing that workload among our program safeguard contractors. This split of functions will enable the carriers and fiscal intermediaries to focus their efforts on educating and providing feedback about Medicare's billing rules and policies to all providers. At the same time, it allows the program security contractors to focus their resources and energies on detecting the true problems in the program: those entities and individuals who are in the program solely to take advantage of the system.

Developing Contractor-Specific Error Rates. In 2000, CMS began developing error rates for each of the private insurance companies that pay Medicare claims. Over time, these error rates will guide error-prevention efforts, such as education and program integrity efforts, at each contractor in more detail than Medicare's overall report can.

Medicare/Medicaid Datamatch Project. CMS entered into a statutorily required Computer Matching Act (CMA) agreement with the State of California to share and compare Medicare and Medicaid data to help find fraudulent or abusive billing patterns. While these may not be evident when billings for either program are viewed in isolation, they can become evident when they are compared. It is expected this project will serve as a model for similar efforts in other states.

Promoting Voluntary Compliance. With extensive input from health care businesses, the OIG has developed a series of voluntary compliance guidelines for hospitals, medical equipment suppliers, clinical laboratories, home health agencies, third-party billers, Medicare+Choice organizations, and other providers.

These guidelines identify reasonable steps to take to improve adherence to Medicare and Medicaid laws, regulations and program directives.

Medicaid Error Rate Project. CMS is working with states to develop Medicaid payment accuracy measurement (PAM) methodologies that can be used both on a state-specific and national basis. In fiscal year 2002, CMS received $2.7 million in Health Care Fraud and Abuse Control (HCFAC) Program funds to continue an initiative that would develop a single payment accuracy measurement methodology appropriate to all states. The nine states that applied and were approved to participate in a pilot program were Louisiana, Minnesota, Mississippi, New York, North Carolina, North Dakota, Texas, Washington and Wyoming. While most of the pilots are focusing on fee-for-service payments, Minnesota will be addressing the validation of managed care encounter data. The initial pilot studies will be completed by the end of 2002. CMS plans to expand the PAM pilot to about 15 states in fiscal year 2003.

Anti-fraud Hotline. The OIG maintains an anti-fraud hotline to report potential fraud and abuse in the Medicare and Medicaid programs. The hotline, 1-800-HHS-TIPS (1-800-447-8477), provides assistance to callers in English, Spanish and Chinese. Tips involving potential errors in beneficiaries' Medicare statements are generally referred to the claims-processing contractors for further review, while suspected fraud is referred to appropriate law enforcement agencies for investigation. The hotline received more than 430,000 calls last year and has fielded about 2.1 million calls since its creation in 1995.

Senior Medicare Patrol Grantees. The HHS Administration on Aging (AoA) provides grants to 52 state and local organizations to help older Americans be better health care consumers and to help identify and prevent fraudulent health care practices. These Senior Medicare Patrol projects teach volunteer retired professionals, such as doctors, nurses, accountants, investigators, law enforcement personnel, attorneys and teachers, to help Medicare and Medicaid beneficiaries to become better health care consumers. Since 1997, these projects and other AoA grants have trained more than 48,000 volunteers, conducted more than 60,000 community education events reaching nearly 10 million people.

Improving Oversight of Medicare Contractors and Strengthening Financial Systems

Strengthening Oversight of Private Contractors. By law, Medicare must rely on private insurance companies to process and pay Medicare claims. In 1999, CMS created national review teams to evaluate contractors' fraud and abuse identification efforts and other key functions, using standardized reporting and evaluation protocols. These teams cut across regions and use their specific expertise to assure more effective evaluations of contractor performance. CMS continues to develop additional defined, measurable standards to support consistent reviews of specific areas of contractor performance.

Upgrading Medicare's Accounting Systems. Medicare's claims-processing contractors do not currently use a uniform financial management system, increasing the risk of administrative and operational errors and misstatements. HHS' proposed fiscal year 2003 budget includes $51 million to continue to develop state-of-the-art accounting systems for Medicare. The funding will help to develop both an Integrated General Ledger Accounting System for CMS to replace the fragmented, outdated systems now in use by CMS's claims-processing contractors, and a new Financial Accounting and Control System to improve internal financial management controls.

Assessing Contractor Customer Service for Program Integrity Activities. Beginning in 2001, CMS began surveying Medicare providers and beneficiaries about their views on how well contractors perform certain program integrity functions, including enrollment, cost report audit, medical review and complaint tracking. The results of these surveys are helping the program direct resources to ensure that contractors are providing the highest quality service in these areas.

An earlier fact sheet—reproduced below—specifies some of the "fraud buster" type projects implemented in the 1990s (most of these continue in some form today). On February 10, 1999, the Department of Health and Human Services issued the following fact sheet to illustrate coordinated efforts to fight fraud and abuse.

A Comprehensive Strategy to Fight Health Care Waste, Fraud, and Abuse

Overview

Since 1993, the Clinton Administration has focused unprecedented attention on the fight against fraud, abuse and waste in the Medicare and Medicaid programs. Today, the result is a series of investigations, indictments and convictions, as well as new management tools to identify wasteful mispayments to health care providers. In February 1999, the Office of the Inspector General announced that improper Medicare payments to doctors, hospitals, and other health care providers declined 45 percent from FY 1996 to FY 1998.

A heightened focus on fraud and abuse since 1993 by the HHS Inspector General, the FBI and Department of Justice, CMS and others throughout government is yielding a new, more detailed picture of fraudulent activities aimed at the Medicare and Medicaid systems. New surveys and audits have helped investigators pinpoint areas of vulnerability and ongoing patterns of abuse, which in turn are leading to changes in law enforcement and administrative actions. In addition, beneficiaries themselves are being trained to spot and report fraud and misspending.

At HHS, Secretary Shalala launched Operation Restore Trust, a ground-breaking project aimed at coordinating federal, state, local and private resources and targeting them on areas most plagued by abuse. During its two-year demonstration phase, the project identified $23 in over-payments for every $1 of project costs. In addition, the Secretary led the way toward steady, guaranteed funding for anti-fraud efforts by the HHS Inspector General, included in the Health Insurance Portability and Accountability Act of 1996 (HIPAA).

Under the Health Care Fraud and Abuse Control Program, also created under HIPAA, HHS has reported more than $1.2 billion in fines and restitution returned to the Medicare Trust Fund during fiscal years 1997 and 1998. During these years, HHS also excluded more than 5,700 individuals and entities from doing business with Medicare, Medicaid, and other federal and state health care programs for engaging in fraud or other professional misconduct—up from 2,846 in the previous two years. In addition, HHS increased convictions by nearly 20 percent in 1997 and another 16 percent in 1998. Since 1993, actions affecting HHS health care programs have saved taxpayers more than $38 billion, and have increased convictions and other successful legal actions by more than 240 percent.

In his fiscal year 2000 budget, President Clinton announced an anti-fraud and abuse legislative package that would save Medicare another $2.9 billion over 5 years by eliminating excessive Medicare payments for drugs, ensuring that Medicare doesn't pay for claims owed by private insurers, and other measures.

Fighting Waste, Fraud and Abuse in Medicare and Medicaid

Improper Payments Decline by Half. In 1994, Congress passed the Government Management Reform Act, requiring an annual audit of all government programs according to private sector accounting principles. These annual audits have given CMS a new tool to measure its progress in combating improper payments to Medicare providers. Audits are conducted by the HHS Inspector General with CMS's full cooperation.

In the past two years, according to the Inspector General, the Medicare error rate has declined by almost half, from 14 percent in 1996 to 7.1 percent in Fiscal Year 1998. The Inspector General called this a "truly remarkable improvement" and credited CMS's Medicare Integrity Program, other HHS fraud and abuse initiatives, improved provider compliance with Medicare reimbursement rules, departmental outreach efforts emphasizing Medicare documentation requirements, and implementation of CMS's corrective action plan.

Operation Restore Trust. In May 1995, President Clinton launched Operation Restore Trust (ORT), a comprehensive anti-fraud initiative in five key states designed to test the success of several innovations in fighting fraud and abuse in the Medicare and Medicaid programs. CMS, the HHS Inspector General, and the HHS Administration on Aging are working in partnership to carry out ORT. During the two year demonstration, ORT identified $23 in overpayments for every $1 spent looking at suspected trouble spots in Medicare, including home health care, skilled nursing facilities, and providers of durable medical equipment. In May 1997, Secretary Shalala announced that with its successes demonstrated, ORT techniques would be expanded nationwide and applied to additional areas of fraud and abuse.

Fraud and Abuse Hotline. HHS has expanded the 1-800-HHS-TIPS hotline started in 1995 to report fraud and abuse in Medicare and Medicaid programs. Some 32,000 complaints that warranted follow-up action have been received since it began service. Assistance is available in both English and Spanish.

Administration on Aging Ombudsman Program. As a partner in Operation Restore Trust, the Administration on Aging has trained thousands of paid and volunteer long term care ombudsman and other aging services providers to recognize and report fraud/abuse, including problems in nursing homes and other long term care settings.

Guaranteed and Expanded Funding. In August 1996, President Clinton signed the Health Insurance Portability and Accountability Act (HIPAA) legislation into law, which for the first time created a stable source of funding for fraud control. This law established the Health Care Fraud and Abuse Control Account, a key proposal of the Clinton Administration, to which money is deposited annually from the Medicare Part A Trust Fund to help finance expanded fraud and abuse control activities. The additional funding began with $104 million in FY 1997, and will total $137.5 million in FY 1999, divided between HHS and the Department of Justice. The special funding is used to coordinate federal, state and local health care law enforcement programs, conduct investigations, provide guidance to the health care industry on fraudulent health care practices, and establish a national data bank to receive and report final adverse actions against unscrupulous health care providers and suppliers.

Expanded Office of the Inspector General (OIG). Funding from the Health Care Fraud and Abuse Control Account has enabled the OIG to place personnel in an additional 12 states to carry out enforcement actions, increasing from 26 to 38 the number of states in which the OIG is present.

Increased Efforts by the Department of Justice (DOJ). Funding from the Health Care Fraud and Abuse Control Account has also enabled the Department of Justice, including the FBI, to step up its efforts to investigate health care fraud. DOJ has increased resources, focused investigative strategies, and improved coordination among law enforcement agencies. The number of successful legal actions against fraud and other crimes in the health care field has increased by more than 240 percent since FY 1992.

Rewards for Fraud and Abuse Information. The Incentive Program for Fraud and Abuse Information, which was also created under HIPAA, was implemented in July 1998. Under this program, rewards can be paid to Medicare beneficiaries and others who report fraud and abuse in the Medicare program. Their information must lead directly to the recovery of Medicare money for fraudulent activity, and the provisions can only apply for cases not already under investigation by federal or state agencies or Medicare's contractors. Rewards will be for 10 percent of the recovered overpayment or a $1,000 maximum, and will be financed from collected overpayments.

Tightening Standards for Home Health Care Providers. Because of extensive evidence of abuse, home health was one of the initial targets of Operations Restore Trust.

In September 1997, HHS imposed a four-month moratorium on enrollment of new home health care providers in the Medicare program while new regulations were developed to keep unscrupulous and unqualified providers from entering the program. The new regulations included provisions requiring home health agencies to post surety bonds of at least $50,000 before they can enroll or re-enroll in Medicare, requiring a minimum number of patients to establish an agency's experience prior to seeking Medicare enrollment, and requiring agencies to submit detailed information about all businesses they own to prevent the use of improper financial transactions. With the new regulations in place, the moratorium was lifted in January 1998.

Medicare also has doubled the number of home health audits and increased claims review by 25 percent. It has also increased survey frequency for problem agencies and secured authority to exclude providers convicted of health care-related fraud, as well as establishing minimum capitalization requirements to ensure that new agencies have enough funds on hand to operate responsibly. HHS also now requires home health agencies to be more accountable for the care they provide, and to conduct criminal background checks on the aides they hire.

HHS is also developing a new payment system for home health services that includes incentives to provide for care efficiently and avoid unnecessary visits. The new system will pay providers prospectively, similar to the way Medicare pays hospitals.

Savings from home health anti-fraud initiatives have been projected by the Congressional Budget Office at $8.8 billion over five years, in addition to further savings to be realized from payment reforms.

New Requirements for Durable Medical Equipment Suppliers. Payment for durable medical equipment was another area targeted by Operation Restore Trust because of evidence of extensive abuse. In 1998, HHS proposed new regulations for suppliers of DME (including wheelchairs, canes, and other medical supplies), aimed at assuring that beneficiaries would be served by legitimate businesses. The new regulations would require suppliers to obtain surety bonds and would ban DME supplier telemarketing. It would also require suppliers to have a physical office and a listed phone number, and would codify a requirement that suppliers re-enroll in Medicare every three years. In addition, it would prohibit suppliers from reassigning a supplier number, and would apply criminal and civil sanctions for misrepresentations on billing number applications. At the same time, Medicare began conducting on-site inspections of all medical equipment suppliers when they apply to participate in the program and when they re-enroll, to assure that beneficiaries are served by legitimate businesses.

Targeting Fraud in Community Mental Health Centers. In September 1998, HHS announced new actions to ensure that Medicare beneficiaries with acute mental illness receive quality treatment in community mental health centers and that Medicare pays appropriately for those services. As part of a comprehensive action plan, HHS began termination actions against centers that were unable to provide Medicare's legally required core services, and required others to come quickly into compliance.

HHS also demanded repayment of money that had been paid inappropriately for non-covered services or ineligible beneficiaries. The actions came after CMS and the HHS Inspector General found providers enrolled in the program who were not qualified to deliver psychiatric services, as well as enrollment of patients who were ineligible for the Medicare benefit, and services billed to Medicare

that were not appropriate. As part of Operation Restore Trust, CMS/HCFA had begun in 1997 to identify patterns of fraud and abuse of the benefit at community mental health centers. In 1998, CMS/HCFA followed up with site visits to about 700 Medicare-participating centers and applicants. Many met few, if any, of the statutory requirements for Medicare participation, raising doubts about their ability to care properly for beneficiaries.

The Medicare Integrity Program (MIP) and Payment Safeguards. This system of payment safeguards, also authorized by HIPAA, identifies and investigates suspicious claims throughout Medicare, and ensures that Medicare does not pay claims other insurers should pay. MIP also ensures that Medicare only pays for covered services that are reasonable and medically necessary. CMS's current payment safeguards are already paying dividends in cost savings. These safeguards comprise a comprehensive system which attempts to identify improper claims before they are paid, to prevent the need to "pay and chase."

CMS's current strategy for program integrity focuses on prevention and early detection. Some of the payment safeguard activities include the Medicare Secondary Payer Program, medical review, cost report audits and anti-fraud activities. The payment safeguard activities returned $14 for every $1 spent, and saved an estimated $7.5 billion for FY 1997. The Secondary Payment Program alone, which is identifying whether insurers should pay claims that in the past have inappropriately been paid by Medicare, saved more than $3 billion in 1997.

Improving Health Care Industry Compliance. The HHS Office of the Inspector General has issued compliance program guidance for hospitals to assist in developing measures to combat fraud and abuse in the hospital industry. In addition, the OIG released guidelines identifying steps for clinical laboratories, hospitals, home health agencies, and third-party billers to undertake to improve adherence to Medicare and Medicaid statutes, regulations, and program directives. The guidelines are part of the Inspector General's continuing efforts to work with health care providers to promote voluntary compliance with the applicable statutes, regulations, and program requirements pertaining to federal and other health care programs. In addition, the OIG has issued fraud alerts, advisory opinions and other guidance as part of an ongoing effort to promote the highest level of ethical and lawful conduct by the health care industry.

Correct Coding Initiative. In 1994, CMS/HCFA began the Correct Coding Initiative by awarding a contract for the development of correct coding policy for all physician billing codes referred to as current procedural terminology (CPT®) codes. Implemented in 1996, this enhanced pre-payment, control and associated software update resulted in $215 million in savings in FY 1997. So far, Medicare has developed more than 100,000 edits to detect improper claims. In addition, CMS has begun using commercial off-the-shelf data processing products.

Substantive Claims Testing. CMS is now working to develop a substantive testing process to help determine not only whether claims are paid properly, but also whether services are actually rendered and medically necessary.

Education Efforts. CMS's contractors educate the provider billing community, including hospitals, physicians, home health agencies and laboratories about Medicare payment rules and fraudulent activity. This education covers current payment policy, documentation, requirements and coding changes through quarterly bulletins, fraud alerts, seminars and, more importantly, through local medical review policy.

Tough New Requirements for Medicare and Medicaid Participants. President Clinton's FY 1998 budget proposal included several additional anti-fraud provisions. In addition, President Clinton introduced new legislation in March 1997, the "Medicare/Medicaid Anti-Waste, Fraud and Abuse Act of 1997," that established tough new requirements for individuals and companies that wish to participate in Medicare and Medicaid. Most of the Clinton Administration's recommendations were included in the budget bill signed by the President on August 5, 1997, including:

- Penalties for services billed by a provider who has been excluded by Medicare and Medicaid.

- Penalties for hospitals who contract with providers who have been excluded by Medicare and Medicaid.

- Civil monetary penalties levied on providers that violated the anti-kickback statute, under which the physician received some kind of incentive for referring patients.

- Requiring health care providers applying to participate in Medicare or Medicaid to provide their Social Security numbers and their employer identification numbers so CMS can check an applicant's history for past fraudulent activity.

- Barring convicted felons from participating in Medicare and Medicaid.

Budget 2000 Anti-Fraud and Abuse Legislative Package. To build on unprecedented success in fighting health care fraud, waste, and abuse, President Clinton's FY 2000 budget proposal will include further anti-fraud and abuse legislative package that would save Medicare some $2.9 billion over five years.

The package includes measures that would eliminate current requirements in federal law which require Medicare to make excessive payments for certain drugs; prevent abuse of Medicare's "partial hospitalization" benefit; ensure that Medicare does not pay for claims owed by private insurers; expand CMS contracting authority to purchase high-quality and cost-effective health care; and expanding CMS's authority to terminate contractors who do not perform effectively.

Administration on Aging "Fraud Buster Projects." The Administration on Aging (AoA) has trained thousands of paid and volunteer long-term care ombudsman, insurance counselors and other aging service providers to recognize and report fraud and abuse in nursing homes and other service settings.

The AoA also awarded $2 million in grants to 12 states to recruit and train thousands of retired professionals to serve as health care "fraud busters" who work with older persons in their communities to review benefits statements and report potential cases of waste, fraud, and abuse. Millions of persons have been reached through the projects' public service announcements, community education events, training sessions, and informational materials.

Recent government programs have been initiated to encourage Medicare beneficiaries to help identify fraudulent activities by physicians and others. Although beneficiaries are in a position to report obvious instances of fraud and abuse, these new initiatives—including fraud alerts—could easily be misinterpreted if not adequately communicated.

Outreach Program—Beneficiary Awareness of Medicare Fraud

The OIG described the Outreach program in its *Semiannual Report—March 1998* as follows:

> In 1996, OIG launched an initiative called "Outreach" whose primary goal is to combat Medicare fraud, waste and abuse. The initiative involves three activities: creation of a more user-friendly hotline; establishment of partnerships with CMS, the Administration on Aging and the American Association of Retired Persons; and inauguration of a nationwide outreach campaign to educate beneficiaries and other citizens on Medicare fraud.

> As part of that campaign, OIG conducted a telephone survey to assess current beneficiary knowledge and awareness of Medicare fraud. **The OIG found that more than half of beneficiaries believe that Medicare fraud is common**, and they overwhelmingly agree that it is their personal responsibility to report suspected cases of Medicare fraud. [boldface added]

> Further, beneficiaries appear to be well-positioned to identify potential Medicare fraud with three out of four saying that they "always" read their Explanation of Medicare Benefit (EOMB) statements. However, beneficiaries believe that recognizing fraud is difficult and most have never received information on Medicare fraud.

> They are not aware of agencies working to stop Medicare fraud nor of the toll-free number to report Medicare fraud. Finally, most beneficiaries agree that they would be more likely to report Medicare fraud if they knew more about it. The survey findings not only confirm the need for a campaign to educate beneficiaries, but also provide OIG with baseline data on Medicare beneficiaries' current awareness of Medicare fraud. The survey will be repeated in 1 to 2 years to assess the effectiveness of the outreach campaign. (OEI-12-97-00440)

The "Who Pays? You Pay" Campaign

In February 1999, a campaign was initiated as described in the announcement below from the Department of Health and Human Services. Readers might also want to review the comments on fraud and abuse on the AARP Web site: www.aarp.org/confacts/health/medfraud.html.

Campaign to Fight Fraud and Abuse

The Department of Health and Human Services has joined with the Department of Justice and AARP to launch a new national initiative against fraud, waste, and abuse in the Medicare program.

The campaign is titled, "Who Pays? You Pay." It is aimed at both waste, including simple billing errors as well as unnecessary or excessive spending, and at criminal fraud and abuse against the Medicare program.

The campaign asks beneficiaries to raise most billing questions first with their provider or Medicare insurance company, since most problems can be resolved there. If beneficiaries believe they may be aware of fraud, or if they are not satisfied with the explanation of the Medicare carrier, they are asked to call the HHS Inspector General Hotline at 1-800-447-8477 (1-800-HHS-TIPS).

The initiative was launched on February 24, with a 5-city press conference and training sessions in 31 cities for 10,000 Medicare beneficiaries and AARP volunteers. HHS Secretary Donna E. Shalala said that the Medicare program needs its 39 million beneficiaries to act as "eyes and ears" in spotting mispayments. "We need a new kind of partnership with our beneficiaries," she said. "We need our beneficiaries to watch for mispayments, and for possible fraud, just as they would look for mis-charges on their own bills."

Shalala said Medicare is phasing in a monthly state-ment for all beneficiaries that will show the claims and payments that have been made for the beneficiary. By reviewing the statement, beneficiaries will be able to determine whether payments appear accurate, whether there are questions or problems, or whether claims may have been paid for services that were never delivered.

Helpful Materials

As part of the campaign, the partners in this effort have developed a public service announcement to help get the message to the public; it was produced in both English and Spanish. Using the common theme of "Who Pays? You Pay," most of the partners have developed their own written materials, from pamphlets and brochures, to posters and "fraud fighter" kits. They can be found on the web sites of those individual agencies . . . .

A Team Effort

The "Who Pays? You Pay" campaign represents an unprecedented effort between three organizations who are acutely concerned with fraud, waste, and abuse in the Medicare program: the Department of Health and Human Services, which administers the Medicare pro-gram, ensures its integrity, and looks out for the Medicare beneficiary; the Department of Justice, which helps investigate Medicare fraud and bring those crimi-nals to justice; and the AARP, which acts as an advocate for the elderly and those millions of Americans who are beneficiaries of the Medicare program.

Within HHS, three main agencies have been working together to fight Medicare fraud and abuse and have helped develop this campaign from the ground up: The Health Care Financing Administration, which oversees and administers the Medicare program; the Office of Inspector General, which investigates, audits, and evalu-ates Medicare to insure its integrity; and the Administration on Aging, which works on behalf of Medicare beneficiaries and all the elderly. Each of these three agencies has developed pamphlets, brochures, fact sheets, and other helpful information on this cam-paign for the public.

The government is producing various fraud pamphlets, fraud alerts, and other information encouraging Medicare beneficiaries' assistance in reporting potential fraudulent activity. The illustration below is from CMS's Web site at www.cms.hhs.gov/providers/fraud/DEFINI2.ASP.

Medicare Definition of Fraud

Fraud is an intentional representation that an individual knows to be false or does not believe to be true and makes, knowing that the deception could result in some unauthorized benefit to himself/herself or some other person. The most frequent kind of fraud arises from a false statement or misrepresentation made, or caused to be made, that is material to entitlement or payment under the Medicare program.

The violator may be a physician or other practitioner, a hospital or other institutional provider, a clinical laboratory or other supplier, an employee of any provider, a billing service, beneficiary, Medicare carrier employee or any person in a position to file a claim for Medicare benefits.

Under the broad definition of fraud are other violations, including the offering or acceptance of kickbacks, and the routine waiver of co-payments. Fraud schemes range from those perpetrated by individuals acting alone to broad-based activities by institutions or groups of individuals, sometimes employing sophisticated telemarketing and other promotional techniques to lure consumers into serving as the unwitting tools in the schemes. Seldom do perpetrators target only one insurer or either the public or private sector exclusively. Rather, most are found to be defrauding several private and public sector victims, such as Medicare, simultaneously.

According to a 1993 survey by the Health Insurance Association of America of private insurers' health care fraud investigations, overall health care fraud activity broke down as follows:

- 43% Fraudulent diagnosis
- 34% Billing for services not rendered
- 21% Waiver of patient deductibles and co-payments
- 2% Other

In Medicare, the most common forms of fraud include:

- Billing for services not furnished
- Misrepresenting the diagnosis to justify payment
- Soliciting, offering, or receiving a kickback
- Unbundling or "exploding" charges
- Falsifying certificates of medical necessity, plans of treatment, and medical records to justify payment
- Billing for a service not furnished as billed; i.e., upcoding

In 2001, the following letter was written to the health care community:

An Open Letter to Health Care Providers
Office of Inspector General

330 Independence Ave., SW
Washington, DC 20201
An Open Letter to Health Care Providers
November 20, 2001

In the three months since I was sworn in as Inspector General of the Department of Health and Human Services (HHS), I have seen firsthand the importance of the work done by the Office of Inspector General (OIG) in ensuring the integrity of our Federal health care programs. As the HHS Inspector General, I have become aware of ways in which existing OIG policies can be modified to better serve both providers and those charged with protecting the Federal health care programs. For these reasons, I am pleased to announce modifications to OIG policies and practices that are responsive to concerns that we have heard from the provider and enforcement community regarding the civil settlement process.

In an effort to improve the corporate integrity agreement and voluntary compliance initiatives, our office has been engaged in an ongoing dialogue with the provider community. For example, we recently completed a survey of providers and held a roundtable discussion with compliance officers from providers operating under corporate integrity agreements. With the help of the provider community, the OIG has been working to promote the adoption of voluntary compliance programs, including issuing compliance program guidances, special fraud alerts, and advisory opinions. The OIG will continue to be a leader in promoting voluntary compliance.

As a result of the OIG's outreach efforts, we recognize the provider community's interest in streamlining the civil recoveries process. The OIG and the Department of Justice will continue to seek to resolve a provider's permissive exclusion liability concurrently with its False Claim Act liability. However, we recognize there may be a limited number of cases where it would be appropriate to resolve a provider's permissive exclusion liability separately or subsequent to resolution of the False Claims Act case. We also recognize that in certain cases it may be appropriate to release the OIG's administrative exclusion authorities without a corporate integrity agreement. I have directed my staff to consider the following criteria when determining whether to require a corporate

integrity agreement, and, if so, the substance of that agreement: (1) whether the provider self-disclosed the alleged misconduct; (2) the monetary damage to the Federal health care programs; (3) whether the case involves successor liability; (4) whether the provider is still participating in the Federal health care programs or in the line of business that gave rise to the fraudulent conduct; (5) whether the alleged conduct is capable of repetition; (6) the age of the conduct; (7) whether the provider has an effective compliance program and would agree to limited compliance or integrity measures and would annually certify such compliance to the OIG; and (8) other circumstances, as appropriate.

Through our communications with providers, we have also become aware of and are concerned about the financial impact of corporate integrity agreements on providers. To address this concern, the OIG is modifying the provisions of our corporate integrity agreements that address billing reviews and the use of independent review organizations to reduce their financial impact, without weakening the integrity of a provider's compliance program. Specifically, the corporate integrity agreement billing review requirements will, in the future, require the use of a full statistically valid random sample only in instances where the initial claims review (which we will call a discovery sample) identifies an unacceptably high error rate.[1] This modification, once finalized, will be incorporated into future corporate integrity agreements, and, where appropriate, will be made available to providers currently operating under a corporate integrity agreement. We will also be exploring ways to increase reliance on providers' internal audit capabilities, and offer additional flexibility in other corporate integrity agreement requirements, such as employee training.

The OIG will be reviewing each provider's corporate integrity agreement to determine whether it is appropriate to incorporate the new claims review procedures into the provider's existing corporate integrity agreement. Our office will contact providers regarding amendments to existing corporate integrity agreements. A further explanation of this amendment process is more fully set forth in a series of frequently asked questions, which will be posted on the OIG's website[2] at http://oig.hhs.gov or from the OIG's Public Affairs office at 202/619-1343.

In conclusion, I think you will see many positive changes in the way the OIG approaches its civil enforcement initiatives and corporate integrity agreements. We will continue to balance our enforcement initiatives with provider outreach and education in order to ensure the integrity of our Federal health care programs.

Sincerely,
Janet Rehnquist
Inspector General

1. For a more detailed explanation of this proposal see the summary.
2. See http://oig.hhs.gov/cia/ciafaqcr.pdf.

Examples of Potentially Fraudulent or Abusive Billing Practices

Some categories of fraud and abuse are as follows:

1   Billing for services that were not rendered (including situations where a higher-paying service is billed when a less extensive service was actually provided, ie, upcoding).

2   Billing for services that would likely be denied as "medically unnecessary" or "non-covered" for the patient's condition under a health plan by using covered diagnoses or other documentation that misrepresents the patient's condition.

3   Paying or receiving remuneration or kickbacks for referrals.

4   Violation of federal and state statutes relating to self-referrals (Stark I and II and various state laws).[6]

5   Other schemes that may misrepresent the facts of patient encounters or services provided, or fail to follow coverage and billing requirements.

Anyone familiar with billing for medical services realizes that the rules are quite complex. In fact, knowledgeable coders often disagree as to the appropriate way to code claims for similar services. Payers are often confused as well. Such complexity increases the likelihood of honest mistakes. Payer communications and newsletters are often ambiguous and even misleading at times. It is very easy to make a legitimate error under a system that is this complex. It is not unusual for billing errors to result in less than appropriate payment.

Of course, there has always been some tolerance for occasional, legitimate billing errors. With legitimate errors, detection by payers usually results in a request to return overpayments and perhaps some interest. Despite assurances from CMS and the OIG that fraud and abuse prosecution will not be initiated in response to billing errors, there is still a concern in today's environment that activities that might have been deemed legitimate billing errors in the past could now be construed as abusive or even fraudulent billing and may be referred to law enforcement officials as a matter of course.

Physicians and other health care professionals are not always aware of what happens in their billing departments. While most billing staffs work hard to ensure that claims are submitted appropriately, there are situations where well-meaning staff purposely upcode insurance claims—above what the physician marked on the patient's encounter form—to improve collections. In other instances, billing staff used ICD-9 diagnostic codes that they knew the carrier would cover, even though the condition did not reflect the patient's condition. Those are false claims and can be prosecuted as such under the False Claims Act.

Sometimes, everyone knows the services are legitimate, but the billing staff may not know the "secret" to getting the claims paid because payers have failed to communicate billing rules effectively. The point here is that there are better ways to ensure that claims are paid properly without resorting to billing practices that could be questioned.

Potentially, false claims and abusive billing practices subject a physician to significant sanctions and penalties and exclusion from Medicare and other government health care programs. In an environment with heightened sensitivity to the implications of noncompliance, conviction of health care fraud carries a number of adverse implications:

- Fines, exclusion from Medicare and other government health care programs, imprisonment, etc

- Seizure of assets

- Action by private insurers

- Qui tam suits where employees may be entitled to a portion of any judgment, or employees turning state's evidence

- Significant defense costs (which are usually not insured)

- Expulsion from group practice, networks, etc[7]

- "Adverse Action Report" to National Practitioner Data Bank if action is taken by hospital, managed care plan, liability insurer, licensing board, etc (and possible investigations by entities and regulatory agencies that review data bank reports)

The mere fact that a physician is being investigated may result in:

- Tarnished professional reputation

- Restriction or revocation of hospital privileges

- Loss of patients

- Loss of referrals from colleagues and other sources

- Stress, loss of time, etc

- Stress among partners in a group where one physician is suspected of billing irregularities

Chapter 2 provides detailed descriptions of activities that could be classed fraudulent or abusive.

Reporting of Government Sanctions

The OIG maintains a Web site that includes a Cumulative Sanction Report that reflects the status of physicians and others who have been excluded from participation in the Medicare and Medicaid programs (www.oig.hhs.gov/fraud/exclusions/listofexcluded.html). The listing is introduced with the following comments:

> The Office of Inspector General's (OIG) List of Excluded Individuals/Entities (LEIE) provides information to health care providers, patients, and others regarding individuals and entities that are excluded from participation in Medicare, Medicaid, and other Federal health care programs. Information is readily available to users in two formats on over 15,000 individuals and entities currently excluded from program participation through action taken by the OIG.

> The on-line searchable database allows users to obtain information regarding excluded individuals and entities sorted by 1) the legal bases for exclusions; 2) the types of individuals and entities excluded by the OIG; and 3) the States where excluded individuals reside or entities do business. . . .

In the past, noncompliance was primarily an issue for those participating in government programs. In recent years, private payers have become increasingly concerned about compliance issues. The HIPAA includes provisions that may be used by private payers to prosecute those suspected of illegal billing activities.

Other risks include termination from key managed care plans and loss of hospital privileges. While there are usually some appeals available, many managed care plans will simply terminate physicians or others suspected of improper billing practices. The credentialing process followed by hospitals and many managed care organizations includes checking for government sanctions.

According to the October-March 1996 Semiannual Report of the OIG, Department of Health and Human Services:

> The actions taken by the Office of Inspector General to exclude individuals and entities have made it a focal point in the credentialing of health care providers. As a means of safeguarding the provision of health care in the private sector, a number of hospitals and others in the health care industry have established a routine practice of querying OIG to ensure that individuals they are considering hiring have not been excluded from Medicare and State health care program participation. In fact, the National Committee on Quality Assurance (NCQA) has mandated that any HMO seeking accreditation by it must credential all of their health care professionals.
>
> **The NCQA has included in this credentialing process the requirement that the Department of Health and Human Services' OIG specifically be queried to determine if any of the HMO's health professionals have been excluded from program participation.**
>
> As more and more HMOs have sought accreditation and the practice of credentialing has grown, the number of queries to OIG for exclusion information has increased substantially. During this 6-month period, OIG responded to credentialing requests from HMOs, hospitals, medical societies, licensing boards, etc., to certify the exclusion status of over 11,000 individuals.

In any event, these implications further illustrate the need for some type of effort to ensure compliance in every medical practice and health care facility. Additional information on the effect of exclusion is available in the OIG's September 1999 special advisory opinion entitled "The Effect of Exclusion From Participation in Federal Health Care Programs." This document is available at Web site www.oig.hhs.gov/fraud/docs/alertsandbulletins/effected.htm.

Statistics on Noncompliance

Everyone has favorite estimates that purport to demonstrate how noncompliance pervades the health care systems. Broad generalizations that approximately 10% of our nation's annual health care expenditures is lost to fraud and abuse unfairly implicate the vast majority of physicians and other health care professionals. If that figure is true, approximately $100 billion is paid to undeserving entities or individuals. Detection of health care fraud and abuse has now become a top enforcement priority of the Department of Justice, ranking behind violent crime and drugs.

Although it is not always clear from media accounts, fraud and abuse are not limited to hospitals or physicians. Business persons, beneficiaries and their relatives, nurses, physical therapists, laboratories, medical equipment suppliers, and nursing homes and their administrators have all been the subject of federal and state investigations.

Even Medicare contractors and their employees have been convicted and assessed penalties for defrauding the government. A Medicare carrier/intermediary agreed to pay $27.6 million to settle a qui tam suit initiated by a former employee. Apparently, the carrier provided false reports to CMS to cover up shoddy work related to cost report audits designed to detect overpayments to hospitals. This same carrier was also found liable for an additional $24 million for inappropriate payments made when Medicare beneficiaries had other insurance coverage. Carrier employees were not, however, subjected to criminal prosecution.

Another Medicare carrier paid $2.75 million for submitting false reports to CMS containing inflated information that enabled the carrier to receive larger payments from Medicare. Once again, carrier personnel were spared criminal prosecution.

According to the FBI, physicians are the least likely to be involved in fraud. In preparing this guide, we reviewed a substantial amount of material, including indictments, grand jury testimony, FBI investigative reports, and court transcripts. In some instances, the physician's involvement occurred without his or her knowledge of any wrongdoing, and physicians have often been instrumental in reporting fraudulent activity.

Durable medical equipment companies, home health agencies, and nursing homes are three of the entities most often involved in multimillion-dollar Medicare or Medicaid fraud schemes. These schemes often involve the purchase of signed certificates of medical necessity, forged certifications, and fraudulent use of beneficiary identifiers.

Some of the largest fraud settlements have occurred through so-called qui tam (ie, whistle-blower) suits filed against independent clinical laboratories. (We will discuss qui tam suits later in this book.)

One source of information on fraud and abuse prosecutions is the OIG's Semiannual Report. These reports are available, at no cost, to the general public (they are even available on the Internet at www.oig.hhs.gov). These publications include facts related to OIG fraud and abuse activities, including studies that may lead to future audit targets.

The summary to the OIG's *Semiannual Report* for the period ending September 2001 includes the following comments:

Message from the Inspector General

Recently sworn in as the Inspector General of an office known for the dedication of its employees and the success of its endeavors, I am honored to have this opportunity to serve as a member of the Department of Health and Human Services team.

I am especially proud of the work of this office during FY 2001 and pleased to announce record breaking accomplishments. This year OIG has achieved a savings of over $18 billion, the greatest ever savings to the tax payer. We have achieved the most significant health care settlement in the history of our organization, totaling over $800 million, and recorded $1.5 billion in investigative receivables, the highest figure to date. In addition, we excluded 3,756 individuals and entities from participation in the Federal health care programs, a greater number than in any prior fiscal year.

As we face the challenge of maintaining this level of success, it is my goal to work with the service provider community by generating information, advice and compliance guidance to ensure their successful participation in HHS programs. We will rededicate our efforts to provide the best service possible to our beneficiaries and strengthen our efforts to prevent and respond to intentional fraud or abuse of our programs.

I look forward to working with Secretary Thompson, his senior Department officials and members of Congress so that we can continue meeting the needs of our program beneficiaries and the service provider community— all the while anticipating and preparing for the needs of the future. Through our joint efforts, HHS programs can work more effectively, at less cost, and with reduced risk to fraud and abuse.

Janet Rehnquist
Inspector General

Statistical Accomplishments

For Fiscal Year (FY) 2001, OIG reported savings of $18.011 billion comprised of $16.1 billion in implemented recommendations and other actions to put funds to better use, $411 million in audit disallowances and $1.5 billion in investigative receivables.

Also for FY 2001, OIG reported exclusions of 3,756 individuals and entities for fraud or abuse of the Federal health care programs and/or their beneficiaries, 423 convictions of individuals or entities that engaged in crimes against departmental programs, and 417 civil actions. . . .

The OIG's *Semiannual Report* for the period October 2001 to March 2002 included the following statements:

During this semiannual reporting period, OIG investigations resulted in 250 successful criminal actions. Also during this period, 696 cases were presented for criminal prosecution to DOJ and, in some instances, to state and local prosecutors. Criminal charges were brought by prosecutors against 312 individuals and entities.

In addition to terms of imprisonment and probation imposed in the judicial processes, over $780.8 million was ordered or returned as a result of OIG investigations during this reporting period. Civil settlements from investigations resulting from audit findings are included in this figure.

During the six month reporting period, OIG administered 1,472 sanctions, in the form of program exclusions or civil actions, on individuals and entities for alleged fraud or abuse or other activities that posed a risk to federal health care programs and/or their beneficiaries. During this reporting period, OIG excluded 1,366 individuals and entities.

The OIG also assists DOJ in bringing (and settling) cases under the False Claims Act. Many providers elect to settle their cases prior to litigation. As part of resolving these cases, providers often agree to put compliance measures in place to avoid exclusions and to remain a provider in the Medicare program. The integrity programs established by these agreements are designed to prevent a recurrence of the fraudulent activities that gave rise to the case at issue.

The government, with the assistance of OIG and often the FBI and other law enforcement agencies, recouped more than $728.7 million through both Civil and Monetary Penalties Law and False Claims Act civil settlements related to the Medicare and Medicaid programs during this reporting period.

In keeping with a longstanding commitment to assist providers and suppliers in detecting and preventing fraudulent and abusive practices, on October 21, 1998,

OIG issued a set of comprehensive guidelines for voluntary self-disclosures titled, "Provider Self-Disclosure Protocol." The Protocol is available on the Internet at http://oig.hhs.gov in the "Compliance Tools" section. In addition, it can be found in 63 *Federal Register* 58,399 (October 30, 1998).

Essentially, the Protocol guides providers and suppliers through the process of structuring a disclosure to OIG of matters uncovered that are believed to constitute potential violations of federal laws (as opposed to innocent mistakes that may have resulted in overpayments). Pursuant to the Protocol, an appropriate submission would include a thorough internal investigation as to the nature and cause of the matters uncovered and a reliable assessment of their economic impact (e.g., an estimate of the losses to the federal health care programs). The OIG evaluates each submission to determine the appropriate course of action. To date, OIG has received 131 submissions.

Among the benefits experienced by disclosing providers is the allocation of investigative resources that can contribute to an expeditious inquiry and a prompt resolution of the matter. Additionally, disclosing providers that demonstrate the effectiveness of their compliance programs and that, as part of the resolution of the matter, agree to continue such compliance activities may avoid entering into a corporate integrity agreement with OIG. In those cases where objective evidence of a comprehensive compliance program exists and OIG believes an agreement is necessary, OIG may make significant modifications in the term of an agreement or the role of the independent review organization.

Overall, the Protocol provides helpful guidance to providers and the community at large concerning how to achieve resolution of identified misconduct through a cooperative and open relationship with the government. To date, selfdisclosure cases have resulted in 30 recoveries and 15 settlements collectively totaling over $46.5 million.

The above statistics regarding the number of individuals and entities sanctioned are related to actions by the OIG. They do not include audits that were settled at the carrier level through an overpayment request rather than being referred to law enforcement agencies.

Another report, issued jointly by the Department of Justice and the Department of Health and Human Services, included the following comments[8]:

The Department of Health and Human Services and the Department of Justice Health Care Fraud and Abuse Control Program Annual Report for FY 2001

April 2002

Executive Summary

The detection and elimination of health care fraud and abuse is a top priority of Federal law enforcement. Our efforts to combat fraud were consolidated and strengthened considerably by the Health Insurance Portability and Accountability Act of 1996 (HIPAA). HIPAA established a national Health Care Fraud and Abuse Control Program (HCFAC or the Program), under the joint direction of the Attorney General and the Secretary of the Department of Health and Human Services (HHS), acting through the Department's Inspector General (HHS/OIG), designed to coordinate Federal, state and local law enforcement activities with respect to health care fraud and abuse. The fifth year of operation under the Program saw a continuation of the collaborative efforts of Federal and state enforcement and oversight agencies to identify and prosecute the most egregious instances of health care fraud, to prevent future fraud or abuse, and to protect program beneficiaries.

Monetary Results

In 2001, the Federal government won or negotiated more than $1.7 billion in judgments, settlements, and administrative impositions in health care fraud cases and proceedings. As a result of these activities, as well as prior year judgments, settlements, and administrative impositions, the Federal government collected more than $1.3 billion. More than $1 billion of the funds collected and disbursed in 2001 were returned to the Medicare Trust Fund. An additional $42.8 million was recovered as the Federal share of Medicaid restitution. This is the largest return to the government since the inception of the Program.

Enforcement Actions

Federal prosecutors filed 445 criminal indictments in health care fraud cases in 2001. A total of 465 defendants were convicted for health care fraud-related crimes in 2001. There were also 1,746 civil matters pending, and 188 civil cases filed in 2001. HHS excluded 3,756 individuals and entities from participating in the Medicare and Medicaid programs, or other federally sponsored health care programs, most as a result of convictions for crimes relating to Medicare or Medicaid, for patient abuse or neglect, or as a result of licensure revocations. This record number of exclusion actions is the result of successful collaboration with state Medicaid Fraud Control Units (MFCUs) and state licensure boards.

. . . The Social Security Act section 1128C(a), as established by the Health Insurance Portability and Accountability Act of 1996 (P.L. 104-191, HIPAA or the Act), created the Health Care Fraud and Abuse Control Program, a far-reaching program to combat fraud and abuse in health care, including both public and private health plans. The Act requires that an amount equaling recoveries from health care investigations—including criminal fines, forfeitures, civil settlements and judgments, and administrative penalties, but excluding restitution, compensation to the victim agency, and relators' shares—be deposited in the Medicare Trust Fund. All funds deposited in the Trust Fund as a result of the Act are available for the operations of the Trust Fund.

As stated above, the Act appropriates monies from the Medicare Trust Fund to an expenditure account, called the Health Care Fraud and Abuse Control Account (the Account), in amounts that the Secretary and Attorney General jointly certify as necessary to finance anti-fraud activities. The maximum amounts available for certification are specified in the Act. Certain of these sums are to be available only for activities of HHS/OIG, with respect to Medicare and Medicaid programs. In 2001, the Secretary and the Attorney General certified $181 million for appropriation to the Account.

Accomplishments

2001 marked the fifth year of the Program. During those five years, the Program's accomplishments have been impressive. Over $2.9 billion has been returned to the Medicare Trust Fund. In 1999, the Trustees of the Medicare Trust Fund extended their estimate of the financial life of the fund by 30 years. One of the primary contributing factors cited by the Trustees was "the continuing efforts to combat fraud and abuse." (Trustees Annual Report, 1999).

Returns to the Federal government as a whole are even larger, over $3 billion. In addition, more than 2,000 defendants were convicted for health care fraud-related offenses. Over 15,000 entities or individuals were excluded from participating in Medicare, Medicaid and other federally sponsored health care programs.

The Healthcare Integrity and Protection Data Bank is "up and running" and industry guidance and beneficiary outreach have been greatly expanded. These continuing accomplishments of DOJ and HHS and other partners in the coordinated anti-fraud effort, as well as the extensive preventive activities, demonstrate that the increased funds to address health care fraud and abuse are sound investments.

Collections

During this year, the Federal government won or negotiated more than $1.7 billion in judgments, settlements, and administrative impositions in health care fraud cases and proceedings. As a result of these activities, as well as prior year judgments, settlements, and administrative impositions, the Federal government collected $1.3 billion in cases resulting from health care fraud and abuse, of which more than $1 billion was returned to the Medicare Trust Fund, and $42.8 million was recovered as the Federal share of Medicaid restitution. It should be emphasized that some of the judgments, settlements, and administrative impositions in 2001 will result in collections in future years, just as some of the collections in 2001 are attributable to actions from prior years.

. . . Corporate Integrity Agreements. Many health care providers that enter agreements with the government in settlement of potential liability for violations of the FCA also agree to adhere to a separate CIA. Under this agreement, the provider commits to establishing a program or taking other specified steps to ensure its future compliance with Medicare and Medicaid rules. The duration of most CIAs is 5 years, during which time the provider must submit periodic reports to HHS/OIG. These agreements require a substantial effort by the provider to ensure that the organization is operating in accordance with Federal health care program requirements and the parameters established by the CIA. At the close of 2001, HHS/OIG was monitoring more than 300 CIAs. . . .

In response to feedback received from the Provider Roundtable and the survey of providers subject to CIAs, the HHS/OIG developed a plan to modify its role in the civil settlement process. First, the HHS/OIG developed criteria for the provider community as to those situations which would not require a CIA to resolve a provider's liability under the FCA. Second, the HHS/OIG modified the claims review procedures contained in CIAs, and revised the CIA requirement with respect to the use of independent review organizations.

Both changes are intended to reduce the financial impact of these requirements without weakening the integrity of a provider's compliance program. These modifications will be offered both to providers which negotiate future CIAs, as well as those with existing CIAs.

Medicare Error Rate. The HHS/OIG reported that improper payments under Medicare's fee-for-service system totaled an estimated $11.9 billion during 2000. That estimate was the lowest to date and about half of the $23.2 billion that was estimated for 1996, when HHS/OIG developed the first national error rate. The HHS/OIG developed the estimate of improper payments with the support of medical experts who together reviewed a comprehensive statistical sample of Medicare fee-for-service claims expenditures and supporting medical records to determine the accuracy and legitimacy of the claims.

The HHS/OIG believes that since the first error rate of 1996, CMS has demonstrated continued vigilance in monitoring the error rate and developing corrective action plans. Clearly these corrective actions have been successful. The majority of health care providers now submit claims to Medicare for services that are medically necessary, billed correctly, and documented properly. As in past years, HHS/OIG estimated that over 90 percent of the 2000 fee-for-service payments met Medicare reimbursement requirements. The HHS/OIG's 5-year analysis indicates that over 70 percent of the claims that did not meet reimbursement requirements were attributable to unsupported and medically unnecessary costs—two areas that will receive ongoing monitoring. . . .

Civil and Criminal Enforcement Actions

Accomplishments—Criminal Prosecutions

The primary objective of criminal prosecution efforts is to ensure the integrity of our nation's health care programs and to punish and deter those who, through their improper activities, adversely affect the health care system and the taxpayers. Each time a criminal case is referred to a USAO from the FBI, HHS/OIG, or another law enforcement agency, it is opened as a matter pending in the district. A referral remains a matter until an indictment or information is filed or the case is declined for prosecution. In 2001, the USAOs had 1,791 criminal matters pending involving 2,733 defendants, a 7 percent decrease in the number of criminal matters over 2000. During 2001, 445 cases were filed involving 601 defendants. This represents a 2 percent increase over cases filed in 2001. A total of 465 defendants were convicted for health care fraud-related crimes in 2001. Health care fraud convictions include both guilty pleas and guilty verdicts . . .

Accomplishments—Civil Cases

Civil health care fraud efforts constitute a major focus of Affirmative Civil Enforcement (ACE) activities. The ACE Program helps ensure that Federal laws are obeyed and that violators provide compensation to the government for losses and damages they cause. Civil health care fraud matters ordinarily involve the United States utilizing the FCA, as well as common law fraud remedies, payment by mistake, unjust enrichment and conversion to recover damages from those who have submitted false or improper claims to the United States.

Each time a civil referral is made to a USAO it is opened as a matter pending in the district. Civil health care fraud matters are referred directly from Federal or state investigative agencies, or result from filings by private persons known as "relators," who file suits on behalf of the Federal government under the 1986 qui tam amendments to the FCA. Relators may be entitled to share in the recoveries resulting from these lawsuits.

[NOTE—Interestingly, the report noted that a total of $83,335,798 was paid to private parties to qui tam actions.]

At the end of 2001, the USAOs had 1,746 civil health care fraud matters pending. A matter becomes a case when the United States files a civil complaint, or intervenes in a qui tam action, in United States District Court. The vast majority of civil health care fraud cases and matters are settled without a complaint ever being filed. In 2001, 188 civil health care fraud cases were filed . . .

Civil Division

Civil Division attorneys vigorously pursue civil remedies in health care fraud matters, working closely with the USAOs, the FBI, the Inspectors General of the Department of Health and Human Services and the Department of Defense, CMS, and other Federal and state law enforcement agencies. Cases involve providers of health care services, supplies and equipment, as well as carriers and fiscal intermediaries, that defraud Medicare, Medicaid, the TRICARE program of the Department of Defense, the FEHBP, and other government health care programs. . . .

Final Comments

We are at a point where those who provide health care are expected to know what constitutes appropriate billing practices. Consequently, physicians and other health care professionals and entities should seriously consider implementing programs to ensure compliance.

One of the primary goals of this book is to help physicians identify reasonable ways to monitor compliance in their organization. Compliance programs will vary by the type of entity and its size. A solo physician is not in a position to implement as extensive a compliance program as a hospital or large multispecialty group. However, the essential elements of an effective compliance program are the same for all physician practices.

This book focuses on the aspects of health care fraud and abuse related to inappropriate billing for services rendered and some of the sanctions and penalties under so-called antikickback and self-referral legislation (Stark).[9] Potentially fraudulent activities include a wide range of situations, such as inappropriate use of controlled substances; fraudulent provision of defective or previously used medical supplies and equipment; selling pharmaceuticals intended as samples; schemes to defraud insurance companies by patients or insureds; and practicing medicine without a license.

Please realize that it is impossible to discuss all the risks. There are any number of situations that carriers and other investigators could begin targeting tomorrow. There are new laws, and new and sometimes controversial interpretations of existing laws. The rules are often complex, ambiguous, and difficult—if not seemingly impossible—to communicate and implement. There are also a number of state laws, rules, and regulations related to health care fraud. Some states have enacted special provisions that may apply to situations not addressed directly in federal law.

New risks arise as physicians and others merge into larger groups or participate in networks to compete under managed care. Larger medical groups, hospitals, and other organizations become bigger targets. One or two seemingly minor infractions could prompt expensive and time-consuming investigations that affect the whole entity.

Corporations and other business organizations face liability for the actions of their officers and even line employees, especially where the business and individuals benefited from the illegal action and made little attempt to ensure proper billing practices (ie, there were no sincere compliance efforts). Fortunately, larger organizations also should have the resources to implement an effective compliance program to manage risks.

We have attempted to avoid becoming too bogged down in citing laws, proposed legislation, potential fines under each statute, and lengthy details of court cases and administrative penalties. There are several books available for those interested in a detailed discussion of the statutory provisions and precedent-setting cases. Most hospitals will have some books available that discuss these topics.

Endnotes

1. There is always the danger that enforcement agencies could allege there is sufficient evidence of fraudulent intent to pursue criminal sanctions.

2. Obviously, there are cases where physicians and others have defended themselves by demonstrating that laws, rules, or guidelines applicable to specific allegations of fraudulent billing were ambiguous, too complex, not sufficiently communicated, etc. However, one should not rationalize possible fraudulent billing activities by relying on such a defense.

3. 42 USC §1128A(a)(1) 1320a-7a(a)(1).

4. Attorneys and consultants who assist physicians in overpayment requests report recoupments of $100,000 to $300,000 or more in a number of cases involving a single physician. Thus, the financial impact of improper billing can be serious (not to mention the emotional stress, attorney and consultant fees, and the possibility of civil or criminal action).

5. Unfortunately, it may be difficult to resolve all criminal and civil causes of action at one time. It is a little easier coordinating government administrative remedies, such as "exclusion" from Medicare, Medicaid, and other federal health care programs, since such action usually comes through the OIG. Now, HIPAA could result in private payers taking action against a person convicted of Medicare fraud if they can show similar fraudulent filing of claims.

6. Antikickback and self-referral legislation is included in this document because it is closely related to fraudulent and abusive billing practices.

7. The types of fraudulent activity that could occur in capitated plans are different from those that occur with plans that use fee schedules or a combination of capitation and fee schedules. For example, it may be fraudulent or abusive activity to withhold necessary care under a capitated contract. Regardless of whether fraud could be proved in criminal or civil proceedings, a managed care plan that strives for high-quality ratings will often terminate physicians from participation if it suspects that they are not providing the level of care and services contemplated in contracts. (There is usually some contractual appeal mechanism available to physicians.)

8. A complete copy of this report is available at Web site www.usdoj.gov/dag/pubdoc/hipaa01fe19.htm.

9. The term *compliance* is also used with respect to laws unrelated to the billing process. However, this document does not address non-billing-related topics, such as the Clinical Laboratory Improvement Act, Occupational Safety and Health Administration, antitrust, employment/benefit laws, the Americans With Disabilities Act, standards of clinical practice, sexual harassment, moral issues, tax issues, building codes, credit/collection policies, licensing requirements, etc.

Chapter 2

Examples of Fraud and Abuse

One of the keys to avoiding noncompliance is to develop an understanding of what may be deemed improper billing. Depending on the nature, the intent, and the extent of a billing irregularity, the examples in this chapter could result in a fraud investigation by law enforcement agencies or may remain at the carrier level as an audit to determine whether an overpayment request should be issued.

Categories of potentially fraudulent or abusive billing practices include the following:

- Intentional misrepresentation of services rendered, such as (1) using covered CPT® codes for noncovered services; (2) misuse of modifiers; (3) improper use of place-of-service indicators to achieve payments for services that might not be covered in the actual setting (such as using a physician's office as the place of service, when it was actually provided in an inpatient setting or hospital emergency department)[1]; (4) using a covered ICD-9 code when it does not reflect the patient's condition, rather than a noncovered diagnosis code[2]; or (5) otherwise altering claim forms to obtain a higher payment amount

- Upcoding evaluation and management (E/M) codes or other CPT® codes that include various levels or designations, such as simple vs complex, deep vs superficial, open vs closed, with vs without, individual vs group, etc. In the past few years, some Medicare carriers have begun looking closely at 99214 and 99233 because CMS/HCFA believes these codes account for a high percentage of coding errors

- Billing for services not rendered or supplies not provided[3]

- Routine foot care (such as trimming of normal nails) billed as covered nail debridement

- Billing an E/M code in the place of a minor surgical code or other minor procedure that would likely be denied (such as a lesion removal, routine foot care, and the like)

- Billing for services that were performed, but that may be questioned as to medical necessity (see Chapter 8)

- Unbundling or fragmenting CPT® codes[4]

- Billing cosmetic surgery—which is often noncovered under insurance plans—as a procedure that is more likely to be covered, such as surgery to decrease pain or irritation, reduce swelling, or restore field of vision. Removal of nonmalignant skin lesions that do not cause the patient physical problems is a common example

- Billing E/M codes in addition to minor surgical procedures when a significant, separately identifiable E/M service is not performed (ie, inappropriately appending the -25 modifier to the E/M code when documentation does not indicate a separately identifiable E/M service was performed)

- Billing preventive care as a covered service to health benefit plans that do not normally cover preventive care (such as Medicare). Often this is accomplished by using ICD-9 diagnostic codes that are not reflective of the patient's condition, issues addressed during the encounter, or documentation in the medical record[5]

- Billing for procedures to malignant lesions, when the lesions were known to be benign[6]

- Misrepresenting time for anesthesia, psychotherapy, various testing, E/M counseling, etc, where time is a component of the CPT® code description

- Overutilization of laboratory testing and billing for screening laboratory tests that may be noncovered by means of covered diagnostic codes

- Improper billing with individual psychotherapy codes when group psychotherapy was performed

- Improper billing with CPT® code 90862 (pharmacologic management) when Medicare's special code M0064 (brief office visit for the sole purpose of monitoring or changing drug prescriptions used in treatment of mental, psychoneurotic, and personality disorders) is descriptive of the services performed. Make sure payer guidelines are followed when pharmacologic management is billed

- Referrals billed with higher-paying CPT® consultation codes, rather than office or hospital visit codes; however, physicians should watch for announcements from their carriers that may liberalize the use of consult codes when Medicare services are billed[7]

- Deliberate false diagnosis coding to obtain payment. This has been a common problem with reference laboratories or diagnostic screening tests that may not be covered by a given health plan. Misrepresentation of a diagnosis code may result in noncovered screening tests or routine physicals being reimbursed improperly

- Inappropriate billing of the number of nurse anesthetists supervised by an anesthesiologist[8]

- Not complying with new anesthesia guidelines. The November 2, 1998, Federal Register provides some clarifications, including various conditions for payment for medically directed anesthesia services; documentation entries the physician must make personally; functions or services that the physician must perform; and those limited activities permitted during medical direction. While there are no major changes from past rules, this is a good time for physicians to make sure their standard documentation thoroughly addresses these requirements

- Fee splitting, such as a chiropractor splitting payment with a physician for E/M codes billed under the physician's provider number

- Falsifying medical records to justify payments. Sometimes physicians find themselves in a situation where patients pressure them to be creative in documenting diagnoses and other care elements to get claims paid. Again, payers are becoming much more sensitive to this type of activity

- Billing a noncovered service—by using covered CPT® and ICD-9 codes—provided to patients in nursing homes or other facilities by podiatrists, psychologists, psychiatrists, ophthalmologists, optometrists, or others: routine eye examinations, routine foot care, what authorities may deem as unnecessary services being billed as psychotherapy, and social services billed as group psychotherapy

- Billing based on what is often referred to as "gang visits" (eg, a physician visits a nursing home and bills an E/M code for each of 20 patients without furnishing any specific service to, or on behalf of, each patient)

- Significant occupational therapy, physical therapy, speech therapy, psychiatric services, and various forms of psychotherapy for patients with senile dementia or Alzheimer's disease who are deemed to be unable to benefit from the service. Admittedly, it is difficult to know when such services are not of benefit to the patient; therefore, it is vital to document records thoroughly. Check with payers—such as Medicare carriers—that may have documentation guidelines including requirements for documenting the patient's progress, care plans and assessments, and specific services to be provided

- Billing services of a teaching physician when not all supervisory requirements have been met or documented appropriately

- Misuse or misrepresentation of modifiers, or other codes, to circumvent carrier payment edits[9]

- Billing daily visits for patients in a rehabilitation unit when payers question medical necessity of too frequent encounters. Document signs, symptoms, conditions, and circumstances that require encounters

- Filing two or more claims for same date of service (without -51 or similar modifier) in an attempt to achieve greater payment for multiple surgical procedures (from payers that reduce payments for multiple procedures)

- Alteration of claims to obtain payment

- Deliberately changing dates of service to circumvent correct coding edits

- Deliberately applying for duplicate payment, eg, billing both Medicare and the beneficiary for the full amount for the same service or billing Medicare and another insurer in an attempt to get paid twice

- Completing certificates of medical necessity for patients not personally and professionally known by the physician (and signing blank prescriptions or certificates of medical necessity for durable medical equipment or home health services)[10]

- Billing for a more costly procedure, when a less costly one is considered a prerequisite to the more costly one. For example, with certain exceptions, many payers have rules regarding billing standard x-ray procedures before resorting to computed tomography or magnetic resonance imaging, or certain endoscopic procedures

- Being associated with an organization or individual who has been prosecuted or cited for fraudulent activity.[11] The OIG Web site www.oig.hhs.gov/fraud/exclusions/listofexcluded.html provides a database search for individuals and organizations excluded from Medicare participation

- Misrepresenting the identity of the person receiving the services

- Participating in schemes that involve collusion with a beneficiary or a supplier that results in higher costs or charges to the Medicare program

- Billing laboratory tests incorrectly, including unbundling, manual vs automated tests, or failure to use panel codes when appropriate[12]

- Hospitals, nursing homes, and similar facilities filing cost reports that inappropriately include expenditures that are not payable by Medicare, Medicaid, etc

- Billing for services rendered under another physician's provider number.[13] Physicians should always inform their Medicare carriers and other payers in writing when they change location or sell their practice

- Acceptance of kickbacks, bribes, rebates, or other remuneration in exchange for referrals; payments made by hospitals, nursing homes, durable medical equipment suppliers, home health agencies, laboratories, or others for referrals; soliciting, offering, or receiving a kickback, bribe, rebate, or other remuneration (eg, paying for a referral of patients in exchange for the ordering of diagnostic tests and other services or medical equipment). Such kickbacks or bribes do not have to be made directly in cash. Examples of noncash payments for referrals include rent below fair market value, vacations, computer systems, free supplies, providing a phlebotomist who helps with other tasks in a physician's office, or discounts on some services that might influence referrals.[14] (See Chapter 4 for more information on kickbacks)

- Routine waiver of coinsurance and deductibles. Under Medicare, failure to attempt to collect copayments and deductibles could be deemed an inducement to generate referrals, thereby violating the antikickback statute. There are some exceptions when the patient is indigent or the cost of collections is more than the copayment.

Check your carrier's bulletins. (Potentially, law enforcement agencies may view "insurance-only" claims as improper because the charge is being overstated if there is no intention to collect copayments or deductibles; see Chapter 3)

- Falsely applying for Medicare or Medicaid certification by falsification of address, or misrepresentation of credentials or other pertinent facts

- Billing for services rendered to one beneficiary under the Medicare number of another. It is a good idea to obtain photographic identification—such as driver's license—for new patients in case they are using a stolen Medicare or other insurance card. This is a good idea from a collection standpoint as well. Physicians and staff should be aware that there have been cases of patients who sold their Medicare or Medicaid numbers for profit

- Presentation of a claim for physician services performed by a nonphysician (unless the "incident to" provisions apply)[15]

- Billing for services to additional family members present when a patient encounter was almost entirely related to one family member. (This is a common warning in Medicaid programs)

- Reporting an incorrect place of service (one with a greater allowance) when providing medically necessary care to a patient could be considered intentional fraud. Under Medicare, for example, many surgical procedures have significantly greater allowances when performed in a physician's office rather than at a facility

- A training site sponsored by CMS/Medicare states that keeping an overpayment received from a government program could be considered fraud because "intentional withholding of an identified overpayment may be considered fraud" (Source: www.cms.hhs.gov/medlearn/medicare_fraud.pdf)

- Referrals to certain entities providing ancillary services where the physician or an immediate family member has a financial relationship. See Chapter 5 for a discussion of what is commonly called "Stark" legislation. This legislation includes a list of services—such as x-rays, clinical lab, home health, durable medical equipment, and other specifically identified services—that may violate self-referral regulations (there are exceptions). The government has recently started enforcing certain provisions under this self-referral legislation

Actions Taken by the Office of Inspector General

Physicians are all familiar with some of the large, well-publicized fraud and abuse cases, such as the recent investigation of Columbia/HCA for Medicare overpayments. Below are a few examples of less publicized criminal and civil actions cited in reports published by the Office of Inspector General (OIG), Department of Health and Human Services, for the period March 1995 through April 2002. Please refer to Appendix A for an extensive list of examples.

- A physician was sentenced to 6 months of house arrest, 2 years of probation, and payment of a $20,000 fine. The physician had previously pled guilty to mail fraud in connection with defrauding the Medicare and Medicaid programs. As part of his criminal plea, he agreed to surrender his medical license for life and to pay $26,112 in criminal restitution. A psychiatrist in practice for 30 years, he falsely represented that he treated patients when a licensed professional counselor actually provided the services. He also engaged in improper billing practices related to the treatment of his patients during hospitalization; for example, he submitted claims to Medicare for individual psychotherapy services and psychiatric evaluations not rendered. In addition, the investigation uncovered allegations that the psychiatrist used treatment of an unconventional and sexually inappropriate nature.

- A laboratory owner was sentenced to 3 years of probation, with a special condition that he serve 4 months in a special treatment center, followed by 8 months of home confinement, for conspiracy to submit false claims. The man paid kickbacks to local physicians and clinic owners in return for their referring clinical laboratory services to his laboratory. Moreover, he actively solicited clinics and encouraged them to order certain tests, with a higher Medicare reimbursement rate, for which he could bill the program. In order to have the cash necessary to pay these kickbacks, the laboratory owner engaged in an elaborate money laundering scheme. Two codefendants, who participated in the money laundering scheme by cashing checks under the $10,000 Internal Revenue Service reporting requirement, were sentenced as well. One was sentenced to 60 days of home confinement, 2 years of probation, and participation in an approved outpatient mental health program. The other was sentenced to 3 months of home confinement and 4 years of probation, with a special condition that he serve 4 months in a special treatment center. (Note: It may also be a crime to accept kickbacks.)

- A physician and his oncology clinic jointly agreed to pay the government $963,736 to resolve their civil liability for submitting false claims and entered into a corporate integrity agreement with OIG. Between 1992 and 1997, the physician and his clinic allegedly submitted improper claims to Medicare and the state Medicaid program for services rendered at the clinic by nonphysicians without a physician's supervision or presence. The corporate integrity agreement applies to all entities in which the physician has an ownership or management interest and that submit claims for reimbursement to any federal health care program.

- A physician, who also owned and operated a clinic, was sentenced to 5 years in prison and ordered to pay $2.87 million in restitution. The physician was convicted of multiple felony counts, including mail fraud, wire fraud, bankruptcy fraud, and making false statements. Evidence proved the physician deliberately misdiagnosed patients as suffering from a rare vascular disease that requires patients to obtain expensive pumps, braces, and other medical devices. The physician was also convicted of making false statements when he filed for bankruptcy in 1996.

- A neurologist was sentenced for his part in a scheme to defraud the Medicare and Medicaid programs. He had previously pled guilty to four felony counts of mail fraud. The physician submitted claims for nerve conduction studies and upcoded claims for office visits and electromyograms. He was sentenced to 6 months of home detention and 3 years of probation. He was also ordered to pay $118,750 in restitution and perform 3,000 hours of community service.

- A husband and wife were sentenced for stealing health care funds from their former employer. The husband was sentenced to 19 months incarceration and his wife to 13 months. The couple was also ordered to pay a total of $189,304 in restitution and to undergo drug treatment and counseling. While working for a company that provides billing and other management services to health care providers, the couple engaged in a scheme through which they diverted health care payment checks to accounts established for their own personal use.

- A physician agreed to pay the government $225,000 to settle allegations that his practice upcoded office visits and angioplasty consultations. This settlement figure represents approximately treble damages. The physician also agreed to enter into a 3-year corporate integrity agreement.

- A physician agreed to pay the government $23,041 to settle allegations related to improper billing practices. Between August 1991 and December 1996, the physician allegedly billed Medicare for certain arthroscopy surgical procedures as if they were more complex surgical procedures than those actually performed. As a result, he received an approximate overpayment of $14,127. As part of the settlement, the now-retired physician agreed to permanent exclusion from Medicare, Medicaid, and other federal health care programs.

- An OB-GYN practice and several individual physicians paid $109,900 to resolve their civil monetary penalty liability for violations of the physician self-referral (Stark) statute and the kickback provisions of the Civil Monetary Penalties Law. From 1997 through 2000, the physicians had a financial relationship with a mobile ultrasound company from which they received referral fees "ostensibly in the form of rent" in return for referring Medicare beneficiaries to the company for ultrasound studies and diagnostic testing.

- A physician and his clinic agreed to pay the government $1.7 million to settle allegations of violating the federal physician self-referral prohibition and federal health care program regulations. The physician allegedly participated in a scheme to circumvent prohibitions against the referral of patients to a home health agency in which the physician had a significant ownership interest. The physician violated these statutes by indirectly referring his patients to a home health agency owned by his wife. In settling this case, the OIG waived its permissive exclusion authority and imposed a corporate integrity agreement requiring outside audits, reporting, and other compliance measures during the next 5 years. One factor considered in the OIG's decision to waive its permissive exclusion authority involved the essential specialized services the physician provided to indigent patients in an underserved area. This investigation arose out of a civil lawsuit involving allegations of cost report fraud against the physician's wife.

- With the expansion of exclusion authority under the Health Insurance Portability and Accountability Act of 1996 (HIPAA) to include the sanctioning of individuals controlling previously sanctioned entities, a physician was excluded from program participation for 10 years. The physician was the owner of a methadone clinic that had been convicted of knowingly and willfully making false statements in applications for payment to Medicaid. The clinic paid restitution in the amount of $290,000, based on an overpayment of $95,000, and was excluded for 10 years.

- The HIPAA of 1996 also expanded the mandatory exclusion authority to exclude any individual convicted of a felony relating to health care fraud. A certified provider for the developmentally disabled was excluded for 5 years after being found guilty of a felony related to health care fraud. The provider submitted documents for reimbursement claiming that she had purchased clothing for a patient in the disability home in which she worked. She had purchased clothing; however, it was actually for herself.

- A hospital agreed to pay $45,000 to resolve two allegations of "patient dumping." The hospital failed to provide an appropriate medical screening examination and stabilizing treatment to a psychiatric patient. In addition, an on-call surgeon refused to accept an appropriate transfer of an individual who required the hospital's specialized facilities when the hospital had both the capacity and capability to treat the individual.

- An occupational health care firm agreed to pay $306,670 to resolve its liability for submitting false claims to Medicare. The firm submitted claims as though physical therapy services were incident to professional services of the physician, although the physician provided no professional services. When therapy was performed, the physician had no initial or subsequent contact with the beneficiaries.

- A pain control center and its president agreed to pay the government $75,215 to settle allegations of submitting false Medicare claims. During the period 1991 through 1994, the center and its president falsely represented acupuncture services provided to beneficiaries as physical therapy treatments in claims submitted to Medicare; Medicare does not cover acupuncture. They also submitted claims for physical therapy that was not medically necessary or not authorized and prescribed by a physician. The settlement additionally called for a 5-year exclusion of the codefendants.

- An emergency department physician agreed to pay $15,000 to resolve one dumping allegation. The incident involved the inappropriate transfer of a gunshot victim to a trauma center approximately 30 miles away. The patient was thought to be stabilized; however, immediately before transfer, the patient began to bleed heavily. Nonetheless, the physician transferred the patient by ambulance but without blood, even though blood was available and the patient had been prepped to receive blood. Shortly after arriving at the trauma center, the patient died of blood loss and a heart attack.[16]

See Appendix A for additional examples of actions taken by the OIG.

Examples of Improper Billing Identified by Others

- A federal jury convicted an OB-GYN and the anesthesiologist who worked with him of falsely billing insurance companies for covered gynecological procedures as a way of getting payment for uncovered fertility procedures. The physicians were convicted of conspiracy, health care fraud, and mail fraud in 2000. Prosecutors said the false billing went on for 10 years and that the OB-GYN made at least $2.5 million in that time. The state is one of about 15 states with laws requiring insurance companies to cover or to offer coverage for infertility treatment; however the law requires that insurers pay only for the diagnosis and treatment of medical conditions that result in infertility. It doesn't require insurers to pay for in vitro fertilization or other procedures that induce pregnancy. (News in brief. *AMNews*, Feb. 12, 2001.)

- An article in *AMNews* provided several examples of physicians having to repay funds to Medicare carriers for claims that were inappropriately submitted by the physicians' contracted billing services. In one case, six psychiatrists had to repay funds paid for some 4,800 claims submitted for services when only about 600 were documented in the physicians' records. Another example related to a billing company that upcoded physicians' claims. The physicians could not bring action against the billing service because it had closed. Several government officials expressed opinions that the physicians should monitor billing companies closer, make sure the company has an ongoing compliance program, and require contracts to define each party's responsibilities. (Landers SJ. Doctors warned of fraud liability. *AMNews*, April 24, 2000.)

- A physician repaid substantial billings to a Medicare HMO for services that the insurance company stated were included in the payment for the primary procedure. The physician argued that the services were noncovered and could, therefore, be billed directly to the patient (because the patient had signed a notice similar to the Advanced Beneficiary Notice). The HMO argued that the services were not noncovered—they were covered in the payment for another procedure.

- A study of Medicare payments for mental health services revealed that 39 percent of psychiatric services in nursing homes were medically unnecessary, had no mental health documentation, or were questionable. An area of particular vulnerability was psychological testing. Nearly one third of the tests were too frequent, medically unnecessary, or utilized questionable testing instruments. CMS has agreed to develop guidelines in these areas, which will both protect the quality of mental health services and could result in a potential savings of $30 million a year.[17]

- In a western state, two medical practice groups agreed to pay $10.25 million to settle allegations that they knowingly defrauded Medicare, TRICARE, and Medicaid from 1992 to 1999 by submitting numerous false claims to inflate reimbursement payments from Medicare, TRICARE, and Medi-Cal. The false billings alleged included: (1) billing for nonreimbursable annual physical exams; (2) billing for routine doctor "referrals" as more highly reimbursable consultations; (3) exaggerating the complexity of "evaluation and management" office visits to obtain greater reimbursement; and (4) billing for undocumented lab work and other ancillary services.[18]

- A number of Medicare audits involve alleged upcoding of Evaluation and Management (E/M) CPT® codes. The government's criteria used to determine whether a selected code is the proper level is very complex and ambiguous—there are even several sets of documentation requirements and the government is attempting to garner acceptance of a new set of guidelines to improve the selection process.

- There are software programs and other tools available that were designed by private companies to help physicians select the level of E/M codes. Some of these are helpful tools, but others may actually encourage physicians to upcode services—increasing audit liability—by performing or at least documenting unnecessary portions of higher code's selection criteria related to examinations, history taking, or medical decision making. One fault common to many of these tools is that the tool may show what documentation needs to be added to justify the higher level—and higher paying—code, but it does not consider that the medical necessity for those components may not be present in the patient encounter. That is, one can document all the components of the highest paying level of E/M code, but that may not justify billing the service if the patient's only complaint and problem addressed during the encounter is a "stubbed toe." The point is, one should not rely totally on these tools for code selection. Similarly, an article in the July 23, 2001, *AMNews* discusses recommendations made by coding seminar instructors and consultants that may suggest inappropriate upcoding. (Albert T. Consultants' bad billing advice may elicit fraud investigation. *AMNews*, July 23, 2001.)

OIG's Work Plans—1998 through 2002

Each year the OIG submits a work plan. The items below were selected from the OIG's 1998, 1999, 2000, 2001, and 2002 work plans. Most of these studies are ongoing and are not necessarily concluded during a specified time period. The work plan indicates some situations that are or could become audit targets in the future (however, these situations do not always become audit targets).

Physicians at Teaching Hospitals (PATH)

This initiative is designed to verify compliance with Medicare rules governing payment for physician services provided in the teaching hospital setting and to ensure that claims accurately reflect the level of service provided to patients. Previous OIG work in this area suggested that many providers were not in compliance with applicable Medicare reimbursement policies. *OAS; W-00-99-30021; Various CINs Year 2000, 2001, and 2002*

Billing for Resident Services

We will assess the extent of improper Medicare billings resulting from the issuance of provider billing numbers to resident physicians at teaching hospitals. In general, Medicare regulations do not allow residents to bill Medicare for their services. The exception is if the billable services are related to "moonlighting" activities unrelated to the resident's training program. Our work at one carrier found that a hospital had requested and received over 40 billing numbers for its residents over a 6-year period. The residents were not involved in "moonlighting" activities, and the hospital used the numbers to improperly bill Medicare for services provided by the residents. We will determine the extent of this condition at the carrier in this State and at other carriers. *OAS; W-00-98-30003; A-05-98-00053 Year 2000, 2001, and 2002*

Accuracy of and Carrier Monitoring of Physician Visit Coding

We will determine whether physicians correctly coded evaluation and management services in physician offices and effectively used documentation guidelines. We will also assess whether carriers identified any instances of incorrect coding and what corrective actions they took. Medicare payments for evaluation and management codes total approximately $18 billion per year and account for almost half of Medicare spending for physician services. Since 1992, Medicare has used visit codes developed by the American Medical Association to reimburse physicians for evaluation and management services. Generally, the codes represent the type and complexity of services provided and the patient status, such as new or established. Revised guidelines were issued in 1995 and again in 1997. Following the issuance of the 1997 guidelines, providers were told that they could use either the 1995 guidelines or the 1997 guidelines. Revised guidelines are again under development. *Year 2000–2002*

Consultations

This study will determine the appropriateness of billings for physician consultation services and the financial impact on the Medicare program from any inaccurate billings. In addition, we will determine the primary reasons for any inappropriate billings. In 2000, total allowed charges to Medicare for consultations were $2 billion. *OEI; 00-00-00000 Year 2001 and 2002*

Use of Surgical Modifier -25

We will determine whether physicians are improperly using modifier 25 on their Medicare Part B claims to increase reimbursements. Modifier 25 is for physicians to claim "Significant, Separately Identifiable Evaluation and Management Service on the Day of Surgery"—the key words being "Separately Identifiable." *OAS; W-00-98-30021; A-04-98-00000*

Physician and Other Provider Use of Diagnosis Codes

This review will examine a sample of services paid by Medicare. By comparing Medicare claims to beneficiary medical records, a medical reviewer will determine the extent to which diagnosis codes on claims match the reason for ordering and providing various services.

In a previous report entitled "Imaging Services for Nursing Facility Patients: Medical Necessity and Quality of Care" (OEI-09-95-00092), we found that physicians and other providers of imaging services do not follow CMS/HCFA's guidance on use of diagnosis codes. *OEI; 00-00-00000*

Anesthesia Services

This review will identify anesthesiologists who bill for personally performed services and determine if these services were in compliance with Medicare regulations. We found several instances where anesthesiologists were improperly billing for supervising residents in three or more operating rooms at the same time. *OAS; W-00-98-30021; A-03-98-00000*

Inappropriate Anesthesiology Claims

This review will assist Office of Investigations to determine whether the Medicare program has been inappropriately charged for anesthesiology services. The intermediary is concerned that a provider's billing practices for services furnished by Certified Registered Nurse Anesthesia (CRNA) and related costs included in its cost reports has resulted in double billing to the Medicare program. *OAS; W-04-97-30018; A-04-97-01167*

Critical Care Services

This review will focus on those providers who incorrectly bill Medicare for critical care based on the location of the patient and not the actual services provided by the physician. Critical care is that requiring the constant attention of the physician. It is usually, but not always, provided in a critical care area, such as a coronary care unit, intensive care unit, respiratory care unit or an emergency care facility. Physician services for patients who are not critically ill but happen to be in a critical care unit are to be claimed using "subsequent care" hospital codes. *OAS; W-00-98-30021; A-03-98-00-00000*

Billing for Services Rendered by Physician Assistants

We will determine whether physicians are improperly billing for services rendered by physician assistants. Medicare allows physician assistants to render certain services as "incident to" services, which are billed by the employing physician as if the service was personally rendered by the physician. However, if the services do not fall under the "incident to" criteria, the employing physician must bill using a modifier which reduces the Medicare payment. Medicare is overpaying physicians who improperly bill physician assistant services as "incident to" rather than using the proper modifiers. *OAS; W-00-97-30021; A-06-97-00047*

Billing Service Companies

This review will determine whether: (1) Medicare claims prepared and submitted by billing service companies are properly coded in accordance with the physician services provided to beneficiaries; and (2) the agreements between providers and billing service companies meet Medicare criteria. Medicare allows providers to contract with billing service companies that provide billing and payment collection services. The contractual agreements between the provider and the billing service company must meet certain Medicare criteria and a copy of the agreement must be provided to the applicable Medicare Carrier. Past OIG investigations have shown that billing service companies may be upcoding and/or unbundling procedure codes to maximize Medicare payments to physicians. The CMS/HCFA officials have expressed concern that the agreements may not meet the required criteria. *OAS; W-00-97-30021; A-06-97-00044*

Services and Supplies Incident to Physicians' Services

We will evaluate the conditions under which physicians bill 'incident-to' services and supplies. Physicians may bill for the services provided by allied health professionals, such as nurses, technicians, and therapists, as incident to their professional services. Incident-to services, which are paid at 100 percent of the Medicare physician fee schedule, must be provided by an employee of the physician and under the physician's direct supervision. Because little information is available on the types of services being billed, questions persist about the quality and appropriateness of these billings. OEI; 00-00-00000 *Year 2002*

Improper Billing of Psychiatric Services

We will determine whether providers are properly billing Medicare for psychiatric services in the following three areas: (1) providers' billing Medicare for individual psychotherapy rather than inpatient hospital care, resulting in Medicare overpayments, (2) providers' billing Medicare for a psychological testing code on a per test basis rather than a per hour basis, as required, or (3) providers' billing Medicare for group psychotherapy in cases which do not qualify for Medicare payment because either the group sessions do not involve actual psychotherapy services or the patients cannot benefit by group psychotherapy. Improper billing of these psychiatric services results in Medicare overpayments. *OAS; W-00-97-30021; A-06-97-00045* [Also suggests reviewing the use of CPT® code 90862 (pharmacologic management) and M0064 (brief office visit sole purpose of monitoring or changing drug prescription. . . .)]

Outpatient Hospital Psychiatric Claims

We will review outpatient psychiatric services rendered by both acute care and psychiatric hospitals to Medicare beneficiaries. Our reviews will determine whether the claims were for services actually provided and whether all Medicare billing and reimbursement requirements were met. *OAS; W-00-00-30026; Various CINs Year 2000*

Automated Encoding Systems for Billing

We will determine if errors found in Medicare billings for physician services are associated with providers' use of automated encoding software. Using billing errors identified in recent audits of CMS/HCFA's financial statements, we will contact providers to determine if automated software was used to prepare the billing. By comparing providers known to have submitted erroneous records with those that did not, we can take a first step in identifying any adverse effect of this software. Results of this work may lead to further reviews. *OEI; 00-00-00000*

[In 2000, the work plan included this statement.] We will determine whether errors found in Medicare billings for physician services are associated with providers' use of automated encoding software. We will also examine billing processes to identify vulnerabilities that occur when physician offices bill independently or through use of a third party system. *OEI; 05-99-00100*

Physician Case Management Billings

This review will determine if, when a home health claim has been denied by the regional home health intermediary, the Part B carrier also denies any related payments submitted by the physician for oversight of the plan of care. Payment to physicians for plan care oversight is to be recovered when a claim did not meet Medicare criteria for home health services. The intermediaries and carriers should be interacting with regard to such claims. Based on our early survey work, physician billings for plan care oversight could be substantially reduced based on the potential denial rate that should have taken place. *OAS; W-00-98-30009; A-06-98-00000*

Physicians With Excessive Nursing Home Visits

We will identify and audit physicians with excessive visits to Medicare patients in skilled nursing facilities (SNF). The OIG nursing home project identified trends in Medicare and Medicaid payments and populations and identified aberrant providers of nursing home services by type of service. Using this data as well as other computer screening techniques, we identified physicians with aberrant billing patterns for visits to SNF patients, such as an excessive number of visits in a given day and excessive visits to the same beneficiaries. Individual reviews will be conducted for those physicians with the most egregious billing patterns. We also plan to determine how the carriers could better identify and prevent such billings. *OAS; W-00-96-30015; A-09-97-00062; A-06-97-00050*

Physician Routine Nursing Home Visits

This review will assess whether CMS/HCFA needs to establish controls over Medicare payments for routine nursing home visits. Currently, physicians bill one of three possible procedure codes, depending on the level of care, when providing services to nursing home residents. The CMS/HCFA allows payments for physicians' routine monthly examinations, in addition to other medically necessary services. Our analysis in five States revealed that physicians sometimes billed for more services than they could perform in a normal workday. In these States, Medicare paid over $120 million for nursing home visits in FY 1998. Based on the level of care required for the codes billed, we have concerns about the quality of care provided to beneficiaries and the payments allowed for these services. *OAS; W-00-00-30014; A-06-00-00000 Year 2000*

Financial Conflicts of Interest

We will examine nursing homes purchased, either partially or wholly, by durable medical equipment supplier chains and/or physician groups. This review will look at claims submitted for Medicare beneficiaries in these homes and identify any aberrant billing patterns for services and supplies provided by owners with a substantial financial interest. *W-00-98-30014; A-03-98-00000*

Therapy in Nursing Facilities

A series of OIG reviews will evaluate the reasonableness of and costs associated with therapy services provided in skilled nursing facilities. The Medicare skilled nursing facility benefit is intended to provide post-hospital care to persons requiring intensive skilled nursing and/or rehabilitative services. These rehabilitative services may include physical and occupational therapy which may be paid by either Medicare Part A or Part B: Part A if the services are provided by nursing home staff or by outside staff paid by the nursing facility; Part B if the outside provider bills Medicare Part B directly. Past OIG work has found that services purchased under arrangement with outside providers were significantly higher than salaried therapy costs. We will examine a number of issues connected with these services and payment arrangements, including medical necessity and excessive costs. *OAS; W-00-98-30014; A-04-98-00000 OEI; 09-97-00120*

Therapy Services in Skilled Nursing Facilities

We will determine the medical necessity of physical and occupational therapy services provided to patients of skilled nursing facilities. The Medicare skilled nursing facility benefit is intended to provide post-hospital care to persons requiring intensive skilled nursing and/or rehabilitative services, including physical and occupational therapy. A probe sample in one State revealed significant evidence of medically unnecessary therapy services and

other issues related to the provision of therapy services. Because of these findings, we plan to conduct a national review. *OEI; 09-97-00121 Year 2000*

Beneficiary Access to Preventive Services

This study will evaluate beneficiaries' access to the expanded preventive services offered by Medicare since the passage of the Balanced Budget Act of 1997. The act created four classes of covered preventive services: annual screening mammography for all women aged 40 and over; screening pap smear and pelvic exams every 3 years; colorectal screening; and bone mass measurements to identify bone mass, detect bone loss, or determine bone quality. *OEI; 00-00-00000 Year 2002*

Advance Beneficiary Notices

We will examine the use of advance notices to Medicare beneficiaries and their financial impact on beneficiaries and providers. Physicians must provide advance notices before they provide services that they know or believe Medicare does not consider medically necessary or that Medicare will not reimburse. Beneficiaries who are not notified before they receive such services are not responsible for payment. Indications are that practices vary widely regarding when advance beneficiary notices are provided, especially with respect to noncovered laboratory services. *OEI; 00-00-00000 Year 2000, 2001 and 2002*

Hyperbaric Oxygen Treatment

We will examine the extent and appropriateness of hyperbaric oxygen treatment provided to Medicare beneficiaries. Medicare covers treatment for 14 different conditions, though effectiveness for many of these and other conditions is controversial. There are concerns that some physicians may be using the treatment for noncovered conditions or conditions for which the appropriate traditional treatments have not been tried. For example, though not covered, hyperbaric oxygen treatments for decubitus ulcers and diabetic foot wounds have been revealed through medical review. We will analyze payment and utilization trends, assess medical appropriateness, and examine the qualifications of hyperbaric oxygen treatment chambers and providers. *OEI; 06-99-00090 Year 2000*

Podiatry Services

This study will review podiatry claims to determine if the services met CMS/HCFA coverage policy. From 1992 through 1995, Medicare expenditures for nail debridement increased 46 percent, while Medicare expenditures for all other Part B services increased only 18 percent. We will examine a national sample of podiatry claims to gain a better understanding of the possible factor(s) affecting the extreme variation in allowed charges per thousand beneficiaries. *OEI; 00-00-00000 Year 2000*

Myocardial Perfusion Imaging

We will assess the medical appropriateness of myocardial perfusion imaging and explain the high increase in utilization since 1997. Myocardial perfusion imaging is a cardiac imaging procedure that is used to detect coronary artery disease and determine prognoses. This type of imaging procedure accounted for a large portion of the 23 percent increase in billing for all nuclear imaging services between 1997 and 1998. *OEI; 00-00-00000 Year 2000*

Reassignment of Physician Benefits

We will evaluate the practice of allowing physicians to reassign their billing numbers to clinics. Clinics that employ more than one doctor may accept a "reassignment" of the physicians' billing numbers, allowing the clinic to handle all billing and keep all fees for services provided by the physicians, usually in exchange for paying a flat fee or salary to the physicians. This practice, known as reassignment of benefits, provides considerable convenience to both physicians and the clinic business offices. Typically, in these instances, the physician never sees what is billed under his or her physician number. This practice shifts the accountability and liability for billing abuses away from the physician to the clinics. We will examine past reassignment abuses to determine specific vulnerabilities. *OEI; 00-00-00000 Also in year 2000*

Reassignment of Benefits II

We will examine the use of staffing companies and how this practice affects emergency room physicians. We will also identify any vulnerabilities in relation to Medicare reassignment rules. Hospitals commonly contract with billing and staffing companies to handle administrative functions. Over 50 percent of the hospitals in the United States use practice management or staffing companies to administer the daily operation and coverage of emergency room departments. Under these arrangements, emergency room physicians work for the staffing companies as either employees or independent contractors. These physicians may reassign their Medicare benefits only if they are employees of the staffing company. *OEI; 04-01-00080 Year 2002*

Physician Perspectives on Medicare HMOs

This study will determine the experiences and perspectives of physicians who work with Medicare health maintenance organizations (HMOs). The OIG has issued numerous reports on Medicare HMOs over the past several years. Some of these reports have raised concerns with the impact of HMOs on the access and quality of health care provided to Medicare beneficiaries. These previous studies have surveyed only Medicare HMO enrollees and administrators. This study will obtain the perspectives of another important player in the Medicare HMO industry, the physician. *OEI; 02-97-00070*

Physician Incentive Plans

We will review physician incentive plans included in contracts between physicians and managed care plans. In March 1996, CMS/HCFA published its final rule requiring managed care plans to disclose any arrangements that financially reward or penalize physicians based on utilization levels. It also requires plans to disclose these arrangements to beneficiaries. As part of this review, we will also look at other clauses in these contracts that may affect the quality of care provided. *OEI; 00-00-00000 Year 2000*

Managed Care Health Plan Data

We will assess how CMS/HCFA uses and ensures the quality of Health Plan Employers Data and Information Set data submitted by Medicare managed care organizations. The CMS/HCFA required managed care organizations to submit these data, which provide encounter-level health care quality information, for the first time in 1997 and annually thereafter. In addition to reviewing the accuracy of the data, we will analyze how CMS/HCFA uses the data to assess the performance of managed care organizations and how plans are held accountable for poor performance. *OEI; 00-00-00000 Year 2000*

Credentialing Medicaid Providers

This study will identify effective practices used by States in credentialing Medicaid providers. Some States are very careful about who can participate in the Medicaid program. They employ a variety of credentialing practices, including bonding, certification, background checks, and other activities to ensure that providers are reputable, competent, and accountable. We will also assess steps taken by States to credential Medicaid providers and to address the supply and availability of each type of provider within a State. *OEI; 00-00-00000 Year 2000*

Physician Certification of Durable Medical Equipment

This study will assess how effectively physicians are meeting Medicare expectations that they act as controls against unnecessary use of non-physician services and supplies. This study will build on our work assessing the physician's role in home health (OEI-02-94-00170) and in completing certificates of medical necessity (OEI-03-96-00010). We will identify common obstacles and successes in ensuring that physicians perform this important service. *OEI; 00-00-00000; 00-00-00000*

Medical Necessity of Durable Medical Equipment

We will determine the appropriateness of Medicare payments for certain items of durable medical equipment, including wheelchairs, support surfaces, and therapeutic footwear. We will assess whether the suppliers' documentation supports the claim, whether the item was medically necessary, and whether the beneficiary actually received the item. *OEI; 00-00-00000 Year 2002*

Physician Involvement in Approving Home Health Care

This follow-up review will determine the current extent of physician involvement in approving and monitoring home care for Medicare beneficiaries. Earlier OIG work found that physicians often did not have a relationship with their home health patients and relied extensively on home health agencies to determine the care needed. As part of our review, we will look at how frequently physicians examine home care patients and identify obstacles to physician involvement in monitoring their patients. *OEI; 00-00-00000 Year 2000*

Hospital Ownership of Physician Practices

We will assess Medicare billing practices and utilization when hospitals own physician practices. In recent years, integration in the health care marketplace has included hospital purchases of physician practices. Vulnerabilities may include inappropriate referrals (in either direction) between hospitals and physicians, excessive costs and billings, and overutilization of services when hospitals bill the Medicare program through physician practices they own. *OEI; 04-97-00090*

Physician Credit Balances

This review will determine whether physicians are reviewing their records for Medicare credit balances and refunding to their carriers those indicating an overpayment. A credit balance occurs when a provider receives and records higher reimbursement than the amount actually charged to a specific Medicare beneficiary. Some credit balances result from duplicate payments and in these cases a Medicare overpayment exists. Past OIG work which identified credit balances at hospitals resulted in significant recoveries for the Medicare program. *OAS; W-00-98-30021*

Multiple Discharges

We will determine whether duplicate payments have been made for day of discharge patient management services. Discharge day management can only be billed by the admitting physician. In one State, we have noted examples where two or more physicians are billing for discharge day management for the same beneficiary admission. We will develop a computer application to identify those beneficiaries whose discharge day management was billed by more than one physician during a single inpatient stay. *OAS; W-00-98-30021; A-03-98-00000*

Experimental Drug Trials

We will conduct two reviews to determine whether hospitals and other providers are inappropriately billing Medicare for items or services provided to beneficiaries as part of research grants and experimental drug trials. Many research projects are funded by the Public Health Service and private foundations, whereas experimental drug trials are usually paid by pharmaceutical companies. We will determine if claims for these projects are also being paid by Medicare. *OAS; W-00-98-30010; A-06-98-00000*

Duplicate Billing of Outpatient Hospital Services

We will compare the billing practices of hospital-based outpatient clinics and physicians who bill for similar services in the clinics. Services rendered in a hospital-based outpatient clinic are billed under Medicare Part B but through a fiscal intermediary. The physicians providing services in these clinics may be billing for the same services under Part B, but submitting their claims to the carrier. If both are billing for and receiving reimbursement for the same services, then duplicate payments result. These types of duplicate payments would be hard to routinely detect because bills are sent to different contractors. *OAS; W-00-98-30010; A-03-98-00000*

Mental Health Services in Nursing Facilities: A Follow Up

We will determine the continued existence of vulnerabilities to Medicare resulting from the expanded provision of mental health services to nursing facility residents. In a 1996 OIG study, we found medically unnecessary or questionable Medicare mental health services in nursing facilities in addition to a number of other vulnerabilities. We recommended that CMS/HCFA take steps to prevent inappropriate payments for these services, such as developing guidelines for carriers, developing screens to implement these guidelines, and conducting focused medical review and providing physician educational activities. This study will determine whether mental health services in nursing facilities continue to be inappropriately billed. Our work will be coordinated with that on outpatient mental health care. *OEI; 00-00-00000*

Part B Payments

We will determine the appropriateness of payments made to physicians, durable medical equipment suppliers and other providers of Part B services on behalf of hospice patients. Separate Part B payments for hospice beneficiaries are appropriate only for conditions unrelated to the patient's terminal illness. A recent nationwide review disclosed significant problems in Part A payments to hospitals and skilled nursing facilities for hospice patients; a similar situation appears to be occurring on the Part B side. *OAS; W-00-96-30015*

Identifying and Collecting Overpayments

We will assess the effectiveness of contractor activities to identify and collect Medicare overpayments. Providers are often paid more than the appropriate amount for services they bill. Although contractors use a variety of methods to identify, quantify, and recover overpaid trust fund amounts, some types of overpayments may never be identified. Further, once overpayments are identified, contractor efforts and success in recovering them vary widely. *OEI; 04-98-00530, -00531, -00532; 03-98-00520 Year 2000*

Medicare Provider Numbers and Unique Physician Identification Numbers

We will determine whether information associated with Medicare provider numbers and unique physician identification numbers is accurate and up to date. A number of OIG reports have identified deficiencies in the issuance of provider numbers for specific areas of the program, such as durable medical equipment providers and independent physiological laboratories. Other studies have noted that unused provider numbers are not deactivated timely and thus constitute a potential fraud vulnerability. In recent years, CMS/HCFA has taken a number of actions to standardize Medicare enrollment and has required providers to submit more information to ensure compliance with Social Security Act reporting requirements. We will assess the current condition of this information. *OEI; 07-98-00410 Year 2000*

Reimbursement for Diabetic Shoes

This review will determine the appropriateness of supplier billings for diabetic shoes. Medicare beneficiaries with diabetes have an increased risk of developing foot problems which could lead to amputation. Effective May 1, 1993, Medicare covers therapeutic shoes and related footwear designed to prevent the occurrence of serious foot problems. Medicare payments for such footwear have been increasing rapidly. Preliminary allowances for 1996 climbed to more than $12 million, an increase of over 20 percent from 1995 figures. Because of this rapid increase, we will review program expenditures in this area to determine if abusive billings are occurring. *OEI; 03-97-00300*

Medical Necessity of Oxygen

This review will assess Medicare beneficiaries' self-reported use of home oxygen therapy compared with documentation supporting the medical need for such therapy. We will assess the prescribing practices of physicians who order the systems and how Medicare monitors utilization and medical necessity for the systems. Allowances for oxygen equipment increased from about $835 million in 1992 to over $1.6 billion in 1995. *OEI; 03-96-00090*

Orthotic Body Jackets

In 1993, the OIG issued a report on Medicare payments for orthotic body jackets and found 95 percent of claims submitted should not have been paid because the "body jackets" did not meet construction and medical necessity criteria. Many of the devices were primarily used to keep patients upright in wheel chairs. A follow-up study will be done to determine if suppliers are still billing for "non-legitimate" orthotic body jackets. *OEI; 04-97-00390*

Clinical Laboratory Improvement Amendments

This study will determine how CMS/HCFA is enforcing the numerous provisions of the Clinical Laboratory Improvement Amendments of 1988; determine the relative strengths and weaknesses of its enforcement strategy; and recommend improvements if needed. The 1988 amendments strengthened quality standards under the Public Health Service Act and extended these requirements to all entities performing laboratory testing, including those in physicians' offices. *OEI; 05-92-01020*

[2002 OIG's Work Plan included this statement] We will determine whether laboratories conduct tests and bill Medicare within the scope of their certifications under the Clinical Laboratory Improvement Amendments (CLIA) of 1988. Laboratories with certifications of waiver or physician-performed microscopy procedures may perform only a limited menu of test procedures. Moderate- and high-complexity laboratories are also restricted to testing certain preapproved specialty groups and must meet CLIA standards. We will use CLIA certification and Medicare billing records to assess compliance with these requirements. *OEI; 05-00-00050*

Medicare Billings for Cholesterol Testing

We will determine whether cholesterol tests billed to Medicare are medically necessary and accurately coded. Although total cholesterol testing can be used to monitor many patients, Medicare claims reflect a preponderance of claims for lipid panels, which include HDL cholesterol and triglycerides also. Systems capable of doing all three tests, plus glucose, are advertised on the Internet as CLIA-waived. We will examine Medicare claims for the frequency of testing and the medical necessity of lipid panels. *OEI; 00-00-00000*

Clinical Laboratory Proficiency Testing

We will determine whether clinical laboratories that serve the Medicare population participate in proficiency testing programs and take appropriate action in response to failures. The Clinical Laboratory Improvement Amendments of 1988 established quality standards for all laboratory testing. A key condition of participation is proficiency testing in which a lab is sent samples for analysis and is graded on its performance in each testing specialty. This review will assess how well laboratories perform on these tests and what actions are taken in the case of unsatisfactory test results. *OEI; 00-00-00000 Year 2000*

[2002 OIG's Work Plan included this statement] We will assess the policies and procedures used for proficiency testing under CLIA and examine the quality of the testing results. The CLIA requires all moderate- and high-complexity laboratories to enroll with an approved proficiency testing agency for certain tests. These agencies are responsible for grading the accuracy of a laboratory's results; repeated failures can cause the laboratory to lose approval to perform those and similar tests. Because of the critical importance of proficiency testing, we will examine the testing and grading process. *OEI; 00-00-00000*

Utilization of Laboratory Services

This study will review trends in utilization of Medicare laboratory services. We will review these changes in light of the Clinical Laboratory Improvement Amendments of 1988, new laboratory test procedures, changes in physician fee schedules and growth in managed care. We will also look at possible mechanisms that can be effectively used to control utilization, including bundling of services into physician office visit reimbursement.

Such a proposal was advocated in a 1991 OIG report and was estimated to save $12 billion over 5 years. *OEI; 00-00-00000*

Fraud and Abuse in Cytology Laboratories

This review will assess the extent that cytotech workload records may be falsified and the reliability of laboratory procedures in workload record keeping. The Clinical Laboratory Improvement Amendments of 1988 imposed strict limits on the number of cytology slides that could

be read in a day. No more than 100 slides can be read by one person in a 24-hour period. This review is being undertaken at the request of CMS/HCFA officials because they have found through their inspection activity that the limit is being circumvented. *OEI; 02-95-00290*

Claims for Outpatient Hospital Laboratory Services

This follow-up review will determine the adequacy of procedures and controls used by fiscal intermediaries to process Medicare payments for clinical laboratory services performed by hospital laboratories on an outpatient basis. Clinical laboratory services include chemistry, hematology and urinalysis tests. The review will focus on whether providers properly bill for tests provided to the same beneficiary on the same day. The need for more effective controls was addressed in our prior review, "Nationwide Review of Laboratory Services Performed by Hospitals as an Outpatient Service" *(A-01-93-00520)*. *OAS; W-00-98-30011; A-01-97-00000*

Independent Physiological Laboratories

This review will identify program vulnerabilities associated with independent physiological laboratories and explore ways to safeguard the Medicare program from fraudulent and abusive providers. Concerns about improper billing by independent physiological laboratories include upcoding, performance of medically unnecessary services, billing for services not rendered and billings by questionable providers. We will analyze claims and related data associated with a sample of providers to determine whether the providers are legitimate and whether the claims meet other criteria for reimbursement. *OEI; 05-97-00240*

External Oversight of Dialysis Facilities

We will assess the extent and nature of CMS/HCFA's monitoring and oversight of quality of care for Medicare beneficiaries on dialysis. We will examine end stage renal disease network activity, State surveys and certification, complaint processes, and data collection and analysis regarding dialysis quality. *OEI; 01-99-00050 Year 2000*

Utilization Service Patterns of Beneficiaries

We will describe the utilization of health care services by end stage renal disease beneficiaries and assess the medical necessity and accuracy of coding of selected categories of services provided outside the composite rate. Recent settlements with major corporations and laboratories that serve end stage renal disease patients have raised questions about Medicare payments for a wide range of services. *OEI; 00-00-00000 Year 2002*

Inpatient Dialysis Services

This review will determine whether Medicare payments for inpatient dialysis services met the billing requirements of Medicare Part B. The Medicare Carrier Manual requires that the physician be physically present with the patient at some time during the dialysis and that the medical records document this in order for the physician to be paid on the basis of dialysis procedure codes. If the physician visits the dialysis inpatient on a dialysis day, but not during the dialysis treatment, physician services are billable under the appropriate hospital visit codes. Fee schedule amounts for inpatient dialysis codes are higher than those for hospital visit codes. *OAS: W-00-01-30021; A-09-01-00068 Year 2002*

Bone Density Screening

We will evaluate the impact of the recent standardization and expansion of Medicare coverage of bone density screening. Bone mineral density studies assess an individual's risk for fracture. Before the Balanced Budget Act of 1997, coverage for bone mass measurements varied by carrier. Effective July 1, 1998, the act standardized coverage of these studies. As the number of claims for bone density screening increases, there are questions about the appropriateness and quality of some services. *OEI; 00-00-00000 Year 2002*

Separately Billable Services

This review will determine the type and extent of separately billable maintenance dialysis services, the Medicare reimbursement for these services, and whether these services were included in the composite reimbursement rate. Under the prospective method of paying for maintenance dialysis, CMS/HCFA uses a composite rate per treatment to reimburse renal dialysis facilities for maintenance dialysis. This is a comprehensive payment for all services related to the dialysis treatment. Only those services whose costs were specifically excluded from the composite rate calculation are separately billable. *OAS; W-00-99-30025; A-01-99-00506 Year 2000*

Method II Billing for End Stage Renal Disease

We will assess method II billing for end stage renal disease services for program vulnerabilities, the adequacy of CMS/HCFA oversight, the impact on nursing home residents, and beneficiary satisfaction. End stage renal disease beneficiaries have the option to elect method II, in which a durable medical equipment supplier provides dialysis supplies, rather than method I, in which an end stage renal disease facility provides supplies and services. The use of method II appears to be growing in some States. A series of reports will look at both financial and quality perspectives of method II. *OEI; 00-00-00000 Year 2000–2002*

Medical Appropriateness of Tests and Other Services

We will assess the medical appropriateness of laboratory tests and other services ordered for end stage renal disease patients. A recent General Accounting Office (GAO) report found that clinically similar patients received laboratory tests at widely disparate rates. It concluded that the wide variation was probably the result of financial incentives, as well as a lack of knowledge and differences in medical practices. We will select a random sample of end stage renal disease beneficiaries and, with the assistance of medical staff where appropriate, conduct medical reviews to determine if laboratory and other services provided to these individuals were medically necessary and provided in accordance with Medicare requirements. *OEI; 04-98-00470 Year 2000*

Questionable Dialysis Claims

We will examine claims for dialysis services to assess the variability in provider billing patterns and to identify any aberrant providers. Dialysis treatments may be provided and billed either as single visits (common procedure codes 90935 and 90945) or, for patients with more complications, as multiple visits (codes 90937 and 90947) which are reimbursed by Medicare at a higher rate. On average, the ratio of services for the high to low codes is approximately 1 to 7.

A fraud alert was issued to carriers to periodically make comparisons in their areas to determine if any nephrologist is extremely deviant from the norm. Aberrant providers would be easy to identify by examining data showing the physicians' billing patterns. *OEI; 00-00-00000 Year 2000*

Duplicate Payments for Office Visits to Nephrologists

This review will identify situations in which Medicare made separate payments to nephrologists for dialysis patients' office visits but the services were already included in the monthly capitation payment for physician services during the same period. *OAS; W-00-00-30025; A-01-00-00000 Year 2000*

Epogen Reimbursement Relating to Hematocrit Levels

This review will determine whether CMS/HCFA's new policy on hematocrit levels will be effective in controlling the escalating cost to Medicare of the drug EPOGEN (EPO). EPO is a Medicare-covered drug used in the treatment of anemia associated with chronic renal failure. The CMS/HCFA recently issued a program memorandum

(AB-97-2) which restricts payments for EPO when a patient's hematocrit reading exceeds a certain level. *OAS; W-00-98-30025; A-01-98-00000*

Medicare Payments for EPOGEN

We will evaluate controls used to adjudicate potentially excessive Medicare claims submitted by dialysis facilities for the drug EPOGEN. The Omnibus Budget Reconciliation Act of 1990 established the EPOGEN reimbursement rate at $11 per 1,000 units administered. Subsequently, the rate was reduced by statute to $10 per 1,000 units administered. During an ongoing review of outpatient services, we identified claims for an excessive number of units; e.g., 7.5 million units were claimed when, in fact, only 75,000 units were administered, resulting in an overpayment of approximately $74,000. *OAS; W-00-02-30025; A-01-02-00000 Year 2002*

Dialysis Supply Kits

This study will determine whether Medicare payments for dialysis supply kits are appropriate. Medicare has created a separate benefit category known as "dialysis supplies and equipment" for beneficiaries who qualify for Medicare because they suffer from end stage renal disease. Such supplies and equipment are covered for patients who receive dialysis at home under the supervision of a Medicare-approved dialysis facility. In 1996, Medicare allowances for the two major procedure codes representing dialysis supply kits are projected to exceed $150 million for the year. *OEI; 00-00-00000*

Bad Debts Nationwide Chain

This review will determine whether home office costs and bad debts reported by a nationwide chain organization are in accordance with Medicare reasonable cost principles, and provisions of the Provider Reimbursement Manual. Under Medicare's composite rate reimbursement system, ESRD facilities are reimbursed 100 percent of their allowable bad debts, up to their unreimbursed Medicare reasonable costs. . . . However, prior reviews have identified unallowable costs in cost reports for facilities claiming bad debts, thus overstating the reimbursable amount. Further, these facilities did not identify unallowable costs on prior cost reports. We will assess the internal controls for Medicare cost reporting, cost allocation, and general ledger maintenance. We will also perform substantive testing to determine whether reported costs are allowable. *OAS; W-00-98-30025; A-01-98-00000*

Dialysis Procedure/Evaluation and Management Code Double Billing

We will determine if renal/nephrology physicians are billing for a dialysis evaluation on the same day that they bill for evaluation and management services. The Medicare Carriers Manual states that a dialysis procedure cannot be paid on the same day as evaluation and management services, unless the services are unrelated to the dialysis, as dialysis and any related physician services are included in the monthly capitation payment. We will study this area to determine the significance of this issue. *OAS; W-00-98-30025; A-03-98-00000*

OIG-Excluded Providers

This review will examine how OIG exclusion data is used outside the OIG and identify improvements needed in the government's ability to protect federally-funded programs and their beneficiaries from fraudulent or poor-performing health care providers. Every year the OIG excludes 1,200-1,500 fraudulent or unqualified practitioners from Medicare and Medicaid participation for varying durations. Interested parties are able to identify these excluded providers by virtue of broad dissemination of OIG exclusion data and other means. However, anecdotal indications are that interested parties other than CMS/HCFA are not using this information, even though these providers are potentially harmful to Federal programs and their beneficiaries. *OEI; 00-00-00000*

Ambulatory Surgery Centers

A series of OIG reports assessed how state agencies and accreditors oversee ambulatory surgical centers (ASCs) and how CMS holds them accountable. The ASCs have experienced explosive growth, more than doubling in number from 1990 to 2000. In the same time period, the volume and complexity of procedures performed in ASCs has increased dramatically, from 12,000 to over 101,000 major procedures annually. However, the OIG believes Medicare's system of quality oversight is not up to the task. States have not recertified nearly a third of ASCs in 5 or more years, and CMS does little to monitor the performance of state agencies and accreditors. The report made recommendations to CMS to strengthen its quality oversight of ASCs. While CMS responded positively to the report, it did not fully commit itself to a number of the recommendations, particularly those calling for a minimum survey cycle and a more accessible complaint process. *OEI-01-00-00450; OEI-01-00-00451; OEI-01-00-00452) Year 2002*

Hospital Privileging Activities

The OIG will review the nature and extent of hospital privileging activities within the context of Medicare conditions of participation. One of the most fundamental internal safeguards in hospitals is the routine practice of granting initial or renewed privileges to physicians. Hospital privileging is the process by which a hospital determines the scope of allowable practice for each physician within that hospital. It occurs at the onset of a physician's relationship with a hospital and on some recurring basis thereafter. *OEI; 00-00-00000 Year 2002*

Quality Assessment and Assurance Committees

The OIG will examine the role and effectiveness of quality assessment and assurance committees in ensuring quality of care in nursing homes. The Omnibus Budget Reconciliation Act of 1987 requires each nursing facility to maintain a committee composed of the director of nursing, a physician, and at least three other staff members. The committee is to meet at least quarterly to identify quality assessment and assurance activities and to develop and implement appropriate plans of action to correct identified quality deficiencies. The CMS requires surveyors to determine whether a facility has such a committee and whether it has a method to "identify, respond to, and evaluate" issues in quality of care. This review is one of a series on the quality of care in nursing homes. *OEI; 01-01-00090 Year 2002*

Medicare Billings for Nebulizer Drugs

This study will determine whether Medicare payments for inhalation drugs are appropriate and whether the drugs are priced appropriately. Medicare covers prescription inhalation drugs used with nebulizers if the nebulizer provides effective therapy for a beneficiary's respiratory illness. Allowances for inhalation drugs have increased steadily, from more than $332 million in 1995 to over $540 million in 1999. We will determine whether suppliers' documentation supports their claims and whether the claims are medically necessary. In addition, we will compare Medicare fee schedules for inhalation drugs with other sources, such as third-party coverage available to beneficiaries and prices paid by other Federal insurers. *OEI; 00-00-00000 Year 2002*

Rural Health Clinics

We will follow up on our previous study of rural health clinics to determine whether our recommendations have been implemented and what changes have occurred as a result of the Balanced Budget Act of 1997. Our study, as well as a review by the General Accounting Office, sparked legislative change that capped provider-based rural health clinic reimbursement and created a triennial certification process to prevent the proliferation of clinics in nonrural areas. Our report offered a number of measures that CMS could take to improve the functioning and oversight of this program. *OEI; 00-00-00000*

Administrative Law Judges' Decisions

We will review the Medicare claims process, including the mechanism by which beneficiary claim denials are aggregated for appeal before Administrative Law Judges. An Administrative Law Judge is empowered to reverse a carrier denial of a claim or group of similar claims, resulting sometimes in substantial post-denial payments to providers and suppliers. Such reversals occur in 70 percent of the appeals submitted to these judges. Under existing laws, the Medicare program has limited recourse to appeal the decision of an Administrative Law Judge. *OEI; 00-00-00000*

Physician Incentive Plans in Managed Care Contracts

We will review physician incentive plans that are included in contracts that physicians enter into with managed care plans. In March 1996, CMS/HCFA published its final rule requiring managed care plans to disclose any arrangement that financially rewards or penalizes physicians based on the utilization levels. It also requires plans to disclose these arrangements to beneficiaries. As part of this review, we will also look at other clauses in these contracts that may impact the quality of care provided. *OEI; 00-00-00000*

Mutually Exclusive Medical Procedures

This review will determine the adequacy of procedures and controls used by Medicare carriers and fiscal intermediaries to prevent payments for mutually exclusive medical procedures. These procedures, based on their definition or the medical technique involved, are impossible or unlikely to be performed at the same session. Reimbursement to providers such as physicians, clinical laboratories, and ambulatory surgical centers are all based on the procedure code submitted to Medicare. The review will focus on whether providers were improperly paid for mutually exclusive procedures provided to the same beneficiary on the same date of service. *OAS; W-00-98-30003*

[The OIG's 2002 Work Plan Stated] We plan to review the procedure coding of outpatient services billed by a hospital and a physician for the same service. In a previous review, we identified a 23-percent nationwide rate of inconsistency between hospital outpatient department procedure coding and physician procedure coding for the same outpatient service. This review will determine whether these coding differences continue and, if so, how they affect the Medicare program. *OAS; W-00-02-30026; A-01-02-00000*

Duplicate Billings for Outpatient Services

We will determine the extent of duplicate billings resulting from outpatient claims being submitted to both intermediaries and carriers. Hospitals, nursing homes and other institutions (Part A providers) certified by the Medicare program submit their claims for reimbursement to intermediaries. Physicians, independent clinical laboratories and other (Part B) suppliers of services submit their claims for reimbursement to carriers. We will assess vulnerabilities in the current systems that may lead to bills for some services being submitted to and paid by both. *OEI; 00-00-00000*

[The OIG's 2002 Work Plan Stated] We plan to review the procedure coding of outpatient services billed by a hospital and a physician for the same service. In a previous review, we identified a 23-percent nationwide rate of inconsistency between hospital outpatient department procedure coding and physician procedure coding for the same outpatient service. This review will determine whether these coding differences continue and, if so, how they affect the Medicare program. *OAS; W-00-02-30026; A-01-02-00000*

Medicare's Correct Coding Initiative

We will evaluate Medicare's correct coding initiative, which is designed to improve the accuracy of Part B claims processed by Medicare carriers. Physicians use the CMS/HCFA common procedure coding system to bill Medicare for services provided to beneficiaries. We will evaluate the effectiveness of the initiative in detecting improper billings, and whether carriers are uniformly adopting practices being promoted by the initiative. *OEI; 00-00-00000*

Provider Billing Numbers Issued to Resident Physicians

We will assess the extent of improper Medicare billings resulting from a control problem we noted at one carrier relative to issuing provider billing numbers to resident physicians at teaching hospitals. In general, Medicare regulations do not allow residents to bill Medicare for their services. The exception is if the billable services are related to "moonlighting" activities at another institution separate from the institution where the resident is pursuing his/her medical studies. We noted that a hospital in one State requested and received over 40 billing numbers for their residents over a 6 year period. The residents were not involved in "moonlighting" activities, and the hospital used the numbers to improperly bill Medicare for services provided by the residents. We will determine the

extent of this condition at the carrier in this State and other carriers. *OAS; W-00-98-30003; A-05-98-00000*

Control of Chiropractic Benefits

Chiropractic claims are one of the more frequently billed services to Medicare. While chiropractic benefits are not currently provided by all State Medicaid programs, an increasing number of States are preparing to offer these benefits. Due to the nature of the services, distinguishing between acute care (which is generally covered) and preventive care (which is not covered by Medicare and seldom covered by Medicaid) is difficult, creating control problems for Medicare carriers, State Medicaid agencies and private insurers. This study will identify the extent and nature of the control problems and identify the mechanisms used by Medicare carriers, Medicaid agencies and private insurers to control the use of chiropractic benefits and to prevent fraud and abuse. In addition, this study will highlight the most effective control mechanisms currently in use. *OEI; 00-00-00000*

Medicare as Secondary Payer

This study will assess the effectiveness of current procedures in preventing inappropriate Medicare payments when beneficiaries have other insurance that is required to pay primary. A 1991 OIG report found that inappropriate Medicare secondary payer payments totaled more than $637 million in 1988 and identified several leading causes. In addition to repeating the 1991 study, we will review the consistency of secondary payer provisions and determine whether standardization would facilitate the implementation of the provisions. *OEI; 00-00-00000*

Medicare Secondary Payer Oversight

We will follow-up on CMS/HCFA's resolution of an OIG recommendation relating to the employer compliance with the Medicare secondary payer (MSP) Data Match Project. Our earlier report recommended that CMS/HCFA take action against employers that failed to provide the necessary employer group health plan information needed for the Data Match Project. In addition, a major insurance association agreed to a global settlement with the Department of Justice and CMS/HCFA to settle disputes over secondary payer claims. As part of the settlement, the association started a 3-year data exchange agreement with CMS/HCFA. Our review will examine what action CMS/HCFA is taking to secure data exchange agreements with the association beyond the 3-year settlement and with other insurance companies not covered by the agreement. *OAS; W-00-98-30003*

Physician Referrals to Self-owned Laboratory Services

This review will analyze CMS/HCFA's enforcement of the self-referral prohibition involving physicians and clinical laboratory services. Medicare law prohibits payment to physicians who have certain proscribed financial relationships with other providers, including entities that provide clinical laboratory services. Other penalties may also apply for violations of this law. We will analyze whether CMS/HCFA has adequate information (i.e., ownership and compensation data) to enforce the law with respect to clinical laboratory services, and document the actions taken to date. *OEI; 09-97-00250*

Medicare Part B Billings By State-Owned Facilities

This review will use computer screens, developed by the OIG, to identify physicians with aberrant billing patterns for visits to patients in State-owned facilities. Prior focused medical reviews by Medicare contractors identified a variety of problems associated with these types of claims related to skilled nursing facilities. We will build on this prior work and determine if all types of State-owned facilities have similar problems. *OAS; W-00-98-30030*

Joint Work With Other Federal and State Agencies

To efficiently use audit resources, we will continue our efforts to provide broader coverage of the Medicaid program by partnering with State auditors, State departmental internal auditors and Inspectors General, Medicaid agencies, and CMS/HCFA financial managers. Since 1994, active partnerships have been developed with States on such issues as prescription drugs, clinical laboratory services, the drug rebate program, and durable medical equipment. Future joint initiatives will cover managed care issues, hospital transfers, prescription drugs, laboratory services, non-physician outpatient services, and nursing home services. In addition, we will continue to work with the National State Auditors Association on a joint audit of long-term care in six States. Potential audit areas include evaluating the licensing and inspection of nursing homes and the reimbursement system. *OAS; W-00-98-30001; Various CINs*

Sharing of Medicaid and Medicare Audit Findings

This review will examine the information sharing process for audits of nursing homes that are conducted by State auditors for Medicaid purposes and by fiscal intermediaries' auditors for Medicare purposes. In a survey in one State, we found that the State's auditors and the intermediary auditors were not consistently sharing audit results. Consequently, overclaims by nursing homes went undetected. We will determine if similar problems are occurring in other States. *OAS; W-00-98-30030*

Pneumonia DRG Upcoding Project

The Pneumonia DRG Upcoding Project was initiated to identify hospitals that falsify the diagnosis and diagnosis related group on claims from viral to bacterial pneumonia. The Office of Investigations is currently working with the Department of Justice to initiate a nationwide project in this area.

Project Bad Bundle

The Office of Investigations launched Project Bad Bundle to identify hospitals that unbundle blood chemistry tests when using automated equipment and then bill for each analysis separately, or bill for an automated test in addition to several of the analyses separately. "Unbundling" refers to the illegal practice of submitting individual bills for separate tests that should be bundled together into a single bill for a group of related tests. The amount allowed under Medicare for this "bundled" amount is considerably lower than the sum of the amount for tests billed separately. Under this initiative, the total civil settlement to date is $8.8 million and involved 24 hospitals.

Private Physician Contracting

This study will review the impact of private contracting between Medicare beneficiaries and physicians. Under the 1997 Balanced Budget Act, physicians and beneficiaries may enter into agreements specifying that the beneficiary will pay out-of-pocket for Medicare-covered services provided by that physician. Physicians who choose to provide covered services under these contracts must "opt out" of the Medicare program for 2 years.

They may not receive payment from Medicare for any service regardless of whether it is provided on a fee-for-service or capitated basis. Though relatively few physicians have chosen this option, its impact on beneficiaries' access to care, as well as other beneficiary protections, is unclear. *OEI; 00-00-00000 Year 2000*

Contractor Fraud Control Units

We will follow up on our previous studies of contractor fraud control units and identify factors that contribute to and work against successful program integrity operations. Our November 1996 report noted deficiencies in carriers' ability to properly identify potentially fraudulent activity and to consistently develop payment information, as well as deficiencies in case documentation and internal and external proactive safeguards. In our November 1998 report, we found that fraud units differed substantially in the number of complaints and cases handled and that some units produced few, if any, significant results. Additionally, half of the units did not open any cases proactively, and more than one-third did not identify program vulnerabilities. *OEI; 00-00-00000 Year 2002*

Review of the OIG's work plan provides insight into areas that may become future audit targets. Of course, the issues raised in the work plan are not the only audit targets. Work plans for 2000, 2001, and 2002 may be viewed at Web site www.oig.hhs.gov.

Also, review the *OIG Compliance Program Guidance for Individual and Small Group Physician Practices* in Appendix C. Appendix A of that document includes a discussion of various compliance risk areas.

Endnotes

1. Under Medicare, the allowable for some CPT® codes is subject to a site-of-service reduction when the service is performed in an outpatient setting. Most Medicare carriers can supply a listing of codes subject to the reduction.

2. Misrepresenting the diagnosis for the patient to justify the services or equipment furnished.

3. This includes things like billing for "no shows," ie, billing Medicare for services that were not actually furnished because the patients failed to keep their appointments. [Billing a cancellation fee for "no shows" is not necessarily inappropriate under non-governmental programs. Check other payers' guidelines.]

4. Medicare's Correct Coding Initiative goes a long way toward defining CPT® codes that might be deemed unbundled, fragmented, or inappropriate coding combinations. Although these coding edits are not perfect, most physicians' offices should maintain a copy of them for reference. While the edits apply to Medicare, they will be used increasingly by private payers to identify potential unbundling and other improper coding combinations.

5. A Medicare carrier representative described this situation as follows: "This is just good medicine. Preventative management is key to good health. The program, however, was never designed or intended to pay for good medicine. The Medicare program was intended to pay only for those services that are reasonable and necessary for the care or treatment of an illness or injury. Preventative maintenance is a non-covered service. Not only is the exam not covered but also any other service performed that day in the course of the exam. That would include EKGs, chest x-rays, and lab services. Although the mindset regarding 'routine' or preventative services is slowly changing, there has not been any legislation that would allow payment for routine physical examinations as a benefit under the program [Medicare]. Physicians' offices often bill these encounters as established patient visits, but the patient's chart clearly states the reason for the encounter is, *Annual physical exam* or *Six month check-up*." In recent years, Medicare coverage has been extended to some screening services such as mammography, Pap smears, colorectal cancer, and prostate cancer.

6. Physicians should carefully review the various CPT® codes for billing skin lesion services. There are codes for excisions, shavings, destruction, etc. Billing for an excision, when a shaving was the surgical method, will usually result in higher reimbursement but could be deemed fraudulent or abusive.

7. In August 1999, the Health Care Financing Administration issued Medicare Carriers Manual Transmittal No. 1644, which included language that appears to expand situations where physicians may use consultation codes. Previous interpretations of guidelines for consultation codes under Medicare required use of office visit or hospital visit codes if care was transferred to the receiving physician. "Care" was usually interpreted by carriers to mean the clinical situation for which the patient was referred (eg, an eye condition or an orthopedic problem). Thus, most carriers would, upon audit, downcode a consultation to an office or hospital visit if it appeared the referring physician's intent was for the receiving physician to handle the condition without the necessity to report back. The new document uses the following language: "A transfer of care occurs when the referring physician transfers the responsibility for the patient's complete care to the receiving physician at the time of referral, and the receiving physician documents approval of care in advance."

Physicians should be cautious in changing past coding practices until the new requirements are released in their carrier's newsletter along with clarifying examples and other requirements for billing a consultation code. Also, note that these are Medicare guidelines and are not necessarily the same guidelines found in CPT®.

8. Sometimes it is difficult to determine the number of concurrent cases, particularly when case times overlap. Another potential problem area is addressed in the Medicare Carrier Manual (section 15018), which indicates that concurrency is not dependent on each case involving a Medicare patient. As one carrier put it: "If an anesthesiologist directs three concurrent procedures, two of which involve non-Medicare patients and the remaining a Medicare patient, this represents three concurrent cases."

9. A Medicare carrier training document cautioned about the improper use of modifiers that designate situations that should not be subjected to "bundling" and duplicate payment edits. Such modifiers include -25 (significant, separately identifiable E/M service by the same physician on the same day of a procedure); -57 (decision for surgery); -59 (distinct procedural service); -76 (repeat procedure by the same physician); and -79

(unrelated procedure or service by the same physician during the postoperative period).

10. *Special fraud alert: physician certifications*: The OIG issued a special fraud alert entitled "Physician Liability for Certifications in the Provision of Medical Equipment and Supplies and Home Health Services." It was published in the Federal Register on January 12, 1999, and is available at the Web site www.oig.hhs.gov/fraud.html. The key portions state: "We [OIG] are issuing this Fraud Alert because physicians may not appreciate the legal and programmatic significance of certifications they make in connection with the ordering of certain items and services for their Medicare patients. While the OIG believes that the actual incidence of physicians' intentionally submitting false or misleading certifications of medical necessity for durable medical equipment or home health care is relatively infrequent, physician laxity in reviewing and completing these certifications contributes to fraudulent and abusive practices by unscrupulous suppliers and home health providers. We urge physicians and their staff to report any suspicious activity in connection with the solicitation or completion of certifications to the OIG.

"Physicians should also be aware that they are subject to substantial criminal, civil, and administrative penalties if they sign a certification knowing that the information relating to medical necessity is false, or with reckless disregard as to the truth of the information being submitted. While a physician's signature on a false or misleading certification made through mistake, simple negligence, or inadvertence will not result in personal liability, the physician may unwittingly be facilitating the perpetration of fraud on Medicare by suppliers or providers. Accordingly, we urge all physicians to review and familiarize themselves with the information in this Fraud Alert. If a physician has any questions as to the application of these requirements to specific facts, the physician should contact the appropriate Medicare Fiscal Intermediary or Carrier."

11. There are a number of defenses for individuals who truly were not aware, or there was no reason for them to be aware, of fraudulent activity. But potentially innocent individuals must recognize the costs of being associated with convicted individuals or entities, which include defense fees, fines, stress, tarnished reputation, and loss of income. This is another reason to insist on compliance programs where you work.

12. The OIG's *Semiannual Report* (October 1997–March 1998) describes an audit of laboratory billings: "The objective of this nationwide audit was to determine the adequacy of procedures and controls used by Medicare carriers to process payments for clinical

laboratory tests performed by independent and physician laboratories. Specifically, the OIG review was designed to determine whether certain chemistry, hematology, and urinalysis tests were appropriately grouped together (bundled into a panel or profile) and not duplicated for Medicare payment purposes and whether certain additional automated hematology indices paid by the Medicare program were ordered by physicians.

"The OIG estimated that, nationwide, Medicare carriers overpaid independent and physician laboratories about $50.2 million for these three types of tests during 1993 through 1995. For the same period, an additional $30.8 million could have been saved if policies had been adopted to preclude payment for additional automated hematology indices. The OIG recommended that CMS/HCFA direct Medicare carriers implement procedures and controls to ensure that clinical laboratory tests are appropriately grouped together, not duplicated for payment purposes and actually ordered by physicians. Also, OIG proposed that CMS/HCFA consider eliminating separate reimbursement for additional indices and that the identified potential overpayments be recovered through coordination with applicable investigative agencies. The CMS/HCFA generally concurred with the recommendations and agreed to take corrective action. (CIN: A-01-96-00509)"

13. Medicare does allow billing under the attending physician's number under reciprocal coverage arrangements and when using locum tenens. There are, however, specific rules for doing so and special modifiers that must be used to designate compliance with the guidelines.

14. Pathologists and similar specialists should review OIG Advisory Opinion No. 99-13, posted December 7, 1999, regarding *account billing*. Without getting into all the details, the term *account billing* as used in the advisory opinion refers to discounting specimen examination services to other physicians in a manner the OIG believes might violate anti-kickback legislation. This advisory opinion is posted on the OIG's Web site, www.oig.hhs.gov/fraud.html. Also, watch for other announcements regarding such services.

15. Under Medicare's rules, the phrase "incident to a physician's professional service" means that services or supplies are furnished as an integral, although incidental, part of the physician's personal professional services in the course of diagnosis or treatment of an injury or illness. The services of employed nonphysicians must be rendered under the physician's *direct* supervision. This does not mean, however, that to be

considered "incident to" each occasion of service by a nonphysician (or furnishing of a supply) need also always be the occasion of the actual rendition of a personal professional service by the physician. Such a service or supply could be considered to be "incident to" when furnished during a course of treatment where the physician performs an initial service and subsequent services of a frequency that reflect his or her active participation in and management of the course of treatment. (However, the direct supervision requirement must still be met with respect to every nonphysician service, with the exception of the provision of certain services to homebound patients and services in a rural health clinic [MCM §2050.1.].)

Expect closer scrutiny of Medicare services performed by physician assistants (PAs) and nurse practitioners (NPs). In 1998, significant changes were made to guidelines for billing PA and NP services. Effective July 1, 1998, physician extenders are required to obtain provider numbers, and claims must be filed identifying the PA or NP as the performing provider.

A physician who bills services performed by a PA or NP as incident to the physician's service will receive a little more reimbursement than if it were billed under the PA's or NP's name. While Medicare rules allow a physician to bill such services as "incident to," Medicare requires the physician to have been involved sufficiently with the patient (this does not necessarily mean the physician had to see the patient on the day of the PA's/NP's encounter). Review your Medicare carrier's bulletins for guidance if you use extenders. Also, the types of services that can be performed by physician extenders vary from state to state. You should watch for changes to Medicare's "incident to" rules.

16. *Civil penalties for patient dumping*: Section 1867 of the Social Security Act (42 USC 1395dd) provides that, when an individual presents to the emergency department for examination or treatment, a hospital that has a Medicare provider agreement is required to provide an appropriate medical screening examination to determine whether that individual has an emergency medical condition or is in active labor. If an individual has such a condition, the hospital must provide, within the capabilities of the staff and facilities available at the hospital, treatment to stabilize the condition, unless a physician certifies that the individual should be transferred because the benefits of medical treatment elsewhere outweigh the risks associated with transfer. Physicians who may be on call also have potential liability if they are unresponsive to a call request.

If a transfer is ordered, the transferring hospital must arrange for a safe transfer, which includes providing stabilizing treatment to minimize the risks of transfer, making sure the receiving hospital has agreed to accept the transfer, and effecting the transfer through qualified personnel and transportation equipment. A hospital is prohibited from delaying provision of examination or treatment for an emergency medical condition to inquire about an individual's method of payment or insurance status. Further, a participating hospital with specialized capabilities or facilities may not refuse to accept an appropriate transfer of an individual who needs those services if the hospital has the capacity to treat the individual.

The OIG is authorized to impose civil monetary penalties (CMPs) of up to $25,000 against small hospitals (less than 100 beds) and up to $50,000 against larger hospitals (100 beds or more) for each instance where the hospital negligently violated any of the section 1867 requirements. In addition, OIG may impose a CMP of up to $50,000 against a participating physician, including an on-call physician, for each negligent violation of any of the section 1867 requirements, and impose a program exclusion in certain cases.

17. The Department of HHS and the Department of Justice, *Health Care Fraud and Abuse Control Program Annual Report for FY 2001*, published April 2002.

18. The Department of HHS and the Department of Justice, *Health Care Fraud and Abuse Control Program Annual Report for FY 2001*, published April 2002.

3

Fraud and Abuse Statutes

Chapter 3 is a summary of various federal laws that are commonly used to prosecute alleged instances of fraud or abuse. This is not intended to be an exhaustive discussion. Many federal laws, state laws, and applications of such laws are not discussed here. Carriers and other payers also promulgate guidelines to determine overpayments and/or abusive billing practices. The examples do not cover all possible instances that could be deemed fraudulent or abusive. As always, the specific circumstances should be discussed with competent legal counsel.

A number of federal statutes may be used as the basis for health care fraud prosecution. In addition, many states have enacted legislation aimed at health care fraud. Even federal legislation such as the Racketeer Influenced and Corrupt Organizations Act (RICO) may be used to prosecute health care fraud. The maximum criminal and/or civil penalties under these laws can be quite severe.

The most commonly used statutes for prosecuting or facilitating the prosecution of health care-related fraudulent or abusive activities are discussed below. They include the Health Insurance Portability and Accountability Act of 1996 (HIPAA), False Claims Act, False Statement Statute, Mail and Wire Fraud Statutes, and Social Security Act civil monetary penalties.

Perhaps the best place to begin discussing the various laws applicable to health care fraud and abuse is the HIPAA, which dramatically changed health care fraud enforcement.

Health Insurance Portability and Accountability Act of 1996

Many readers will be familiar with recently promulgated HIPAA regulations addressing the privacy and security of patient information. In its entirety, the Health Insurance Portability and Accountability Act (HIPAA) of 1996 includes a number of provisions that could be broadly categorized into three sections: (1) directives that improve the "portability" of health insurance when an employee changes or loses their job; (2) those related to transmission and protection of information about patients; and (3) statutes designed to enhance fraud and abuse enforcement. HIPAA also addresses a few other issues such as national "provider numbers" that all payers would recognize, and the like.

Thus, *HIPAA* could mean different things to different people. In this book, we are most concerned about the fraud and abuse provisions.

The law is lengthy and complex. At this time, there are few court decisions to help clarify some of the more ambiguous provisions under HIPAA; however, the intent of the act seems quite clear.

The HIPAA added substantial funding for fraud and abuse activities for several agencies, including the Office of Inspector General (OIG), the FBI, and the Health Care Financing Administration. Additional funding for fraud and abuse prosecutory efforts will be achieved through incentives and recoveries from successfully prosecuted cases. The Act provides incentives for the various enforcement agencies to identify and prosecute fraud cases.

Most of the funding is devoted to the hiring of additional investigators and other enforcement personnel. There are also requirements that all law enforcement agencies coordinate efforts to oppose health care fraud and abuse in the public and private sector. Until now, the Inspector General only dealt with Medicare and Medicaid.

The HIPAA expands the powers of the government with respect to health care fraud and abuse. The Act seems to indicate that the OIG can exclude from Medicare or Medicaid responsible owners, officers, and managing employees of companies who have committed fraud or have been excluded from Medicare, *even if the investor, officer, or employee had no knowledge of the wrongdoing.*[1] The Department of Justice can subpoena records in any health care fraud investigation regardless of whether the investigation is related to Medicare or Medicaid.

One of the key aspects of HIPAA is that it extends fraud and abuse actions to certain offenses against nongovernmental payers. Additionally, it increases penalties for fraud and abuse and offers incentives payable to informants and government departments participating in fraud cases.

Before this act, it was often difficult to prosecute cases involving private payers or insurers. Usually, cases were prosecuted under mail fraud statutes. The HIPAA adds some new criminal provisions that apply to private health plans, but it may be some time before it is clear how far these new provisions go. For example, language in the Act states: "Whoever knowingly and willfully executes, or attempts to execute, a scheme or artifice (1) to defraud any health care benefit program; or (2) to obtain by false or fraudulent pretense . . . shall be fined under this title or imprisoned not more than 10 years, or both . . . ." Imprisonment could be for 20 years, or life, if the violation results in serious injury or the patient's death.

While HIPAA does not explicitly define terms such as *defraud*, it establishes some new federal health care crimes, broadly classified as follows: making materially false statements, health care fraud, embezzlement of monies under control of a health benefit program, obstructing an investigation, and money laundering.

HIPAA creates a new category of offenses—federal health care offenses—which include:

- Health care fraud
- Making false statements
- Theft and embezzlement
- Obstruction of criminal investigations
- Money laundering

Under HIPAA, these categories of crimes apply to private payers, not just Medicare or Medicaid. The crimes are very broad—for example, health care fraud covers a lot of ground. Again, we will have to watch how enforcement unfolds.

Some attorneys are advising their clients that it may now be necessary to review some arrangements that offered services only to non-Medicare/Medicaid patients to avoid violating Medicare and Medicaid rules (ie, those arrangements that avoided Medicare kickback, antireferral, and fraud or abuse implications by providing services only to privately insured patients). Physicians should watch how enforcement under HIPAA unfolds and monitor new legislative proposals.

The HIPAA authorizes the Department of Health and Human Services (HHS) to offer Medicare beneficiaries a "bounty" or reward if they report and HHS recovers any amounts in excess of $100 for services fraudulently billed. The award is capped between $100 and $1,000. This is a significant new inducement for beneficiaries to report suspected cases of fraud. Unfortunately, beneficiaries may report *legitimate* encounters that they simply do not understand, such as bills for anesthesia, pathology, radiology interpretations, and the like; consultations when the patient does not remember seeing the doctor; itemized hospital bills; physician bills for multiple services; and bills to patients for copayments when the patient thought he or she did not owe anything because the services were "assigned." (Encouraging patients to call the physician's office to discuss any billing questions or problems may help prevent unwarranted calls to the hotline.)

Of course, the Medicare program has historically attempted to include beneficiaries in their efforts to identify providers who are billing for services not provided or performing unnecessary services. Medicare has created toll-free hotlines, included messages on explanations of Medicare benefits that explain how to report suspected violations, and issued special fraud alerts.

Penalties for health care fraud and abuse are significantly increased under the Act. Violators may be automatically excluded from Medicare, Medicaid, and other federal health care programs if convicted of a felony dealing with controlled substance abuse or health care fraud regardless of whether the conviction is related to Medicare or Medicaid services.

Some other HIPAA provisions are as follows:

- Medicare and Medicaid exclusion penalties now apply to all other federal health care programs, such as CHAMPUS, Veterans Affairs, black lung, and Federal Employee Health Benefits Program.

- The Act allows imposition of $10,000 per day fines for organizations that continue any "investor" relationship or continue employing a person who has been excluded from any federal health care program.

- It increases civil monetary penalties from $2,000 to $10,000 per infraction plus three times the amount of the overpayment. An infraction could be considered a line item on a claim form resulting in a $10,000 or more penalty every time a fraudulent claim is filed. In other cases, an infraction could result in a $10,000 penalty *per day* that a fraudulent activity is in place.

- The Act requires mandatory exclusion from Medicare for 5 to 10 years for certain offenses.

- The Act describes the level of intent that has to be proved before a physician can be convicted.[2] It makes "deliberate ignorance" or "reckless disregard of the truth" the test as to whether an individual should have known that an activity was fraudulent.

- The Act specifically defines upcoding—of evaluation and management or other services—as a violation (see the next section).

- The legislation authorizes penalties for offering inducements to Medicare beneficiaries or Medicaid recipients to receive care.[3]

- The Act provides language whereby violators could be required to forfeit any assets acquired directly or indirectly from funds related to fraudulent activity. The bill also permits the confiscation of personal property if it is derived from health care fraud.

- The Act establishes a penalty of $5,000 or three times the cost of services for any physician who certifies unneeded home health care.

- Penalties of $25,000 per infraction are available for health maintenance organizations (HMOs) that fail to comply with Medicare contracts or federal regulations.

- The Act makes health care fraud, theft or embezzlement, false statements, money laundering, and obstruction of any health care investigation a federal criminal offense (see the next section).

Upcoding Under HIPAA

In defining persons who have filed a false claim, HIPAA amends previous law as follows:

> Section 1128A(a)(1) (42 USC 1320a-7a[a][1]), Claim for Item or Service Based on Incorrect Coding or Medically Unnecessary Services: ". . . including any person who engages in a pattern or practice of presenting or causing to be presented a claim for an item or service that is based on a code that the person knows or should know will result in a greater payment to the person than the code the person knows or should know is applicable to the item or service actually provided."

> [HIPAA specifically states the term *should know* means that a person] with respect to information—(A) acts in deliberate ignorance of the truth or falsity of the information; or (B) acts in reckless disregard of the truth or falsity of the information, and no proof of specific intent to defraud is required. [italics added]

New Offenses and Crimes

There are new federal health care offenses created under HIPAA. The pertinent language from HIPAA that extends these offenses to nongovernmental programs follows:

> Definitions relating to Federal Health Care Offense—(a) As used in this title, the term 'Federal health care offense' means a violation of, or a criminal conspiracy to violate—(1) section 669, 1035, 1347, or 1518 of this title; (2) section 287, 371, 664, 666, 1001, 1027, 1341, 1343, or 1954 of this title, if the violation or conspiracy relates to a health care benefit program.

> (b) As used in this title, the term 'health care benefit program' means any public or *private plan* or contract, affecting commerce, under which any medical benefit, item, or service is provided to any individual, and includes any individual or entity who is providing a medical benefit, item, or service for which payment may be made under the plan or contract. [italics added]

Each of the new federal health care offenses is briefly discussed below.

Health Care Fraud Under HIPAA

Whoever knowingly and willfully executes, or attempts to execute, a scheme or artifice—(1) to defraud any health care benefit program; or (2) to obtain, by means of false or fraudulent pretenses, representations, or promises, any of the money or property owned by, or under the custody or control of, any health care benefit program, in connection with the delivery of or payment for health care benefits, items, or services, shall be fined under this title or imprisoned not more than 10 years, or both. If the violation results in serious bodily injury (as defined in section 1365 of this title), such person shall be fined under this title or imprisoned not more than 20 years, or both; and if the violation results in death, such person shall be fined under this title, or imprisoned for any term of years or for life, or both.

Theft or Embezzlement

Theft or embezzlement in connection with health care. . . . Whoever knowingly and willfully embezzles, steals, or otherwise without authority converts to the use of any person other than the rightful owner, or intentionally misapplies any of the moneys, funds, securities, premiums, credits, property, or other assets of a health care benefit program, shall be fined under this title or imprisoned not more than 10 years, or both; but if the value of such property does not exceed the sum of $100 the defendant shall be fined under this title or imprisoned not more than one year, or both.

False Statements

False statements relating to health care matters. . . . Whoever, in any matter involving a health care benefit program, knowingly and willfully (1) falsifies, conceals, or covers up by any trick, scheme, or device a material fact; or (2) makes any materially false, fictitious, or fraudulent statements or representations, or makes or uses any materially false writing or document knowing the same to contain any materially false, fictitious, or fraudulent statement or entry, in connection with the delivery of or payment for health care benefits, items, or services, shall be fined under this title or imprisoned not more than 5 years, or both.

Obstruction of Criminal Investigations of Health Care Offenses. There are laws pertaining to obstruction of justice. Revising, concealing, and destroying records are but a few possible violations of these statutes. The HIPAA creates as a federal offense "obstruction of criminal investigations of health care offenses."

Specifically, HIPAA states the following regarding obstruction of an investigation:

(a) Whoever willfully prevents, obstructs, misleads, delays, or attempts to prevent, obstruct, mislead, or delay the communication of information or records relating to a violation of a Federal health care offense to a criminal investigator shall be fined under this title or imprisoned not more than 5 years, or both.[4] (b) As used in this section the term 'criminal investigator' means any individual duly authorized by a department, agency, or armed force of the U.S. to conduct or engage in investigations for prosecutions for violations of health care offenses.

Money Laundering. There are statutes that allow the government to seize assets that can be directly, or in some cases indirectly, tied to fraudulent activities, particularly money laundering schemes. Assets can be seized as part of criminal or civil proceedings. The HIPAA amends section 1956(c)(7) of title 18, USC, by adding language to indicate that it applies to "any act or activity constituting an offense involving a Federal health care offense."

Advisory Opinions in HIPAA

The HIPAA requires the government to issue advisory opinions on a limited list of issues to help physicians and others determine beforehand whether an arrangement might pose a problem. Usually, one would request an advisory opinion—based on complete disclosure of the proposed or current activity—by providing a written explanation of the facts to the OIG.

The OIG advisory opinions are available at the Web site www.oig.hhs.gov/fraud/ advisoryopinions/opinions.html

See Chapter 4 on antikickback statutes for a discussion of advisory opinions.

Health Care Fraud and Abuse Control Program

HIPAA also created a new program—the Health Care Fraud and Abuse Control Program. This program establishes a unique funding source for agencies engaged in health care fraud and abuse. The program is described in a joint report issued by the Department of Justice and HHS as follows:[5]

> The Social Security Act section 1128C(a), as established by the Health Insurance Portability and Accountability Act of 1996 (P.L. 104-191, HIPAA or the Act), created the Health Care Fraud and Abuse Control Program, a far-reaching program to combat fraud and abuse in health care, including both public and private health plans.
>
> The Act requires that an amount equaling recoveries from health care investigations—including criminal fines, forfeitures, civil settlements and judgments, and administrative penalties, but excluding restitution, compensation to the victim agency, and relators' shares—be deposited in the Medicare Trust Fund. All funds deposited in the Trust Fund as a result of the Act are available for the operations of the Trust Fund.

. . . the Act appropriates monies from the Medicare Trust Fund to an expenditure account, called the Health Care Fraud and Abuse Control Account (the Account), in amounts that the Secretary and Attorney General jointly certify as necessary to finance anti-fraud activities. The maximum amounts available for certification are specified in the Act. Certain of these sums are to be available only for activities of HHS/OIG, with respect to Medicare and Medicaid programs. In 2001, the Secretary and the Attorney General certified $181 million for appropriation to the Account. A detailed breakdown of the allocation of these funds is set forth later in this report. These resources generally supplement the direct appropriations of HHS and the Department of Justice (DOJ) that are devoted to health care fraud enforcement, though they provide the sole source of funding for Medicare and Medicaid enforcement by HHS/OIG. (Separately, the Federal Bureau of Investigation [FBI] received $88 million from HIPAA, which is discussed in the Appendix.)

Under the joint direction of the Attorney General and the Secretary, the Program's goals are: to coordinate Federal, state and local law enforcement efforts relating to health care fraud and abuse; to conduct investigations, audits and evaluations relating to the delivery of and payment for health care in the United States; to facilitate enforcement of all applicable remedies for such fraud; to provide guidance to the health care industry regarding fraudulent practices; and to establish a national data bank to receive and report final adverse actions against health care providers. . . .

Federal False Claims Act (31 USC §3729)

The federal False Claims Act allows the government or citizens to bring civil action—rather than a criminal action—against physicians and others filing fraudulent claims.[6] Essentially, the False Claims Act provides for a civil penalty of $5,000 to $10,000 per false claim, plus three times the amount of damages that the government sustains. With respect to health care, the False Claims Act is often used when a physician or other health care provider bills for services not actually rendered.[7] Pertinent language is reproduced below:

1   Any person who knowingly presents, or causes to be presented, to an officer or employee of the United States Government or a member of the Armed Forces . . . a false or fraudulent claim for payment or approval [the term knowingly includes "acting in reckless disregard . . ." or in "deliberate ignorance of the truth or falsity of information"];[8]

2   Knowingly makes, uses, or causes to be made or used, a false record or statement to get a false or fraudulent claim paid or approved by the government;

3   Conspires to defraud the Government by getting a false or fraudulent claim allowed or paid;

4   Has possession, custody, or control of property or money used, or to be used, by the Government and, intending to defraud the Government or willfully to conceal the property, delivers, or causes to be delivered, less property than the amount for which the person receives a certificate or receipt;

5   Authorized to make or deliver a document certifying receipt of property used, or to be used, by the Government and, intending to defraud the Government, makes or delivers the receipt without completely knowing that the information on the receipt is true;

6   Knowingly buys, or receives as a pledge of an obligation or debt, public property from an officer or employee of the Government, or a member of the Armed Forces, who lawfully may not sell or pledge the property; or

7   Knowingly makes, uses, or causes to be used, a false record or statement to conceal, avoid, or decrease an obligation to pay or transmit money or property to the Government, is liable to the US Government for a civil penalty of not less than $5,000 and not more than $10,000, plus three times the amount of damages which the Government sustains because of the acts. Note that the $5,000 to $10,000 penalty is per false claim.

The Act states: "the United States shall be required to prove all essential elements of the cause of action, including damages, by a preponderance of the evidence." Thus, the government does not have to prove its false claims allegations beyond a reasonable doubt.

Qui tam Suits

Private citizens may bring suit on behalf of themselves and the government against fraudulent health care providers by alleging violations of the False Claims Act. *Qui tam* plaintiffs—sometimes referred to as relators and whistle-blowers—may personally receive 10% to 30% of the total recovery plus reasonable attorney fees. The actual percentage is determined by the court, and there are certain maximums depending on whether the government participates in the case.[9]

In certain circumstances where the government has "public information" about potentially fraudulent activity, but the *qui tam* plaintiff is considered an original or significant source of information, the percentage is capped at 10%. Finally, the courts can reduce the payment if the *qui tam* plaintiff was part of the scheme.

Qui tam suits can be filed "in camera," which allows the individual to have the suit reviewed by the Department of Justice or Attorney General to determine whether the government believes the allegations have merit. Generally, the government has 60 days to decide whether it will participate in the case (there may be an extension of the 60 days). If it chooses, the Department of Justice will proceed with the action; if not, the whistle-blower has no exposure. The individual has the option to continue with the suit even if the government declines to participate; however, success in these situations is somewhat rare, and *qui tam* plaintiffs rarely proceed on their own because of the associated expenses and difficulty of proving the case without the government's aid.

Qui tam suits were a by-product of abuses in the defense industry during the Civil War. The vast majority of actions today are brought by disgruntled employees, spouses, or girlfriends or boyfriends. Competitors and patients are also a source of complaints. *Qui tam* actions have even been filed against Medicare carriers by their employees.

The False Claims Act also provides some protection for employees participating in a *qui tam* action from retaliation by an employer. Whistle-blower protection may be available if the employee is discharged because of his or her involvement in the *qui tam* action. Such protection includes reinstatement and damages of double the amount of lost wages. There are other damage awards if the employee is otherwise discriminated against.

According to a report issued by HHS and the Department of Justice in April 2002, $83,335,798 was paid on behalf of "persons who file suits on behalf of the Federal Government under the *qui tam* provisions of the False Claims Act, 31 U.S.C. sec 3730(b)" in fiscal year 2001.[10]

There is currently a Web site for an organization that provides information useful in filing *qui tam* suits.[11] The organization maintains a network of attorneys who have, or are interested in, filing *qui tam* actions. Other attorneys advertise their services on the Internet, in newspapers, and on radio and television.

Qui tam plaintiffs are not without risks. An employer might have some recourse if it were demonstrated that the employee intentionally filed an action knowing that the allegations were not true (although this would probably be difficult to prove). The *qui tam* plaintiff might be responsible for legal fees he or she incurs to the extent that the government does not participate in the case and where the action is not successful. *Qui tam* actions are also likely to take a considerable period of time to complete.

Potentially, the government can minimize the amount of any award in cases where it has already started an investigation. In fact, if the government participates in the suit, it can dismiss or settle the case without the consent of the private party (although the private party is entitled to a hearing).

An obvious danger in these suits is that disgruntled employees can blow things out of proportion, fabricate activities, or notify the government of their own improper activities that occurred without the physician's knowledge. Similarly, patients might pursue a case because they do not understand a billing statement. For example, a patient might call a hotline because he or she received a bill from a pathologist or consulting physician whom the patient does not remember seeing. It is hoped that attorneys soliciting business will weed out the real cases from those without merit.

If you become aware of a potentially fraudulent or abusive billing activity, it is essential that you do something about it. Otherwise, a disgruntled employee's version of your actions may persuade investigators to pursue criminal and/or civil action because it is clear you had knowledge of the issue. Appropriate action may include conducting research to determine whether current billing practices are proper, what changes may need to be made, and whether a repayment is in order.

The real point here is that you should undertake reasonable compliance efforts to identify and resolve situations that could be used in a *qui tam* action by a disgruntled employee. You should create an environment that encourages employees to report any compliance concerns they have by filing a compliance incident report as instructed in your compliance plan. Be sure to investigate compliance incident reports and adopt corrective action, if necessary, in a timely manner.

In 1999, the OIG promulgated the Provider Self-disclosure Protocol. The protocol provides "detailed guidance to health care providers that decide voluntarily to disclose irregularities in their dealings with Federal health care programs." The protocol is posted at www.oig.hhs.gov/authorities/docs/selfdisclosure.pdf.

Unfortunately, the protocol does not include any absolute assurance that would prevent a *qui tam* plaintiff from filing an action, even after repayment has been made subject to the self-disclosure guidelines.

In general, the statute of limitations under the False Claims Act runs for 6 years after commission of an offense. However, cutting through some ambiguity in the act, the statute of limitations may run up to 10 years when certain facts do not come to light within the normal 6-year period.

Conviction of a *criminal* charge of fraud or false statements could be used as irrefutable evidence in a civil action under the False Claims Act.

False, Fraudulent, or Fictitious Claims (18 USC §287)

Section 287 provides for imprisonment of up to 5 years and fines up to $250,000—possibly more if the amount of money gained is large—for individuals who submit to a government agency or contractors any claim "knowing such claim to be false, fictitious or fraudulent." This statute has been used to prosecute physicians for billing services performed when they were out of town and billing diagnostic tests that were not performed. The HIPAA also extends section 287 to private health plans in addition to Medicare, Medicaid, and other federal health care programs.

Under this section, it does not matter if the claim was actually paid. This is an important distinction, because physicians and others are most familiar with Medicare carrier audits of claims for which payment was actually paid. In fact, under audits that remain at the carrier level, paid claims are the only real concern. This provision could be used for actions involving improper claim submissions for which the physician was expecting payment.

False Statements (18 USC §1001)

Section 1001 is similar to section 287 in that it provides for imprisonment of up to 5 years and fines (up to $250,000 for individuals and possibly more if the amount of gain is large). Section 1001 applies to whoever "knowingly and willfully falsifies . . . or makes any false statements. . . ." Again, HIPAA extends section 1001 to private health care plans in addition to government programs.

This section could be used to prosecute physicians for billing services not rendered, knowingly including improper expenditures in hospital cost reports (Medicare Part A), and billing services not personally performed (where no permissible exceptions apply).

In a recent case under this section, the court ruled that the government bears the burden to negate any reasonable interpretation that would make a defendant's claim or statement factually correct where CHAMPUS reporting requirements were ambiguous.[12] We will discuss "intent" with regard to phrases such as *knowingly* and *willfully*.

Mail Fraud (18 USC §1341) and Wire Fraud (§1343)

Mail fraud statutes are commonly used to prosecute fraud cases. Essentially, these statutes allow for imprisonment (up to 5 years) and fines of not more than $1,000 per occurrence for fraudulent schemes in which claims or statements are sent by the mail, telephone, radio waves, etc. Thus, transmittal of almost any fraudulent claim might violate mail or wire fraud provisions (and this applies to using private or commercial interstate carriers).

Once again, HIPAA extends section 1001 to private health care programs in addition to government programs.

Civil Monetary Penalties

Social Security Act Civil Monetary Penalties: Section 1128A (42 USC §1320)

In past semiannual reports, the OIG described its powers with respect to imposing civil monetary penalties (CMPs) as follows:[13]

> Under the CMP authorities enacted by Congress, OIG may impose penalties and assessments against health care providers who submit false or improper claims to Medicare and state health programs. The CMP law allows recoupment of some monies lost through illegitimate claims, and it also protects health care providers by affording them due process rights similar to those available in the program exclusion process. Many providers elect to settle their cases prior to litigation.

The government may impose CMPs of up to $10,000 per claim if the physician knew or should have known the claim was false. HIPAA defines the phrase *should have known* as follows:

> The term 'should know' means that a person, with respect to information—(A) acts in deliberate ignorance of the truth or falsity of the information; or (B) acts in reckless disregard of the truth or falsity of the information, and no proof of specific intent to defraud is required.

A civil monetary action may be brought after successful criminal prosecution.

The discussion of civil monetary penalties that follows is from the *Medicare Carriers Manual* (we have supplied updates where appropriate and omitted certain superfluous information).

Medicare Carriers Manual, Part 3 (HCFA Pub 14-3) 14031
Civil Monetary Penalties Law

The Secretary has the authority to impose civil monetary penalties under the provisions of 1128A of the Act. This authority has been delegated to the OIG. These penalties may be imposed where the Secretary determines that a person presents or causes to be presented a claim for:

- An item or service not provided as claimed;

- An item or service that is false or fraudulent;

- A physician's service provided by a person who was not a licensed physician, whose license had been obtained through misrepresentation, or who improperly represented he/she was a certified specialist; or

- An item or service furnished by an excluded person.

The Secretary may also impose a civil monetary penalty against a person who presents or causes to be presented a request for payment in violation of:

- A Medicare assignment agreement;

- An agreement with State Medicaid agency not to charge a person in excess of permitted limits;

- A Medicare participating physician/supplier agreement; or

- An agreement not to charge patients for services denied as a result of a determination of an abuse of PPS. A person that gives false or misleading information regarding PPS that could reasonably be expected to influence a discharge decision is also subject to imposition of a civil monetary penalty.

Other situations where civil monetary penalties may be applied include:

- Violation of assignment requirements for certain diagnostic clinical lab tests (1833(h));

- Violation of assignment requirements for nurse anesthetist services (1833(1));

- Any supplier who refuses to supply rented DME supplies without charge after rental payments may no longer be made (effective January 1, 1989) (1834(a));

- Nonparticipating physician or supplier violation of charge limitation provisions for radiology services (effective January 1, 1989) (1834(b));

- Violation of assignment requirement for physician assistant services (1842(b));

- Medicare nonparticipating physician's violation of limiting charge limits; Nonparticipating physician's violation of charge limitations (1842(j));

- Physician billing for assistants at cataract surgery without prior approval of PRO (1842(k));

- Nonparticipating physician's violation of refund requirements for medically unnecessary services (1842(l));

- Nonparticipating physician's violation of refund provision for unassigned claims for elective surgery (1842(m)) [where elective surgical form not provided];

- Physician charges in violation of assignment provision for certain purchased diagnostic procedures where mark-up is prohibited or where a payment is prohibited for these procedures due to failure to disclose required information (1842(n));

- Hospital unbundling of outpatient surgery costs (1866(g)); and

- Hospital and responsible physician 'dumping' of patients (1867).

[Carriers are to] take the following action if it appears that the CMPL provisions might apply:

- Promptly telephone OIG upon discovery of any case that may have CMPL aspects, regardless of whether there is any other pending activity, or the case was closed earlier;

- **Before pursuing any sizeable or recurring overpayment demands in any case or any significant cost report adjustment, contact OIG to discuss the possibility of CMPL involvement;** and [boldface added]

- Similarly, in situations where you [carrier] elect to place a practitioner on prepay review or other edit action because upcoding or other forms of misrepresentation of services may be involved, consult OIG immediately to determine CMPL potential.

You are notified on a case-by-case basis when practitioners, providers or suppliers are excluded from the Medicare program. In addition, you will receive a monthly report of sanctioned individuals or entities. (See 14030.13.) You are responsible for ensuring that no payments are made after the effective date of a sanction except as provided for in regulations at 42 CFR 1001.1901(c) and 489.55.

Check payment systems periodically to determine whether any provider, practitioner, or supplier, who has been excluded since January 1982, is submitting claims for which payment is prohibited. If any such claims are submitted by practitioners, providers or suppliers who have been sanctioned under 1128, 1862(d), 1156, 1160(b) or 1866(b), forward them to OIG.

Also, refer all cases to OIG that involve chronic assignment violators. In cases where there is an occasional violation of assignment by a provider, notify the provider in writing that continued violation could result in a penalty under the CMPL. Similarly, refer all cases of misrepresentation (i.e., provider knows or has reason to know items or services were not provided as claimed) to OIG.

Application of CMPs to Waiver of Copayments and Deductibles and Other Beneficiary Inducements

The HIPAA provides that the Secretary of HHS may apply sanctions, such as CMPs up to $10,000 per occurrence, for routine waiver of copayments and deductibles (with a few exceptions) as discussed below (also see the next chapter involving anti-kickback legislation).[14]

Prohibition Against Offering Inducements to Individuals Enrolled Under Programs or Plans[15]

[The Secretary may impose sanctions against a provider who] offers to or transfers **remuneration** to any individual eligible for [Medicare] benefits, or under a State health care program that such person knows or should know is likely to influence such individual to order or receive from a particular provider, practitioner, or supplier any item or service for which payment may be made, in whole or in part. . . .

The term **remuneration includes the waiver of coinsurance and deductible amounts (or any part thereof),** and transfers of items or services for free or for other than fair market value. The term **remuneration does not include** [and a provider would not likely be sanctioned] [boldface added]:

(A) The waiver of coinsurance and deductible amounts, if
   (i)   the waiver is not offered as part of any advertisement or solicitation;
   (ii) the person does not routinely waive coinsurance or deductible amounts; and

(iii) the person (I) waives the coinsurance and deductible amounts after determining in good faith that the individual is in financial need; (II) fails to collect coinsurance or deductible amounts after making reasonable collection efforts; or (III) provides for any permissible waiver as specified in section 1128B(b)(3) or in regulations issued by the Secretary;

(B) Differentials in coinsurance and deductible amounts as part of a benefit plan design as long as the differentials have been disclosed in writing to all beneficiaries, third party payers, and providers, to whom claims are presented and as long as the differentials meet the standards as defined in regulations promulgated by the Secretary not later than 180 days after the date of the enactment of the Health Insurance Portability and Accountability Act of 1996; or

(C) Incentives given to individuals to promote the delivery of preventive care as determined by the Secretary in regulations so promulgated.

Paragraphs (B) and (C) above apply to Medicare HMOs and similar health care benefit plans that may offer such coverage and payment terms.

Medically Unnecessary Services and Upcoding

The HIPAA also includes the following provisions related to the potential for assessing CMPs for billing of medically unnecessary services or upcoding:

> CLAIM FOR ITEM OR SERVICE BASED ON INCORRECT CODING OR MEDICALLY UNNECESSARY SERVICES— . . . including any person who engages in a pattern or practice of presenting or causing to be presented a claim for an item or service that is based on a code that the person knows or should know will result in a greater payment to the person than the code the person knows or should know is applicable to the item or service actually provided; . . . is for a pattern of medical or other items or services that a person knows or should know are not medically necessary.[16]

Home Health Certifications by Physicians

The HIPAA includes the following provisions related to the potential assessment of CMPs for inappropriate home health certifications:

> Any physician who [signs a certification that an individual meets the requirements for coverage of home health services] with respect to an individual knowing that all of the requirements . . . are not met . . . shall be subject to a civil monetary penalty of not more than the greater of—
>
> (i) $5,000, or
>
> (ii) three times the amount of the payments under title XVIII for home health services which are made pursuant to such certification.[17]

Civil Monetary Penalties for "Patient Dumping"

The OIG's *Semiannual Report* for the period October 2001 through March 2002 included the following comments:

Civil Penalties for Patient Dumping

Section 1867 of the Social Security Act (42 U.S.C. 1395dd) provides that when an individual presents to the emergency room of a Medicare-participating hospital, the hospital must provide an appropriate medical screening examination to determine whether that individual has an emergency medical condition. If an individual has such a condition, the hospital must provide either: (1) treatment to stabilize the condition; or (2) an appropriate transfer to another medical facility. If a transfer is ordered, the transferring hospital must provide stabilizing treatment to minimize the risks of transfer and must ensure that the receiving hospital agrees to the transfer and has available space and qualified personnel to treat the individual. In addition, the transferring hospital must effect the transfer through qualified personnel and transportation equipment. Further, a participating hospital with specialized capabilities or facilities may not refuse to accept an appropriate transfer of an individual who needs services if the hospital has the capacity to treat the individual.

The OIG is authorized to collect civil monetary penalties of up to $25,000 against small hospitals (less than 100 beds) and up to $50,000 against larger hospitals (100 beds or more) for each instance in which the hospital negligently violated any of the section 1867 requirements. In addition, OIG may collect a penalty of up to

$50,000 from a responsible physician for each negligent violation of any of the section 1867 requirements and, in some circumstances, may exclude a responsible physician.

Between October 1, 2001, and March 31, 2002, OIG collected $109,000 from 4 hospitals for patient dumping violations. The following is a sampling of the alleged violations involved in the Patient Anti-Dumping statute settlements from this reporting period:

A Victor Valley Community Hospital in California agreed to pay $40,000 to resolve allegations that it had violated section 1867 of the Social Security Act on seven occasions. One patient did not receive stabilizing treatment or an appropriate transfer and another experienced a delay in treatment until her insurance company agreed to pay for treatment. Five patients did not receive appropriate medical screening examinations; four resulting

from the hospital calling the patients' insurance companies for payment authorization which was denied. The settlement amount reflected the hospital's limited ability to pay.

Englewood Hospital in New Jersey agreed to pay $15,000 to resolve allegations that it violated section 1867 of the Social Security Act. The OIG found that the hospital failed to provide medical examinations to Centers for Medicare and Medicaid Services several people who came to the hospital emergency room for evaluation and treatment. The hospital discharged the patients and sent them to private physicians' offices.

In comparison to the amounts collected in the six months ending March 2002 discussed above, the OIG—between April 1, 1999, and September 30, 1999—collected $1.7 million in CMPs from 61 hospitals and physicians.

Gain Sharing Between Hospitals and Physicians

In 1999, the OIG released an advisory bulletin regarding the possibility that CMPs could apply to "gain sharing" arrangements between hospitals and physicians. The advisory bulletin was written after several hospitals requested advisory opinions concerning the legality of "gain sharing" arrangements with physicians on the hospitals' staffs. Such gain sharing arrangements usually involve the hospital giving physicians a percentage share of any reduction in the hospital's costs for patient care attributable in part to the physicians' clinical efforts. In most arrangements, in order to receive any payment, clinical care must not have been adversely affected as measured by selected quality and performance measures.

In July 1999, OIG issued a special advisory bulletin concluding "that gainsharing arrangements violate section 1128A(b)(1) of the Social Security Act, which prohibits a hospital from making a payment, directly or indirectly, to induce a physician to reduce or limit services to Medicare or Medicaid beneficiaries under the physician's direct care. Hospitals and physicians may be liable for CMPs of up to $2,000 per patient covered by the payments. The OIG stated that it will take into consideration whether a gainsharing arrangement was terminated expeditiously in determining whether to prosecute the arrangement."

Civil Monetary Penalties and Managed Care Organizations

The HIPAA also provides that the Secretary of HHS may take actions against managed care organizations, including CMPs, in circumstances discussed below:[18]

In accordance with procedures established under paragraph (9), the Secretary may at any time terminate any such contract or may impose the intermediate sanctions . . . if the Secretary determines that the organization— (A) has failed substantially to carry out the contract; (B) is carrying out the contract in a manner substantially inconsistent with the efficient and effective administration of this section; or (C) no longer substantially meets the applicable conditions of subsections (b), (c), (e), and (f) [regarding services to those enrolled with the HMO].

. . . [T]he Secretary may apply the following intermediate sanctions: (i) Civil money penalties of not more than $25,000 for each determination . . . if the deficiency that is the basis of the determination has directly adversely affected (or has the substantial likelihood of adversely affecting) an individual covered under the organization's contract. (ii) Civil money penalties of not more than $10,000 for each week beginning after the initiation of procedures by the Secretary. . . . (iii) Suspension of enrollment of individuals under this section after the date the Secretary notifies the organization . . . until the Secretary is satisfied the deficiency . . . has been corrected and is not likely to recur. . . .

The Secretary may terminate a contract with an eligible organization under this section or may impose the intermediate sanctions described above in accordance with formal investigation and compliance procedures established by the Secretary under which—(A) the Secretary first provides the organization with the reasonable opportunity to develop and implement a corrective action plan to correct the deficiencies . . . and the organization fails to develop or implement such a plan; (B) in deciding whether to impose sanctions, the Secretary considers aggravating factors such as whether an organization has a history of deficiencies or has not taken action to correct deficiencies the Secretary has brought to the organization's attention; (C) there are no unreasonable or unnecessary delays between the finding of a deficiency and the imposition of sanctions; and (D) the Secretary provides the organization with reasonable notice and opportunity for hearing (including the right to appeal an initial decision) before imposing any sanction or terminating the contract.

Miscellaneous Examples of Civil Monetary Penalties

The examples below were taken from the OIG's Semiannual Reports released between 1998 and March 2002:

Examples of CMP Cases Resolved by OIG

A physician and his oncology clinic jointly agreed to pay the Government $963,736 to resolve their civil liability for submitting false claims, and entered into a corporate integrity agreement with OIG. Between 1992 and 1997, the physician and his clinic allegedly submitted improper claims to Medicare and the Medicaid program for services rendered at the clinic by nonphysicians without a physician's supervision or presence. The corporate integrity agreement applies to all entities in which the physician has an ownership or management interest and that submit claims for reimbursement to any Federal health care program. The physician currently owns two rural oncology clinics.

A physician agreed to pay the Government $225,000 to settle allegations that his practice upcoded office visits and angioplasty consultations. This settlement figure represents approximately treble damages. The physician also agreed to enter into a 3-year corporate integrity agreement. A health care services corporation agreed to pay the Government $195,000 to resolve its liability for submitting claims for poor quality services at one of its nursing facilities. The case stems from a 1996 HCFA survey of several residents' records that uncovered inadequate nutrition care, wound care, incontinence care and supervision at a nursing facility. The poor quality of care alleged was attributed primarily to an inability to control high staff turnover. In addition to the amount paid in damages, the settlement calls for comprehensive compliance provisions that include implementation of a specific quality of care protocol, training and appointment of an independent consultant for 1 year to ensure provision of quality care.

A physician agreed to pay the Government $23,041 to settle allegations related to improper billing practices. Between August 1991 and December 1996, the physician allegedly billed Medicare for certain arthroscopy surgical procedures as if they were more complex surgical procedures than those actually performed. As a result, he received an approximate overpayment of $14,127. As part of the settlement, the now retired physician agreed to permanent exclusion from Medicare, Medicaid and other Federal health care programs.

KPMG, LLP (KPMG), formerly KPMG Peat Marwick LLP, agreed to pay $9 million, plus interest, to the Federal Government to resolve allegations of submitting false hospital cost reports to the Medicare and Medicaid programs on behalf of Basic American Medical, Inc (BAMI) and Columbia Hospital Corporation (now known as HCA, Inc). The government alleged that KPMG, acting as a reimbursement consultant and preparer of the hospital cost reports, knowingly made claims that were false, exaggerated or ineligible for payment and concealed errors from the government, thereby enabling BAMI and HCA to falsely retain funds. KPMG also prepared 'reserve' cost reports detailing non-allowable expenses and allocations contained in the filed cost reports and estimated the reimbursement impact in the event that these nonallowable expenses and allocations were detected on audit.

Raytel Cardiac Services, Inc (RCS) and Raytel Medical Corporation (collectively, Raytel) agreed to pay the government $11.5 million, plus interest, and to enter into a 5-year corporate integrity agreement to resolve the corporation's liability for the submission of false claims and false statements to the government. The $11.5 million settlement figure is comprised of $5 million in restitution based on a guilty plea by RCS to obstruction of a criminal investigation and $6.5 million to resolve Raytel's civil liability under the False Claims Act. A corporation with locations in New York, Connecticut, and New Jersey, Raytel is one of the Nation's largest providers of trans-telephonic pacemaker monitoring. The allegations in the case centered around Raytel's failure to fully complete all necessary steps in performing the monitoring services, as well as conducting the monitoring for the required length of time.

In New York, Impath, Inc (Impath), agreed to pay the government $9 million to settle allegations of improperly billing Medicare for diagnostic pathology services. A qui tam alleged that from 1992 to 1998, Impath, a large clinical laboratory with facilities in New York, California, and Arizona, presented improper Medicare claims and supporting records to the government. The settlement also contains compliance provisions.

Molina Healthcare of California, Inc, doing business as Molina Medical Centers (Molina), a Medicaid managed care plan in California, paid $600,000 to resolve its civil monetary penalty liability for furnishing false and misleading information to Medicaid beneficiaries. Molina sent over 17,000 false and misleading letters stating that if the beneficiaries did not re-enroll with Molina they would lose access to their primary care physicians to Medicaid beneficiaries enrolled in its plan. These letters appeared as though they were sent directly from the beneficiaries' physicians; in reality, they were sent by a mailing house at the request and direction of Molina.

A hospital paid $35,000 in penalties for allegedly discharging an AIDS patient with an unstable emergency medical condition. The patient died approximately 6 hours after being discharged and later taken to another hospital.

Two doctors along with another man and their now-defunct portable x-ray company agreed to pay more than $214,200 to settle civil liabilities for false Medicare and Medicaid claims. They charged $65 each for multiple trips to a nursing home when they only made one trip and took x-rays of multiple patients.

A cardiologist and his office manager agreed to resolve their liability for false Medicare claims, paying $100,000 for penalties and actual damages of $35,792. The office manager submitted claims on behalf of the cardiologist indicating that myocardial perfusion imaging had been performed, when the cardiologist did not even have the necessary equipment. The office manager, who is not a physician and has no Medicare number, claimed he was told by the carrier to bill this code to recover for pharmacological services rendered in conjunction with EKGs.

A physician agreed to pay $30,000 to settle his civil liability for filing improper Medicare claims. He had EKGs and other diagnostic testing equipment installed in his office by a laboratory that provided ultrasound and nuclear imaging diagnostic tests. He performed the diagnostic tests but contracted with another physician to interpret the test results. He then billed Medicare for the interpretations. The loss to Medicare over a 2-year period was more than $19,000 (lab remains under investigation).

A urologist agreed to pay $25,000 and enter a compliance program to resolve civil liability for false Medicare claims. Between 1992 and 1995, the urologist billed Medicare for unnecessary services, falsified documentation, waived beneficiary co-payments and engaged in other violations. The $25,000 is twice the amount he was overpaid.

A nephrologist agreed to pay $20,000 to settle liability for filing false Medicare claims. He had expressed to the Government concerns regarding his Medicare billings and claims. An OIG auditor analyzed the claims and found some false and misleading. He received a monthly "capitation fee" for patients under his care who had end stage renal disease. Nonetheless, he submitted claims for "office visits" and "unrelated services" for these patients, when reimbursement for these services was included in the monthly capitation fee.

Miscellaneous Federal Statutes

Some of the other federal statutes that could be used to prosecute health care fraud and abuse are as follows:

- Laundering of Monetary Instruments (18 USC §1956)

- Conspiracy to Commit Offenses or Defraud the US (18 USC §37)

- Embezzlement, Stealing Public Money, Property, or Records (18 USC §641)

- Criminal Forfeiture (18 USC §982)[19]

- Racketeering (18 USC §1963)

Chapters 4 and 5 include discussion of two other important legislative issues—antikickback and self-referral legislation.

State Laws

State laws vary considerably, but most states have enacted legislation that may be used to bring criminal and/or civil action for fraudulent claims. Many states have statutes falling within the following categories:

- Medicaid fraud

- Conspiracy to defraud the state

- Theft by taking

- False statements

  The penalties can be quite severe. In some states, a violator could be prosecuted under several laws. The fines and penalties are sometimes additive. Because of the increased publicity on fraud and abuse, additional state legislation should be expected.

  Some states have enacted specific antikickback and antireferral legislation, modeled to some extent after federal laws. Some state laws governing self-referral are even more restrictive than Stark legislation and apply to non-Medicaid as well as Medicaid services.

  An article in *AMNews* (Albert T. California Decision Hits Physician for Fraud Against Allstate, *AMNews*, April 2, 2001) stated that "a California jury recently ordered three doctors and nine clinics to pay Allstate Insurance Co. $8.2 million after finding them liable for billing for services they never provided, and for changing bills to justify excessive charges." The author noted that this was the first trial result under a new California law "modeled after the federal False Claims Act . . . that allows insurance companies to pursue civil fraud cases in civil court rather than relying on state authorities to file criminal charges." Three other physicians involved settled prior to trial. It was also reported that "similar to federal law, California allows whistle-blowers to bring lawsuits and to potentially share in a percentage of the money awarded."

  The state medical association is a good source to ask about these laws.

Exclusion From Medicare and Medicaid

Title XI of the Social Security Act provides a number of authorities to exclude physicians, other health care professionals, and entities from programs such as Medicare and Medicaid. For fiscal year 2001, the OIG reported exclusions of 3,756 individuals and entities from participation in federal health care programs.[20]

Those excluded will not receive payment under Medicare, Medicaid, or other federal health care programs. Although this topic is not discussed further here, state Medicaid agencies may exclude physicians and others directly under state law. Exclusions may be imposed for conviction of fraud against a private health insurer, obstruction of an investigation, distribution of a controlled substance, revocation or surrender of a health care license, and failure to pay health education assistance loans. Exclusion is mandatory for certain crimes (see OIG's summary of exclusionary authorities later in this section). The Inspector General of the Department of HHS can exclude a physician or others in certain circumstances even though they have not been convicted in a criminal or civil proceeding.

The length of exclusion varies. Exclusion may be waived completely where a physician is the "sole community physician." Elective exclusions may be for a shorter period, and 3 years is a common exclusionary period.

Obviously, physicians and others are excluded throughout any period their licenses are revoked (although there are some exceptions where one's license is revoked for failure to pay licensure fees, late applications, etc). Exclusions for loss of license may continue even though a provider obtains a license in another state.

The HIPAA extended mandatory exclusions to:

> Any individual or entity that has been convicted for an offense . . . under Federal or State law, in connection with delivery of a health care item or service or with respect to any act or omission in a health care program . . . operated by or financed in whole or in part by any Federal, State, or local government agency, of a criminal offense consisting of a felony relating to fraud, theft, embezzlement, breach of fiduciary responsibility, or other financial misconduct.

> Any individual or entity that has been convicted . . . under Federal or State law, of a criminal offense consisting of a felony relating to the unlawful manufacture, distribution, prescription, or dispensing of a controlled substance.

The HIPAA requires exclusion for a conviction with respect to the "delivery of a health care item or service" whether or not it is financed by a government or private insurance program. Thus, you can now face exclusion from Medicare and Medicaid because of an offense against a commercial insurer.

Also, acceptance of a guilty plea or *nolo contendere* in federal, state, or local courts may be designated as a conviction for imposing exclusionary powers.

The Inspector General may elect to exclude:

> Any individual or entity that has been convicted for an offense . . . (A) of a criminal offense consisting of a *misdemeanor* relating to fraud, theft, embezzlement, breach of fiduciary responsibility, or other financial misconduct (i) in connection with the delivery of a health care item or service, or (ii) with respect to any act or omission in a health care program . . . operated by or financed in whole or in part by any Federal, State, or local government agency; or (B) of a criminal offense relating to fraud, theft, embezzlement, breach of fiduciary responsibility, or other financial misconduct with respect to any act or omission in a program (*other than a health care program*) operated by or financed in whole or in part by any Federal, State, or local government agency. [italics added]

Under HIPAA, the OIG may exclude someone who has an interest in a sanctioned entity:[21]

> Any individual (i) who has a direct or indirect ownership or control interest in a sanctioned entity and who knows or should know . . . (ii) who is an officer or managing employee (as defined in section 1126(b)) of such an entity. . . . the term 'sanctioned entity' means an entity (i) that has been convicted of any offense described in subsection (a) or in paragraph (1), (2), or (3) of this subsection; or (ii) that has been excluded from participation under a program under title XVIII or under a State health care program.

A summary of the OIG's exclusionary authorities is provided below.

Summary of OIG Exclusionary Authorities[22]

Mandatory Exclusions

Conviction of program-related crimes	Minimum period: 5 years
Conviction relating to patient abuse or neglect	Minimum period: 5 years
Felony conviction relating to health care fraud	Minimum period: 5 years
Felony conviction relating to controlled substance	Minimum period: 5 years
Conviction of two mandatory exclusion offenses	Minimum period: 10 years
Conviction on three or more mandatory exclusion offenses	Permanent exclusion
Failure to enter an agreement to repay HEAL loans	Until entire obligation is repaid

Permissive Exclusions

Misdemeanor conviction relating to health care fraud	Minimum period: 3 years
Conviction relating to fraud in non-health care programs	Minimum period: 3 years
Conviction relating to obstruction of an investigation	Minimum period: 3 years
Misdemeanor conviction relating to controlled substance	Minimum period: 3 years
Fraud, kickbacks, and other prohibited activities	Minimum period: None
Failure to grant immediate access	Minimum period: none
Failure to take corrective action	Minimum period: none
Individuals controlling a sanctioned entity	Minimum: same period as entity
License revocation or suspension	Minimum: no less than the period imposed by state licensing authority
Exclusion or suspension under federal or state health program	Minimum period: no less than the period imposed by federal or state health care program

Continued

Claims for excessive charges, unnecessary services or services that fail to meet professionally recognized standards of care, or failure of an HMO to furnish medically necessary services	Minimum period: 1 year
Entities controlled by a sanctioned individual	Minimum period: same as length of individual's exclusion
Entities controlled by a family or household member of an excluded individual and where there has been a transfer of ownership/control	Minimum period: same as length of individual's inclusion
Failure to disclose required information, supply requested information on subcontractors and suppliers, or supply payment information	Minimum period: none
Default on health education loan or scholarship obligations	Minimum: until default is cured or obligations resolved to Public Health Service's satisfaction
Failure to meet statutory obligations of practitioners and providers to provide medically necessary services meeting professionally recognized standards of health care (peer review organization [PRO] findings)	Minimum period: 1 year

The OIG's *Semiannual Report* for October 2001 through March 2002 stated the following regarding exclusion:

Section 1128 of the Social Security Act (42 U.S.C. Section 1320a-7) provides several grounds for excluding individuals and entities from participation in Medicare, Medicaid and other federal health care programs. Exclusions are required for individuals and entities convicted of the following types of criminal offenses: 1) Medicare or Medicaid fraud; 2) patient abuse or neglect; 3) felonies for other health care fraud; and 4) felonies for illegal manufacture, distribution, prescription or dispensing of controlled substances. The OIG has the discretion to exclude individuals and entities on several other grounds, including: misdemeanors for other health care fraud (other than Medicare or Medicaid) or for illegal manufacture, distribution, prescription or dispensing of controlled substances; suspension or revocation of a license to provide health care for reasons bearing on professional competence, professional performance, or financial integrity; provision of unnecessary or substandard services; and submission of false or fraudulent claims to a federal health care program.

During this reporting period, OIG excluded 1,366 individuals and entities . . . . In past years, the OIG has reported examples of exclusion as follows:

A medical clinic was excluded for a period of 20 years due to its affiliation with its excluded owner. The clinic owner,

excluded from participation for the same number of years, was convicted for his involvement in a scheme to defraud the Medicare program by filing approximately $3 million in false claims for physician services, respiratory equipment, related medication and cardiovascular testing. The owner also solicited and received approximately $85,000 in illegal kickbacks for patient referrals and fraudulent prescriptions for cardiovascular testing. He was ordered to pay restitution of almost $3.5 million and is currently serving a sentence of 51 months in Federal prison.

A nurse's aide was convicted of recklessly causing bodily harm to a nursing home patient. While roughly taking the elderly patient out of his wheelchair to a whirlpool, the aide caused the patient's right foot to get caught in his wheelchair, resulting in a fractured ankle. She then dragged the elderly man across the floor, causing him to sustain rug burns. The aide was sentenced to 1 year community supervision and excluded for 10 years.

With the expansion of exclusion authority under the Health Insurance Portability and Accountability Act of 1996 (HIPAA) to include the sanctioning of individuals controlling previously sanctioned entities, a doctor was excluded from program participation for 10 years. The doctor was the owner of a methadone clinic in Maryland which had been convicted for knowingly and willfully making false statements in applications for payment to Medicaid. The clinic paid restitution in the amount of $290,000 based upon an overpayment of $95,000, and was excluded for 10 years.

The HIPAA established OIG mandatory authority to exclude any individual who has been convicted of a felony relating to controlled substance violations. A pharmacist was excluded for a period of 5 years after pleading guilty in a local court to illegally processing drug documents. The pharmacist, a drug user, illegally forged prescriptions for himself. The court ordered that the pharmacist be required to enter into a drug treatment program for 3 years.

The HIPAA also expanded the mandatory exclusion authority to exclude any individual convicted of a felony relating to health care fraud. A certified provider for the developmentally disabled was excluded for 5 years after being found guilty of a felony related to health care fraud. The provider submitted documents for reimbursement claiming that she had purchased clothing for a patient in the disability home in which she worked. She did purchase clothing; however, the clothing was actually for herself and not the intended patient. The provider was placed on supervised probation for a period of 3 years.

An anesthesiologist was indefinitely excluded because his medical license was suspended for reasons bearing on his professional performance. The doctor's license suspension was due to several complaints, including placing an epidural catheter in a patient's abdomen during child birth, instead of properly placing the catheter in the spinal canal. The patient and her unborn child died.

A podiatrist was excluded for a period of 15 years after being found guilty in a local court of unlawful sexual conduct against a patient and tampering with evidence. In addition, the State Medical Board permanently revoked the doctor's license to practice podiatric medicine and surgery. He was sentenced to serve 6 months in a halfway house which included work release.

The Department of HHS may exclude physicians and others from Medicare, Medicaid, and other federal health programs for "rendering excessive, unnecessary, substandard and potentially risky services."

List of Excluded Individuals/Entities

The OIG maintains an exclusion database at the Web site: www.oig.hhs.gov/fraud/exclusions/listofexcluded.html.

According to the OIG, the List of Excluded Individuals/Entities provides information to health care professionals and entities, patients, and others regarding individuals and entities that are excluded from participation in Medicare, Medicaid, and other federal health care programs. Information is readily available to users in two formats on more than 15,000 individuals and entities currently excluded from program participation through action taken by the OIG.

The online searchable database allows users to obtain information regarding excluded individuals and entities sorted by (1) the legal bases for exclusions; (2) the types of individuals and entities excluded by the OIG; and (3) the states where excluded individuals reside or entities do business. In addition, users may query the database to ascertain whether a particular individual or entity is currently excluded from program participation by submitting pertinent information regarding the subject. Users may obtain data sorted by name, profession or specialty, city, state, zip code, or sanction type. Users may input information in any of these fields and receive a list of currently excluded individuals and entities that meet the criteria entered.

In addition to the online searchable database, the OIG continues to provide information on excluded individuals and entities in a downloadable database file format, which will allow users to download the data to their personal computers and either set up their own databases or combine it with their existing data. Monthly exclusion supplements to the downloadable database file will be posted on the OIG's Web site in the same format as the List of Excluded Individuals/Entities, as will separate files containing individuals and entities that have been reinstated each month.

The OIG maintains the sites to "provide information to health care providers who are considering hiring or contracting with an individual or entity, as well as the public in obtaining information about the Medicare or Medicaid participation status of an individual or entity."

In September 1999, the OIG released a Special Advisory Bulletin that discussed the implications of exclusion. Clearly, this is a severe sanction.

Special Advisory Bulletin
The Effect of Exclusion From Participation in Federal Health Care Programs
September 1999

A. Introduction

The Office of Inspector General (OIG) was established in the U.S. Department of Health and Human Services to identify and eliminate fraud, waste, and abuse in the Department's programs and to promote efficiency and economy in Departmental operations. The OIG carries out this mission through a nationwide program of audits, inspections, and investigations. In addition, the OIG has been given the authority to exclude from participation in Medicare, Medicaid and other Federal health care programs individuals and entities who have engaged in fraud or abuse, and to impose civil money penalties (CMPs) for certain misconduct related to Federal health care programs (sections 1128 and 1128A of the Social Security Act (the Act)).

Recent statutory enactments have strengthened and expanded the OIG's authority to exclude individuals and entities from the Federal health care programs. These laws also expanded the OIG's authority to assess CMPs against individuals and entities that violate the law. With this expanded authority, the OIG believes that it is important to explain the effect of program exclusions under the current statutory and regulatory provisions.

The Health Insurance Portability and Accountability Act (HIPAA) of 1996, Public Law 104-191, authorized the OIG to provide guidance to the health care industry to prevent fraud and abuse, and to promote high levels of ethical and lawful conduct. To further these goals, the OIG issues Special Advisory Bulletins about industry practices or arrangements that potentially implicate the fraud and abuse authorities subject to enforcement by the OIG.

In order to assist all affected parties in understanding the breadth of the payment prohibitions that apply to items and services provided to Federal program beneficiaries, this Special Advisory Bulletin provides guidance to individuals and entities that have been excluded from Federal health care programs, as well as to those who might employ or contract with an excluded individual or entity to provide items or services reimbursed by a Federal health care program.

B. Statutory Background

In 1977, in the Medicare-Medicaid Anti-Fraud and Abuse Amendments, Public Law 95-142, Congress first mandated the exclusion of physicians and other practitioners convicted of program-related crimes from participation in Medicare and Medicaid (now codified at section 1128 of the Act). This was followed in 1981 with Congressional enactment of the Civil Monetary Penalties Law (CMPL), Public Law 97-35, to further address health care fraud and abuse (section 1128A of the Act). The CMPL authorizes the Department and the OIG to impose CMPs, assessments and program exclusions against individuals and entities who submit false or fraudulent, or otherwise improper claims for Medicare or Medicaid payment. "Improper claims" include claims submitted by an excluded individual or entity for items or services furnished during a period of program exclusion.

To enhance the OIG's ability to protect the Medicare and Medicaid programs and beneficiaries, the Medicare and Medicaid Patient and Program Protection Act of 1987, Public Law 100-93, expanded and revised the OIG's administrative sanction authorities by, among other things, establishing certain mandatory and discretionary exclusions for various types of misconduct.

The enactment of HIPAA in 1996 and the Balanced Budget Act (BBA) of 1997, Public Law 105-33, further expanded the OIG's sanction authorities. These statutes extended the application and scope of the current CMP and exclusion authorities beyond programs funded by the Department to all "Federal health care programs."

BBA also authorized a new CMP authority to be imposed against health care providers or entities that employ or enter into contracts with excluded individuals for the provision of services or items to Federal program beneficiaries.

In the discussion that follows, it should be understood that the prohibitions being described apply to items and services provided, directly or indirectly, to Federal program beneficiaries. The ability of an excluded individual or entity to render items and services to others is not affected by an OIG exclusion.

C. Exclusion from Federal Health Care Programs

The effect of an OIG exclusion from Federal health care programs is that no Federal health care program pay-

ment may be made for any items or services (1) furnished by an excluded individual or entity, or (2) directed or prescribed by an excluded physician (42 CFR 1001.1901). This payment ban applies to all methods of Federal program reimbursement, whether payment results from itemized claims, cost reports, fee schedules or a prospective payment system (PPS). Any items and services furnished by an excluded individual or entity are not reimbursable under Federal health care programs. In addition, any items and services furnished at the medical direction or prescription of an excluded physician are not reimbursable when the individual or entity furnishing the services either knows or should know of the exclusion. This prohibition applies even when the Federal payment itself is made to another provider, practitioner or supplier that is not excluded.

The prohibition against Federal program payment for items or services furnished by excluded individuals or entities also extends to payment for administrative and management services not directly related to patient care, but that are a necessary component of providing items and services to Federal program beneficiaries. This prohibition continues to apply to an individual even if he or she changes from one health care profession to another while excluded. In addition, no Federal program payment may be made to cover an excluded individual's salary, expenses or fringe benefits, regardless of whether they provide direct patient care.

Set forth below is a listing of some of the types of items or services that are reimbursed by Federal health care programs which, when provided by excluded parties, violate an OIG exclusion. These examples also demonstrate the kinds of items and services that excluded parties may be furnishing which will subject their employer or contractor to possible CMP liability.

Services performed by excluded nurses, technicians or other excluded individuals who work for a hospital, nursing home, home health agency or physician practice, where such services are related to administrative duties, preparation of surgical trays or review of treatment plans if such services are reimbursed directly or indirectly (such as through a PPS or a bundled payment) by a Federal health care program, even if the individuals do not furnish direct care to Federal program beneficiaries;

Services performed by excluded pharmacists or other excluded individuals who input prescription information for pharmacy billing or who are involved in any way in filling prescriptions for drugs reimbursed, directly or indirectly, by any Federal health care program;

Services performed by excluded ambulance drivers, dispatchers and other employees involved in providing transportation reimbursed by a Federal health care program, to hospital patients or nursing home residents;

Services performed for program beneficiaries by excluded individuals who sell, deliver or refill orders for medical devices or equipment being reimbursed by a Federal health care program;

Services performed by excluded social workers who are employed by health care entities to provide services to Federal program beneficiaries, and whose services are reimbursed, directly or indirectly, by a Federal health care program;

Administrative services, including the processing of claims for payment, performed for a Medicare intermediary or carrier, or a Medicaid fiscal agent, by an excluded individual;

Services performed by an excluded administrator, billing agent, accountant, claims processor or utilization reviewer that are related to and reimbursed, directly or indirectly, by a Federal health care program;

Items or services provided to a program beneficiary by an excluded individual who works for an entity that has a contractual agreement with, and is paid by, a Federal health care program; and

Items or equipment sold by an excluded manufacturer or supplier, used in the care or treatment of beneficiaries and reimbursed, directly or indirectly, by a Federal health care program.

D. Violation of an OIG Exclusion By an Excluded Individual or Entity

An excluded party is in violation of its exclusion if it furnishes to Federal program beneficiaries items or services for which Federal health care program payment is sought. An excluded individual or entity that submits a claim for reimbursement to a Federal health care program, or causes such a claim to be submitted, may be subject to a CMP of $10,000 for each item or service furnished during the period that the person or entity was excluded (section 1128A(a)(1)(D) of the Act). The individual or entity may also be subject to treble damages for the amount claimed for each item or service. In addition, since reinstatement into the programs is not automatic, the excluded individual may jeopardize future reinstatement into Federal health care programs (42 CFR 1001.3002).

E. Employing an Excluded Individual or Entity

As indicated above, BBA authorizes the imposition of CMPs against health care providers and entities that employ or enter into contracts with excluded individuals or entities to provide items or services to Federal program beneficiaries (section 1128A(a)(6) of the Act; 42 CFR 1003.102(a)(2)). This authority parallels the CMP for health maintenance organizations that employ or contract with excluded individuals (section 1857(g)(1)(G) of the Act). Under the CMP authority, providers such as hospitals, nursing homes, hospices and group medical practices may face CMP exposure if they submit claims to a Federal health care program for health care items or services provided, directly or indirectly, by excluded individuals or entities.

Thus, a provider or entity that receives Federal health care funding may only employ an excluded individual in limited situations. Those situations would include instances where the provider is both able to pay the individual exclusively with private funds or from other non-federal funding sources, and where the services furnished by the excluded individual relate solely to non-federal program patients.

In many instances, the practical effect of an OIG exclusion is to preclude employment of an excluded individual in any capacity by a health care provider that receives reimbursement, indirectly or directly, from any Federal health care program.

F. CMP Liability for Employing or Contracting with an Excluded Individual or Entity

If a health care provider arranges or contracts (by employment or otherwise) with an individual or entity who is excluded by the OIG from program participation for the provision of items or services reimbursable under such a Federal program, the provider may be subject to CMP liability if they render services reimbursed, directly or indirectly, by such a program. CMPs of up to $10,000 for each item or service furnished by the excluded individual or entity and listed on a claim submitted for Federal program reimbursement, as well as an assessment of up to three times the amount claimed and program exclusion may be imposed. For liability to be imposed, the statute requires that the provider submitting the claims for health care items or services furnished by an excluded individual or entity "knows or should know" that the person was excluded from participation in the Federal health care programs (section

1128A(a)(6) of the Act; 42 CFR 1003.102(a)(2)). Providers and contracting entities have an affirmative duty to check the program exclusion status of individuals and entities prior to entering into employment or contractual relationships, or run the risk of CMP liability if they fail to do so.

G. How to Determine If an Individual or Entity is Excluded

In order to avoid potential CMP liability, the OIG urges health care providers and entities to check the OIG List of Excluded Individuals/Entities on the OIG web site (www.oig.hhs.gov) prior to hiring or contracting with individuals or entities. In addition, if they have not already done so, health care providers should periodically check the OIG web site for determining the participation/exclusion status of current employees and contractors. The web site contains OIG program exclusion information and is updated in both on-line searchable and downloadable formats. This information is updated on a regular basis. The OIG web site sorts the exclusion of individuals and entities by: (1) the legal basis for the exclusion, (2) the types of individuals and entities that have been excluded, and (3) the State where the excluded individual resided at the time they were excluded or the State where the entity was doing business.

In addition, the entire exclusion file may be downloaded for persons who wish to set up their own database. Monthly updates are posted to the downloadable information on the web site.

H. Conclusion

In accordance with the expanded sanction authority provided in HIPAA and BBA, and with limited exceptions, an exclusion from Federal health care programs effectively precludes an excluded individual or entity from being employed by, or under contract with, any practitioner, provider or supplier to provide any items and services reimbursed by a Federal health care program. This broad prohibition applies whether the Federal reimbursement is based on itemized claims, cost reports, fee schedules or PPS. Furthermore, it should be recognized that an exclusion remains in effect until the individual or entity has been reinstated to participate in Federal health care programs in accordance with the procedures set forth at 42 CFR 1001.3001 through 1001.3005. Reinstatement does not occur automatically at the end of a term of exclusion, but rather, an excluded party must apply for reinstatement.

If you are an excluded individual or entity, or are considering hiring or contracting with an excluded individual or entity, and question whether or not the employment arrangement may violate the law, the OIG Advisory Opinion process is available to offer formal binding guidance on whether an employment or contractual arrangement may be in violation of the OIG's exclusion and CMP authorities. The process and procedure for submitting an advisory opinion request can be found at 42 CFR 1008, or on the OIG web site at www.oig.hhs.gov.

Appeal Rights Under an Intent to Exclude

Generally, physicians and others will receive a notice of an intent to exclude. Once a decision has been made to impose an exclusion, the physician may request a hearing before an administrative law judge.[23] If the physician is dissatisfied with the administrative law judge's decision, he or she may request a review by the HHS Departmental Appeals Board.

If the physician is still dissatisfied, the next step is to take the case to federal district court. An appeal generally involves disagreement on whether the exclusion should have been imposed and related issues, and the length of time of the exclusion.

In most cases, those receiving a notice will already have attorneys involved in their case. However, it is essential that an attorney handle these hearings. There are special rules and timetables to meet. Most important, the arguments must be as effective as possible. While it may be difficult to avoid exclusion on appeal, the physician may be able to negotiate for a shorter period, an interim review of progress, or imposition of a voluntary compliance program with periodic reviews.

Intent

A number of possible defenses are available to those charged with fraudulent billings. The specific defense(s) should be determined on the basis of advice of counsel. In keeping with the tenor of this book, we are not going to try to provide specific information regarding the likelihood of success with these defenses. Success with any defense depends on the circumstances of the case, persuasiveness of prosecutors and defense attorneys, recent judicial interpretations, information available to the defendant, billing practices of those in similar situations, attitude of the judge and/or jury, new legislation, and many other factors. Short of criminal prosecution, there are other actions that may be taken—imposition of CMPs, administrative remedies such as exclusion from participation—and one will still have to return monies received in excess of that which should have been paid.

One potential defense relates to the physician's intent with respect to the billing practices in question. The concept of intent, however, and its adequacy as a defense are not straightforward. Some statutes and court decisions indicate that the defendant must have knowingly and willfully acted with an intent to defraud the government or other payer. Other statutes or courts use a test that is best characterized by the phrases *should have known*, *acted in reckless disregard of the truth*, or *acted with deliberate ignorance*.

Other defenses that take into account one's knowledge and/or intent include the following:

- An honest error or mistake was made

- The rules and regulations were simply too confusing and complex, or the carrier applied rules incorrectly or retroactively

- The physician had followed this same billing practice for years without one notice from the payer that it might be inappropriate, or many other payers allow the billing practice in question (but the physician should be very careful with this one—he or she might simply be admitting to additional false claims)

- The physician made a reasonable, although incorrect, interpretation of an overly complex law, regulation, coding guideline, etc

- The physician relied on a payer's advice or other advice that the physician had reason to believe true (preferably such advice was in writing)

- The physician relied on legal advice in structuring arrangements or transactions

On the other hand, the government may counter with arguments that the physician had access to carrier newsletters that adequately explained the billing rules in question; the physician received a copy of the carrier manual; the physician's billing practices changed from previous practices simply to take advantage of the payer; the physician "closed his or her eyes to the rules"; other physicians in similar situations billed correctly; or any reasonable person would have billed differently. The point is, notwithstanding possible defenses like those above, a physician has responsibility with respect to ensuring compliance.

The government may call expert witnesses to testify to their interpretation of correct coding and billing. Imagine the position of a defendant—who is asserting complexity of the billing system as his or her defense—when an "expert" witness testifies that the AMA's CPT® book clearly identifies the correct code and, therefore, the physician billed inappropriately. The defendant's position becomes even more difficult when prosecutors introduce specialty society articles discussing appropriate coding.

The complexity of medical care has necessitated a very detailed coding system, and the added complexity of multiple billing systems often contributes to errors. However, it would be imprudent of physicians to think they are reducing their risk of running afoul of fraud or abuse actions by remaining ignorant of the rules or relying on complexity as a solid defense if a problem arises.

When physicians face prosecution, their attorneys will likely assess the intent of their actions and whether some of the defenses above apply to their specific circumstances. Even if the defense succeeds, they may have incurred substantial defense costs and irreparable damage to their reputation, have become subjected to increased scrutiny, have been put on notice as to the correct billing practice, and still face recoveries for overpayments.

You should not meet with investigators unless your attorney is physically present at the meeting. "Intent" is an important element of the case made against one under investigation for possible fraudulent activity. Any statements made could be used to establish the level of intent necessary to successfully prosecute a case. You must rely on your attorney's advice in these situations.

In fact, be careful what you say to anyone in these situations—not just investigators—because your employees, other physicians, vendors, or patients could testify against you. They may be purposely seeking evidence that proves the level of intent normally needed to convict.

State laws vary widely as to the level of "intent" that must be demonstrated. In some states, legislation seems to indicate that the defendant must have acted with criminal intent and knowledge that claims (or kickbacks, etc) were fraudulent. In other states, the burden of proof is not as difficult. It does appear that many states are taking steps to amend laws to clarify the term *intent*.

Finally, remember that managed care plans—including Medicare and Medicaid managed care organizations—can exclude physicians from participation if they suspect billing irregularities. While the physician may have some appeal rights, appeals may be ineffective when the managed care plan feels it has evidence of fraudulent billing practices.

While there are a number of defenses one may assert upon prosecution, federal laws, state laws, and court interpretations are becoming more restrictive. If a physician is confronted with prosecution, his or her attorney will certainly look at the appropriateness of venue, intent, communication of applicable laws and guidelines, materiality, and other defenses. However, the best way to avoid problems is to stay knowledgeable with respect to rules regarding billing, coding, referrals, and other areas of compliance exposure. Physicians should adopt some compliance efforts that make sense for their practice.

A Word of Caution: Don't Play It Too Loosely Under Managed Care!

Many physicians and their staff have succumbed to wide variance in coding rules among insurance companies. Sometimes physicians guess at appropriate codes, experiment when they are not sure of payer rules, or perhaps stretch the rules a bit when payers cannot or will not help answer coding questions.

This could be very risky. A managed care plan could identify you as a high-cost physician because you are lax in selecting diagnosis codes that clearly indicate the patient's condition (this could affect quality ratings as well). A health plan could brand you as an unbundler or upcoder if you play it too loosely or simply make a lot of errors because you are concentrating on patient care.

If you take too many risks in these respects, you could be terminated from participation in the plan. Perhaps you will have a chance to appeal. However, you might not always get an opportunity to explain your position fully. Finally, it is possible you could be prosecuted for filing false claims.

Federal Sentencing Guidelines

The federal government uses guidelines to help determine a convicted violator's fine. Essentially, the guidelines are a point system with a number of determinants—type of crime, amount of money (if involved), how cooperative the defendant is during an investigation, role of the defendant in the crime vs role of others, risk of injury to patients, any prior convictions, and any other unusual circumstances.

Culpability Score for Organizations Under Sentencing Guidelines

Stripped to basics, the point system works as follows. The ultimate score determines minimum and maximum multipliers to be applied to the base fine. The portion of the fine determined by the multiplier is in addition to the base fine. The base fine is the greatest of the defendant's gain or the government's loss to the extent the loss was caused intentionally, knowingly, or recklessly. The multipliers range from 0.05 to 0.20 for those with a culpability score of 0, to 2.00 to 4.00 for those with a score of 10 or more. The multiplier for 5 points is 1.00 to 2.00.[24, 25]

You begin with 5 points.

Add points for:

- Involvement in or tolerance of criminal activity (points depend on size of organization)

- History (1 to 2 points depending on number/type of convictions)

- Violation of judicial order (1 to 2 points)

- Obstruction of justice (3 points)

Subtract points for:

- Effective compliance plan (ie, subtract 3 points)[26]

- Self-reporting, cooperation, and acceptance of responsibility (2 to 5 points; 5 points for those who voluntarily disclose offenses)[27]

Endnotes

1. Assuming this provision would withstand judicial tests, such powers are a real inducement to implement compliance programs in health care entities. The term *investors* refers to those with a direct or indirect control interest who know or should know. . . .

2. Formerly, the government had interpreted the level of intent to be merely a failure to exercise reasonable diligence. Now it defines *knowingly* and *knows or should know* as acting in deliberate ignorance or reckless disregard of the truth.

3. In some states, most notably Florida, there have been multiple indictments and convictions related to a scam where entities have been established to provide extensive diagnostic workups for Medicare and Medicaid beneficiaries. These companies employed sales forces to market "routine physicals" to Medicare beneficiaries and Medicaid recipients. These clinics were temporarily established, usually for a period of 1 to 2 months, provided the patients transportation in air-conditioned buses, and paid approximately $30 to $150 as an inducement to have the workup.

4. Remember, it appears that the term *federal health care offense* includes actions against private payers, not just government programs.

5. The Department of HHS and the Department of Justice, *Health Care Fraud and Abuse Control Program Annual Report for FY 2001*, published April 2002.

6. It is possible that a violator could be subjected to criminal and civil proceedings; however, some—but certainly not all—civil actions might be deemed "excessive" considering a previous criminal conviction related to the same claims.

7. The physician or other health care professional never saw the patient, billed for a service by using a higher-paying CPT® code than appropriate, or used false documentation to support a service that would likely have been denied.

8. In 1986, the False Claims Act was amended such that the term *knowingly* includes "acting in reckless disregard . . ." or in "deliberate ignorance of the truth or falsity of information." Thus, the standard of intent is not strictly limited to "knowingly" filing false claims. Again, "acting in reckless disregard" might be asserted if one does not take appropriate action for one's type of organization with respect to compliance activities.

9. If the government participates, the potential reward is 15% to 25% (with the 10% cap exception noted above). If the government does not participate, the potential award is 25% to 30%. If the person who brings the action participated in the offense, the court may reduce the share of proceeds. The *qui tam* action does not necessarily protect the person from prosecution if he or she participated in the offense.

10. The Department of HHS and the Department of Justice, *Health Care Fraud and Abuse Control Program Annual Report for FY 2001*, published April 2002.

11. Tax Payers Against Fraud at www.taf.org.

12. *US v Mialiaccio*, 34 F3d (10th Cir 1994).

13. The OIG initiates proceedings before an administrative law judge when assessing civil monetary penalties.

14. See Advisory Opinion No. 99-7, July 8, 1999, which discusses whether an across-the-board waiver of any out-of-pocket beneficiary copayments for medical services covered by the National Eye Care Project®, a public outreach program, constitutes grounds for the imposition of a sanction under section 1128A(a)(5) of the Act. In this case, the unique circumstances of the eye project resulted in an opinion that sanctions would not apply. The opinion is available at www.oig.hhs.gov/fraud/advisoryopinions/opinions.html. Also, see Advisory Opinion No. 98-6, April 24, 1998, whether waiving coinsurance obligations for participants in a clinical study sponsored by the Health Care Financing Administration and the National Heart, Lung, and Blood Institute could be deemed a kickback.

15. 42 USC §1320a-7a.

16. HIPAA amended section 1128 (A)a of the Social Security Act (42 USC §1320a-7a).

17. HIPAA amended section 1128 (A)b of the Social Security Act (42 USC §1320a-7a[b]).

18. We provide this section on HMOs because Medicare managed care plans will be an important source of patients for many physicians in the future. You want to make sure the organizations with which you participate are operating within applicable laws.

19. Technically, this statute is not used to prosecute a person, but to seize any property, real or personal, involved in specified offenses, or any property traceable to such offenses. For specified fraudulent activity, the government can seize property "constituting, or derived from, proceeds the person obtained, directly or indirectly, as result of violation."

20. The Department of HHS and the Department of Justice, *Health Care Fraud and Abuse Control Program Annual Report for FY 2001, published April 2002.*

21. HIPAA also provides for imposition of civil monetary penalties (up to $10,000 per day) should the Secretary of HHS decide to take such action: "In the case of a person who is not an organization, agency, or other entity, is excluded from participating in a program under title XVIII or a State health care program in accordance with this subsection or under section 1128 and who, at the time of a violation of this subsection— (A) retains a direct or indirect ownership or control interest in an entity that is participating in a program under title XVIII or a State health care program, and who knows or should know of the action constituting the basis for the exclusion; or (B) is an officer or managing employee of such an entity."

22. From a table available at the OIG Web site http://www.oig.hhs.gov/fraud/exclusions/exclusionauthorities.html.

23. In some cases, a practitioner facing exclusion may have an opportunity to present additional information and arguments before having to go through a hearing with an administrative law judge. If this additional information is not persuasive, the exclusionary period begins even if you intend to request an administrative law judge hearing. In other cases, the first opportunity to appeal is to an administrative law judge. Depending on the reasons for exclusion, an administrative law judge hearing may be available before the exclusion is imposed. In other circumstances, the exclusion may be imposed before an administrative law judge hearing is available. The notice of intent will address your rights.

24. There are several other factors that the government can use to increase or decrease the fines suggested by the point system. This is an obvious simplification of the point system.

25. Also, the defendant has potential monetary exposure from the civil False Claims Act for treble damages and $5,000 to $10,000 penalty per false claim, and similar exposure under the Social Security Act, as amended in 1996.

26. Notice, only one adjustment for an effective compliance plan would reduce the score by 3 points and the corresponding multiplier by up to 60%. There are, of course, many other reasons to adopt a compliance plan, and reductions in penalties are not necessarily automatic under the point system.

27. Talk to your attorney before turning yourself in. It is important how you do it and what you admit to doing. If possible, it would be desirable to avoid sanctions by returning overpayments and applicable interest.

Antikickback Legislation

A discussion of antikickback legislation and prohibited self-referrals is extremely technical. It is not our purpose here to present all the different ways physicians might violate these laws. In fact, this section is basically a summary of the legislation and related regulatory activity to help physicians realize the importance of having a health care attorney review any arrangement that may trigger these prohibitions.

It is advisable to seek competent counsel because these are relatively new laws, interpretation and enforcement vary, complete regulations have not been issued in all cases, sometimes a potentially illegal arrangement is not readily apparent, and there may be relevant advisory opinions that will be useful in evaluating an arrangement.

The Antikickback Statute

Since the 1970s, there has been federal legislation that prohibits payments for referrals. Early legislation was aimed at outright payments (ie, kickbacks) by clinical laboratories, hospitals, home health agencies, durable medical equipment vendors, and other suppliers. Sometimes, the payments were disguised as grants for which the recipient had to perform very little research (relative to the payments received), provision of significant services that would normally be a cost of business for the recipient, provision of below-market rent to referral sources for space or equipment, and the like.

The antikickback statute prohibits:

1   the knowing and willful offer or making of payment (including a kickback, bribe, or rebate) to induce a referral of a Medicare or Medicaid patient[1]

2   solicitation or receipt of such payments

3   knowingly and willfully inducing, making, or causing to be made any false statement or material misrepresentation in an application for Medicare or Medicaid payment

4   any payment to a physician as an inducement to limit or reduce necessary medical services to Medicare or Medicaid beneficiaries[2]

Violation of the statute is a felony, subject to both criminal and civil penalties and exclusion from Medicare, Medicaid, and other federal health care programs.

There are some exceptions to the general antikickback rules, and the Department of Health and Human Services has issued so-called safe harbors, which specify situations that are unlikely to violate antikickback statutes.[3] Basically, the exceptions recognize that there are legitimate reasons for a health care entity to pay a physician—as a part-time nursing home director, for clinical laboratory oversight, as hospice director, or as hospital medical director. However, when payments exceed what is considered the fair market value for the services provided, there is the possibility that one reason for the payments is to induce a physician to refer patients.[4] A number of safe harbors are discussed later in this chapter, and arrangements falling outside the safe harbors are not necessarily illegal.

Some states have also become involved. In 1997, Florida's medical board indicated that the common method of paying physician practice management corporations (such as PhyCor, MedPartners, FPA, etc) a percentage of revenue might be considered illegal fee splitting. On the basis of the advisory opinion issued by the Office of Inspector General (OIG) on April 15, 1999, these arrangements should be carefully evaluated to ensure compliance with applicable laws. There are advisors who believe Florida's interpretation may be overly restrictive, and there are alternative ways of paying management fees. (We will reproduce a related OIG advisory opinion below.)

The OIG's Semiannual Report for October 2001 through April 2002 describes "kickbacks" as follows:

Many businesses engage in referrals to meet the needs of customers or clients for expertise, services or items which are not part of their own regular operations or products. The medical profession relies heavily upon referrals because of the myriad of specialties and technologies associated with health care. **If referrals of Medicare or Medicaid patients are made in exchange for anything of value, however, both the giver and receiver may violate the Federal anti-kickback statute.** They may also directly or indirectly increase Medicare/caid costs. [boldface added]

The anti-kickback statute authorizes penalties against anyone who knowingly and willfully solicits, receives, offers, or pays remuneration, in cash or in kind, to induce or in return for 1) referring an individual to a person or entity for the furnishing, or arranging for the furnishing, of any item or service payable under the federal health care programs; or 2) purchasing, leasing or ordering, or arranging for or recommending the purchasing, leasing or ordering of any good, facility, service or item payable under the federal health care programs. (Section 1128B(b) of the Social Security Act, 42 U.S.C. 1320a-7b)

The following are examples of anti-kickback enforcement actions [Note: Examples are from various OIG Semi-annual reports]:

An OB-GYN group and several individual physicians paid $109,900 to resolve their civil monetary penalty liability for violations of the physician self-referral (Stark) statute and the kickback provisions of the Civil Monetary Penalties Law. From 1997 through 2000, the physicians had a financial relationship with a mobile ultrasound company from which they received referral fees 'ostensibly in the form of rent' in return for referring Medicare beneficiaries to the company for ultrasound studies and diagnostic testing. (4/2002 Report)

A New York man was ordered to pay $18,000 in restitution and a $5,000 fine for violating the anti-kickback statute. As the security director for a hospital, one of his responsibilities included arranging ambulance transportation for hospital patients. In 1995, the man began accepting kickbacks from the owner/operator of an ambulance company in exchange for Medicare and Medicaid referrals to the company. (4/2002 Report)

Three physicians were sentenced in a northern state. One physician was sentenced to 2 years probation and ordered to pay restitution, fines and penalties totaling $177,000 for tax evasion and accepting kickbacks. The physician entered into a kickback agreement with the owners of a medical supply company through which the physician referred patients to the company in return for Durable Medical Equipment and cash.

The other two, an internist and a cardiologist, were also sentenced for accepting kickbacks in exchange for patient referrals. The internist was sentenced, for illegal kickback activity, to 2 years probation and required to pay a $20,000 fine. The cardiologist was sentenced to 30 months incarceration and ordered to pay a $10,000 fine for conspiracy and illegal kickback activity. (9/2001 Report)

A man was sentenced to 3 years probation, 4 months home detention and a $1,000 fine for conspiracy to commit mail fraud and illegal kickback activity. He engaged in these improper activities while working as the office manager for a physician. From 1990 through 1994, the

two conspired to solicit and obtain kickbacks from specific medical facilities in return for Medicare patient referrals to those facilities for diagnostic services. They then split the kickbacks received. For his part in the scheme, the physician was arrested for mail fraud and sentenced to 2 years probation, 6 months home detention and a $30,000 fine. (9/99 Report)

The faculty practice plan of a hospital agreed to pay $177,000 in settlement of civil monetary liabilities for kickback arrangements by two of the hospital's divisions. Since cardiologists could not bill Medicare for interpretations of coronary angiograms and ventriculograms, but radiologists could, arrangements were made for the radiologists to bill for these interpretations. In return, the radiology group paid kickbacks to the cardiology group. This case is the first civil monetary penalties case to have been based solely on violations of the anti-kickback law. (9/96 Report)

A physician and the owners of two diagnostic companies agreed to settle civil liability for a kickback scheme. The company owners paid $11,000 in kickbacks through a sham lease agreement with the physician and another doctor now deceased. The remaining physician assisted in the prosecution which resulted in the company owners' guilty pleas. The two owners agreed to pay a total of $61,000, and both are permanently excluded from program participation. The physician agreed to pay $18,000 to settle civil liability. (9/97 Report)

The owner of a psychiatric hospital entered for the hospital a plea of guilty to making a false claim to Civilian Health and Medical Plan of Uniformed Services (CHAMPUS). The administrator of the hospital was indicted earlier for paying kickbacks to a physician for referring psychiatric patients to the hospital. The hospital was sentenced to 5 years probation and ordered to pay close to $63,160 in restitution. In lieu of a monetary fine, the hospital must produce a community service plan within 30 days. Both the owner and the hospital agreed to cooperate in the prosecution of the administrator and the physician for Medicare and CHAMPUS fraud. The two had worked together earlier at another hospital, at which the physician was convicted of accepting kickbacks. (3/97 Report)

A physician was sentenced to 18 months in prison and fined $40,700 **for accepting kickbacks for referring patients** to an area cardiologist. The cardiologist, who was sentenced earlier to 6 months in jail and fined $200,000, cooperated in the case against the physician. He had paid the physician more than $50,000 over a 2-year period, basing the amount of each payment an the type and number of procedures for which each patient was referred (for example, he paid $200 for a referral for a treadmill test and $300 for cardiac catheterization). The physician was also given 3 years probation upon release and ordered to perform 1,000 hours community service. [boldface added]

As a result of the ongoing investigation of an impotence clinic company, the owner of a mobile diagnostic laboratory agreed to pay the Medicare Trust Fund $1.77 million and the Internal Revenue Service (IRS) $230,000. The laboratory owner paid kickbacks not only to impotence clinic owners but also to numerous physicians in the area for Medicare patient referrals. During the investigation, $2.3 million of his assets were frozen. (3/98 Report)

Another subject of the impotence clinic case, the owner of a diagnostics service in Florida was sentenced for paying kickbacks for Medicare patient referrals by clinic owners. The kickbacks were disguised as rental or marketing fees paid to the clinics. He was sentenced to 4 months house arrest and 5 years probation, and ordered to make restitution of $106,000 to Medicare. (3/98 Report)

The office manager of a multi-physician practice was sentenced to 21 months in prison and 3 years of supervised release for conspiracy to defraud Medicare. He was also ordered to pay $50,420 in restitution. Between August 1993 and August 1994, he accepted about $23,000 from a clinical laboratory owner in return for referrals. Upon learning of the OIG investigation, he and the laboratory owner drew up a bogus, backdated

consulting contract to give the appearance of its being part of a valid agreement. Despite the contract, the office manager was convicted at trial of all 15 counts of conspiracy and kickbacks. (3/98 Report)

A national corporation agreed to pay over $100 million to settle criminal and civil liabilities for paying kickbacks to physicians for referrals for its home infusion business and growth drug, for improper billings and failing to keep accurate records at some of its Pharmacies. **The company entered criminal pleas, and agreed to cooperate in investigation of individuals involved in the schemes, *including physicians*.** It also entered into a corporate integrity agreement with the Department to maintain a corporate ethics and compliance program for 5 years. The company sold its home infusion business and will no longer be engaged in that field. It also canceled its special arrangements with physicians and HHS, and agreed to address its billing problems. [boldface added]

The parent corporation of a health care provider of inpatient and outpatient services agreed to pay $2 million in settlement of liability for violating the Medicare anti-kickback statute. The company made income guarantees and office rent subsidies to physicians, granted low-interest or no-interest loans, forgave repayment of loans, provided staff support for a physician's private practice and entered 'directorship' contracts in which physicians performed little or no services, to induce them to make referrals to the company. Medicare losses are estimated to total $335,000. The Department, CHAMPUS and the Medicaid program will share the settlement proceeds.

To summarize, the antikickback statute is a criminal statute that applies to those who knowingly and willfully offer, pay, solicit, or receive remuneration to induce the furnishing of items or services under Medicare or state health care programs (including Medicaid). The offense is classified as a felony and is punishable by fines of up to $25,000 and imprisonment for up to 5 years. Violation of the statute is also a basis for exclusion from Medicare, Medicaid, and other federal health care programs.

The following is pertinent language describing "illegal remunerations":[5]

(1) Whoever knowingly and willfully **solicits or receives any remuneration** (including any kickback, bribe, or rebate) directly or indirectly, overtly or covertly, in cash or in kind—[boldface added]

    (A) in return for referring an individual to a person for the furnishing or arranging for the furnishing of any item or service for which payment may be [under Medicare or a state health program], or

    (B) in return for purchasing, leasing, ordering, or arranging for or recommending purchasing, leasing, or ordering any good, facility, service, or item . . . shall be guilty of a felony and upon conviction thereof, shall be fined not more than $25,000 or imprisoned for not more than five years, or both.

(2) Whoever knowingly and willfully **offers or pays any remuneration** (including any kickback, bribe, or rebate) directly or indirectly, overtly or covertly, in cash or in kind to any person to induce such person (A) to refer an individual to a person for the furnishing or arranging for . . . any item or service . . . , or (B) to purchase, lease, order, or arrange for or recommend purchasing, leasing, or ordering any good, facility, service, or item . . . shall be guilty of a felony and upon conviction thereof, shall be fined not more than $25,000 or imprisoned for not more than five years, or both. [boldface added]

(3) Paragraphs (1) and (2) shall not apply to—

    (A) a discount or other reduction in price obtained by a provider of services or other entity under subchapter XVIII of this chapter or a State health care program if the reduction in price is properly disclosed and appropriately reflected in the costs claimed or charges made by the provider or entity under subchapter XVIII of this chapter or a State health care program;

    (B) any amount paid by an employer to an employee (who has a bona fide employment relationship with such employer) for employment in the provision of covered items or services;

    (C) any amount paid by a vendor of goods or services to a person authorized to act as a purchasing agent for a group of individuals or entities who are furnishing services reimbursed under subchapter XVIII of this chapter or a State health care program if—(i) the person has a written contract, with each such individual or entity, which specifies the amount to be paid the person, which amount may be a fixed amount or a fixed percentage of the value of the purchases made by each such individual or entity under the contract, and (ii) in the case of an entity that is a provider of services (as defined in section 1395x(u) of this title), the person discloses (in such form and manner as the Secretary requires) to the entity and, upon request, to Secretary the amount received from each such vendor with respect to purchases made by or on behalf of the entity; . . .

The Health Insurance Portability and Accountability Act of 1996 (HIPAA) extends this legislation to services covered under other federal health care programs, which are defined as "any plan or program that provides health benefits, whether directly, through insurance, or otherwise, which is funded directly, in whole or in part, by the United States Government . . . [other than the Federal Employee Health Benefit Program] or any State health care program."

The HIPAA also allows certain risk-sharing arrangements related to physicians and others providing services financed through managed care organizations.

Waiver of Copayments and Deductibles and Other Inducements

In the previous chapter, we discussed provisions under HIPAA that could be used to apply sanctions, such as civil monetary penalties of up to $10,000 per occurrence for routine waiver of copayments and deductibles (with a few exceptions) as discussed below. It is repeated here because this is a common question in most discussions on fraud and abuse.

Prohibition Against Offering Inducements to Individuals Enrolled Under Programs or Plans[6]

[The Secretary may impose sanctions against a provider who] offers to or transfers **remuneration** to any individual eligible for [Medicare] benefits, or under a State health care program that such person knows or should know is likely to influence such individual to order or receive from a particular provider, practitioner, or supplier any item or service for which payment may be made, in whole or in part. . . . [boldface added]

The **term *remuneration* includes the waiver of coinsurance and deductible amounts (or any part thereof),** and transfers of items or services for free or for other than fair market value. The term **remuneration does not include** [and a provider would not likely be sanctioned]: [boldface added]

(A) The waiver of coinsurance and deductible amounts, if
  (i)   the waiver is not offered as part of any advertisement or solicitation;
  (ii) the person does not routinely waive coinsurance or deductible amounts; and
  (iii) the person (I) waives the coinsurance and deductible amounts after determining in good faith that the individual is in financial need; (II) fails to collect coinsurance or deductible amounts after making reasonable collection efforts; or (III) provides for any permissible waiver as specified in section 1128B(b)(3) or in regulations issued by the Secretary;

(B) Differentials in coinsurance and deductible amounts as part of a benefit plan design as long as the differentials have been disclosed in writing to all beneficiaries, third party payers, and providers, to whom claims are presented and as long as the differentials meet the standards as defined in regulations promulgated by the Secretary not later than 180 days after the date of the enactment of the Health Insurance Portability and Accountability Act of 1996; or

(C) Incentives given to individuals to promote the delivery of preventive care as determined by the Secretary in regulations so promulgated.

Paragraphs (B) and (C) above apply to Medicare HMOs and similar health care benefit plans that may offer such coverage and payment terms.

Potentially Illegal Hospital-Physician Incentives

In the mid-1990s, the OIG published a pamphlet that delineated some potentially illegal hospital kickback incentives. Some of these are not necessarily illegal if structured correctly and provided for reasons not associated with inducing referrals (nor does this list cover all potentially illegal arrangements). These are the areas of concern in the OIG's list:

- Payment or incentive of any sort by the hospital each time a physician refers a patient to the facility

- The use of free or significantly discounted office space or equipment (in facilities usually located near the hospital). Always insist on a lease agreement at fair market value for similar office space in the same area

- Provision of free or significantly discounted billing, nursing, or other staff services; such services should be set in an "at arm's-length" transaction priced at fair market value

- Payment for physicians' continuing education courses

- Free training for a physician's office staff in areas such as management techniques, CPT® coding, and laboratory techniques

- Guarantees that provide that, if a physician's income fails to reach a predetermined level, the hospital will supplement the remainder up to a certain amount

- Low-interest or interest-free loans, or loans that may be forgiven if a physician refers patients (or some number of patients) to the hospital

- Payment of the cost of physicians' travel and expenses for conferences that do not directly benefit the hospital

- Coverage on hospitals' group health insurance plans at an inappropriately low cost to the physician

- Payment for services (which may include consultations at the hospital) that require few, if any, substantive duties by the physician, or payment for services in excess of the fair market value of services rendered

In the *Compliance Program Guidance for Hospitals* issued in 1998, the OIG discussed some illegal arrangements between physicians and hospitals:

> . . . Excessive payment for medical directorships, free or below market rents or fees for administrative services, interest-free loans and excessive payment for intangible assets in physician practice acquisitions are examples of arrangements that may run afoul of the anti-kickback statute. See 42 U.S.C. § 1320a-7b(b) and 59 Fed. Reg. 65372 (12/19/94). [Arrangements that may violate the antikickback statutes] are generally established between those in a position to refer business, such as physicians, and those providing services for which a federal health care program pays. Sometimes established as joint ventures, these arrangements may take a variety of forms.

The hospital should have policies and procedures in place with respect to compliance with federal and state anti-kickback statutes, as well as the Stark physician self-referral law.

Such policies should provide that:

A. all of the hospital's contracts and arrangements with referral sources comply with all applicable statutes and regulations;

B. the hospital does not submit or cause to be submitted to federal health programs claims for patients who were referred to the hospital pursuant to contracts and financial arrangements that were designed to induce such referrals in violation of the anti-kickback statute, Stark physician self-referral law or similar federal or state statute or regulation; and

C. the hospital does not enter into financial arrangements with hospital-based physicians that are designed to provide inappropriate remuneration to the hospital in return for the physician's ability to provide services to federal program beneficiaries at that hospital.

Regarding item C above related to hospital-based physicians, the OIG released a report in 1991 that addresses this issue and included comments from the American Hospital Association and College of American Pathologists. The report, entitled *Financial Arrangements Between Hospitals and Hospital-Based Physicians*, is available at the OIG Web site www.oig.hhs.gov/fraud/fraudalerts.html.

Safe Harbors

The term *safe harbors* is used to describe activities in which one can safely engage without violating antikickback laws. In 1991, regulations were published that defined activities that would not be deemed a violation of the antikickback statutes. There were some proposed additions to the safe harbors in 1993 and 1994, but publication of a final rule did not occur until November 19, 1999.[7]

What constitutes the safe harbors will likely remain in a state of flux. The HIPAA requires the government to solicit proposals annually for modifying existing safe harbors and adding new ones. The OIG will publish an announcement annually in the Federal Register soliciting new proposals.[8] Physicians involved in activities with antikickback implications should monitor future announcements and recognize that each safe harbor includes very specific requirements that must be met.

The following is a summary of the status of safe harbors at the end of 1999 from a fact sheet published by the OIG in November 1999.

Federal Antikickback Law and Regulatory Safe Harbors

Overview: On the books since 1972, the federal anti-kickback law's main purpose is to protect patients and the federal health care programs from fraud and abuse by curtailing the corrupting influence of money on health care decisions. Straightforward but broad, the law states that anyone who knowingly and willfully receives or pays anything of value to influence the referral of federal health care program business, including Medicare and Medicaid, can be held accountable for a felony. Violations of the law are punishable by up to five years in prison, criminal fines up to $25,000, administrative civil money penalties up to $50,000, and exclusion from participation in federal health care programs.

Because the law is broad on its face, concerns arose among health care providers that some relatively innocu-ous—and in some cases even beneficial—commercial arrangements are prohibited by the anti-kickback law. Responding to these concerns, Congress in 1987 author-ized the Department to issue regulations designating specific "safe harbors" for various payment and busi-ness practices that, while potentially prohibited by the law, would not be prosecuted.

The Office of Inspector General has previously published 13 regulatory safe harbors, 11 in 1991 and two in 1992. A new final rule scheduled for publication in the Nov. 19, 1999, Federal Register will establish eight new safe-harbor provisions and clarify six of the original 11 safe harbors published in 1991. These proposals were pub-lished in the Federal Register in 1993 and 1994 and have been significantly modified in response to voluminous public comments.

Additionally, an interim final rule establishing a safe har-bor for shared-risk arrangements is scheduled for publi-cation in the Nov. 19, 1999, Federal Register. After publication of the two new rules, there will be a total of 23 anti-kickback safe harbors consolidated in the Code of Federal Regulations in 21 subparagraphs.

Safe Harbors Generally

Safe harbors immunize certain payment and business practices that are implicated by the anti-kickback statute from criminal and civil prosecution under the statute. To be protected by a safe harbor, an arrangement must fit squarely in the safe harbor. Failure to comply with a safe harbor provision does not mean that an arrangement is per se illegal. Compliance with safe harbors is voluntary, and arrangements that do not comply with a safe harbor must be analyzed on a case-by-case basis for compliance with the anti-kickback statute. Parties who are uncertain whether their arrangements qualify for safe harbor pro-tection may request an advisory opinion. Instructions on how to request an advisory opinion are available on the Internet at www.oig.hhs.gov/fraud/advisoryopinions.html.

The following is a listing of Medicare antikickback safe harbors (ie, arrangements the government believes do not violate antikickback laws if all requirements are satisfied).

This list is only a brief summary of the safe harbors. If you are involved in any arrangement with antikickback implications, you must carefully analyze your situation—with your attorney—to make sure you fall within the safe harbors or that you have otherwise structured the arrangement to avoid violating antikickback legislation. You may still be on safe ground, even if your particular arrangement does not fall within the safe harbors. However, analyze and periodically review the situation carefully.

The first 13 safe harbors were originally promulgated in 1991 and 1992. In 1999, some of the original ones were clarified or modified slightly. After these 13 are summarized, the discussion will turn to the additional and revised safe harbors formally published in a final rule in 1999.

Original Safe Harbors

1. Investment Interests in Large Publicly Held Health Care Companies

2. Investments in Small Health Care Joint Ventures.

In general, the OIG is concerned about arrangements where a physician or other health care provider invests in a medical entity such that the return on investment is tied to the physician/investor's referrals. Investments acquired through a registered national securities exchange through a broker are generally "safe." A number of requirements must be met. For example, the safe harbor is not met if physicians and other providers who are in a position to refer patients own a high percentage of any class of investment in a small publicly traded company (the 60-40 rule, where 60% of the investors must not be providers). The 60-40 rule and other aspects of this safe harbor were clarified in the November 19, 1999, *Federal Register*.

3. Space Rental.

A kickback could be disguised as an inflated rental payment (eg, a diagnostic testing entity pays a physician a rental payment based on referrals) or as a reduced rental rate (eg, a hospital charges a physician zero rent to induce referrals). The safe harbors are designed to allow arrangements in which one entity rents space or equipment from another entity receiving referrals provided the lease has a commercially reasonable business purpose, is in writing, is signed by all parties, is for a term of 1 year or more, and reflects fair market value.[9] The provision related to a term of at least 1 year is designed to prevent physicians and others in a position to refer from receiving kickbacks by having their lease renegotiated to take into account the value of referrals.

In February 2000, the OIG released a "Special Fraud Alert" that addresses its concerns related to "rental of space in physician offices by persons or entities to which physicians refer." In this alert, the OIG summarized its concerns as follows:

> A number of suppliers that provide health care items or services rent space in the offices of physicians or other practitioners. Typically, most of the items or services provided in the rented space are for patients, referred or sent, either directly or indirectly, to the supplier by the physician-landlord. In particular, we are aware of rental arrangements between physician-landlords and comprehensive outpatient rehabilitation facilities (CORFs) that provide physical and occupational therapy and speech-language pathology services in physicians' and other practitioners' offices; mobile diagnostic equipment suppliers that perform diagnostic related tests in physicians' offices; and suppliers of durable medical equipment, prosthetics, orthotics and supplies (DMEPOS) that set up "consignment closets" for their supplies in physicians' offices.

The OIG is concerned that in such arrangements, the rental payments may be disguised kickbacks to the physician-landlords to induce referrals. We have received numerous credible reports that in many cases, suppliers, whose businesses depend on physicians' referrals, offer and pay "rents"—either voluntarily or in response to physicians' requests—that are either unnecessary or in excess of the fair market value for the space to access the physicians' potential referrals.

The alert goes on to explain in detail how the OIG would review such arrangements to determine if they violate the antikickback statute. The complete document is available at www.oig.hhs.gov/fraud/fraudalerts.html. These type arrangements have resulted in a number of convictions under the antikickback statute.

4. Equipment Rental. See discussion above. Safe harbors 2 and 3 were clarified in the November 19, 1999, *Federal Register*.

5. Personal Services and Management Contract. Directorships, employment arrangements, and the like can be legitimate provided there is a commercially reasonable business purpose and a legitimate contract and compensation is considered at fair market value for services provided (ie, not linked to referrals).

In OIG Advisory Opinion 98-4 issued in April 1998 (this advisory opinion is produced later in this chapter), it is noted that:

> The personal services and management contracts safe harbor provides protection for personal services contracts if all of the following six standards are met: (i) the agreement is set out in writing and signed by the parties; (ii) the agreement specifies the services to be performed; (iii) if the services are to be performed on a part-time basis, the schedule for performance is specified in the contract; (iv) the agreement is for not less than one year; (v) the aggregate amount of compensation is fixed in advance, based on fair market value in an arms-length transaction, and not determined in a manner that takes into account the volume or value of any referrals or business otherwise generated between the parties for which payment may be made by Medicare or a State health care program; and (vi) the services performed under the agreement do not involve the promotion of business that violates any Federal or State law.

6. Sales of Retiring Physicians' Practices to Other Physicians. The original safe harbors only addressed sales between physicians who are not in a position to refer patients. This safe harbor does not specifically address practices purchased by hospitals. The purchase must be completed within 1 year. This safe harbor does not, however, mean that other practice sales are prohibited, but one must be very careful how the purchase is structured to avoid antikickback implications. Competent legal advice is extremely important for a number of reasons. (As discussed in the next section, new safe harbors include provisions related to practice purchases and sales in health professional shortage areas.)

7. Patient Referral Services (Such as Those Maintained by a Hospital). To fall within this safe harbor, requirements must be met that include equal rates for all participating providers; rates must be based on the cost of operation, not on the value or volume of referrals; the referral service must not dictate how the physician will render services; and the referral service must disclose information to patients about the arrangement with physicians and others.

8. Discounts. The government realizes that there are discount arrangements with commercially reasonable business purposes that should be encouraged under federal health programs. The OIG is concerned about arrangements where a discount is given on nongovernmental business with the intent to induce, directly or indirectly, the referral of Part B Medicare or other federal health care program business.[10] Safe harbors were developed to allow nonabusive discount arrangements. Generally, discounts for goods and services must be known at the time of sale; the discounts are fully disclosed on claim forms (if a separate claim is submitted); etc. There are safe harbor requirements that apply to hospitals and other providers who file cost reports. Health maintenance organizations (HMOs) acting under risk contracts generally will not violate the safe harbor. There are certain requirements placed on sellers, such as including the discount on invoices.[11] If the seller files claims, they must reflect the discount.

9. Warranties. Warranties for medical equipment are acceptable as long as they are not disguised as a kickback. For example, at one time some medical equipment companies paid physicians for replacing a defective item—such as a pacemaker—that was then billed to Medicare. Buyers must disclose any reduction in price (on claim forms or cost reports). In other words, it would be inappropriate to charge Medicare the full cost of a pacemaker if it malfunctioned, and an allowance was due, during the warranty period. Nor is it appropriate to accept payment from a supplier for replacing a device, such as a pacemaker, that may be under warranty.

10. Employee Compensation. Amounts paid to employees under a bona fide employment arrangement and that are considered reasonable or fair market compensation are generally within the safe harbors. Contractual arrangements with independent contractors are not covered by the safe harbors but may be legal, depending on how the contract is structured.

11. Group Purchasing. Group purchasing arrangements are generally within the safe harbors as long as there is a written contract or agreement between the parties, the purchasing organization discloses to physicians and other health care providers the amounts it receives from vendors, and the amount paid by vendors to the purchasing organization is 3% or less (there are some exceptions allowing higher amounts).

12. Hospitals Waiving Coinsurance and Deductibles for Indigents. Hospitals cannot report the waiver as a bad debt on cost reports. They cannot offer the waiver on selected diagnosis-related groups (ie, those that are profitable to the hospital) or based on length of stay.

13. Inducements Offered to Potential Enrollees by HMOs and Similar Discounts Offered to HMOs, etc, by Participating Providers. This safe harbor protects certain arrangements between physicians and managed care organizations, and between managed care organizations and enrollees or insureds. For example, certain price reductions offered to health plans are considered to fall within the safe harbors (section 1001.952[m]). In addition, Congress enacted in HIPAA a statutory shared-risk exception for certain managed care plans and arrangements that put individuals or entities at substantial financial risk.

Additional Safe Harbors

In addition to clarifying or modifying some of the original safe harbors, the OIG formally added the following safe harbors in the final rule published in the November 19, 1999, *Federal Register*:

- Investments in ambulatory surgical centers

- Joint ventures in underserved areas

- Practitioner recruitment in underserved areas

- Sales of physician practices to hospitals in underserved areas

- Subsidies for obstetric malpractice insurance in underserved areas

- Investments in group practices

- Specialty referral arrangements between providers

- Cooperative hospital services organizations

Again, the following discussion is merely a brief summary of these safe harbors. Very specific requirements determine whether a set of circumstances falls within the applicable safe harbor. Refer to the *Federal Register* for complete details.

The OIG's fact sheet, published in November 1999, summarizes these safe harbors as follows:

The preamble to the new final rule [published in the November 19, 1999, Federal Register] includes a summary of each proposal from 1993 and 1994, a summary of each new safe harbor, and the Office of Inspector General's response to public comments on each topic area. The new safe harbors address the following areas: investments in underserved areas; practitioner recruitment in under served areas; obstetrical malpractice insurance subsidies for underserved areas; sales of practices to hospitals in underserved areas; investments in ambulatory surgical centers; investments in group practices; referral arrangements for specialty services; and cooperative hospital service organizations.

1) Investments in Ambulatory Surgical Centers (ASCs)

The original proposal protected only Medicare-certified ASCs wholly owned by surgeons. Many in the industry urged that the original proposal be broadened. The expanded final rule protects certain investment interests in four categories of freestanding Medicare-certified ASCs: surgeon-owned ASCs; single-specialty ASCs (e.g., all gastroenterologists); multi-specialty ASCs (e.g., a mix of surgeons and gastroenterologists); and hospital-/physician-owned ASCs. In general, to be protected, physician investors must be physicians for whom the ASC is an extension of their office practice pursuant to conditions set forth in the safe harbor. Hospital investors must not be in a position to make or influence referrals. Certain investors who are not existing or potential referral sources are permitted. The ASC safe harbor does not apply to other physician-owned clinical joint ventures, such as cardiac catheterization labs, end-stage renal dialysis facilities or radiation oncology facilities.

Note: The OIG issued an advisory opinion on November 16, 2001 addressing certain issues regarding a medical center's proposed acquisition of an investment interest in a currently operating ambulatory surgical center. See OIG Advisory Opinion Request No. 01-21 at the Web site www.oig.hhs.gov.

2) Joint Ventures in Underserved Areas

Often health care ventures in medically underserved areas have difficulty attracting needed capital, and, often, the best available sources of capital are local physicians. Many underserved area ventures cannot fit in the existing safe harbor for small entity joint ventures because that safe harbor limits physician ownership and the revenues that can be derived from referrals from physician investors. The underserved area joint venture safe harbor relaxes several of the conditions of the existing joint venture safe harbor. The new safe harbor permits a higher percentage of physician investors—up to 50 percent—and unlimited revenues from referral source investors. The new safe harbor expands on the 1993 proposal by including joint ventures in underserved urban, as well as rural, areas. To qualify, a venture must be located in a medically underserved area, as defined by Department regulation, and serve 75 percent medically underserved patients.

3) Practitioner Recruitment in Underserved Areas

This safe harbor protects recruitment payments made by entities to attract needed physicians and other health care professionals to rural and urban health professional shortage areas (HPSAs), as designated by the Health Resources and Services Administration. The safe harbor requires that at least 75 percent of the recruited practitioner's revenue be from patients who reside in HPSAs or medically underserved areas or are members of medically underserved populations, such as the homeless or migrant workers. The safe harbor limits the duration of payments to three years. The safe harbor does not prescribe the types of protected payments, such as income guarantees or moving expenses, leaving that determination to negotiation by the parties.

Because of the risk of disguised payments for referrals, the safe harbor does not protect payments made by hospitals to existing group practices to recruit physicians to join the group, nor does it protect payments to retain existing practitioners. Such arrangements remain subject to case-by-case review under the anti-kickback statute.

4) Sales of Physician Practices to Hospitals in Underserved Areas

This safe harbor protects hospitals in HPSAs that buy and "hold" the practice of a retiring physician until a new physician can be recruited to replace the retiring one. To qualify for safe harbor protection, the sale must be completed within three years, and the hospital must engage in good faith efforts to recruit a new practitioner.

5) Subsidies for Obstetrical Malpractice Insurance in Underserved Areas

This safe harbor protects a hospital or other entity that pays all or part of the malpractice insurance premiums for practitioners engaging in obstetrical practice in HPSAs. To qualify for protection, at least 75 percent of the subsidized practitioners' patients must be medically underserved patients.

6) Investments in Group Practices

This safe harbor protects investments by physicians in their own group practices, if the group practice meets the physician self-referral (Stark) law definition of a group practice. The safe harbor also protects investments in solo practices where the practice is conducted through the solo practitioner's professional corporation or other separate legal entity. The safe harbor does not protect investments by group practices or members of group practices in ancillary services' joint ventures, although such joint ventures may qualify for protection under other safe harbors.

7) Specialty Referral Arrangements Between Providers

The safe harbor protects certain arrangements when an individual or entity agrees to refer a patient to another individual or entity for specialty services in return for the party receiving the referral to refer the patient back at a certain time or under certain circumstances. For example, a primary care physician and a specialist to whom the primary care physician has made a referral may agree that, when the referred patient reaches a particular stage of recovery, the primary care physician should resume treatment of the patient. The safe harbor does not protect arrangements involving parties that split a global fee from a federal program. The safe harbor requires that referrals be clinically appropriate, rather than based on arbitrary dates or time frames.

8) Cooperative Hospital Services Organizations

This safe harbor protects cooperative hospital service organizations (CHSOs) that qualify under section 501(e) of the Internal Revenue Code. CHSOs are organizations formed by two or more tax-exempt hospitals, known as "patron hospitals," to provide specifically enumerated services, such as purchasing, billing, and clinical services solely for the benefit of patron hospitals. The safe harbor will protect payments from a patron hospital to a CHSO to support the CHSO's operational costs and payments from a CHSO to a patron hospital that are required by IRS rules.

Safe Harbors for Shared-Risk Arrangements

An interim final rule, also published in the November 19, 1999, *Federal Register* (pages 63503–63515), provides two safe harbors from the antikickback law (section 1128B[b] of the Social Security Act) for certain managed care arrangements. A few corrections were made to this interim final rule in the December 22, 1999, *Federal Register*.

The first safe harbor protects certain financial arrangements between managed care plans and individuals or entities with whom they contract for the provision of health care items and services, where federal health care programs pay such plans on a capitated basis.

The second safe harbor protects certain financial arrangements between managed care plans (including employer-sponsored group health plans) and individuals or entities with whom they contract for health care items and services with respect to services reimbursed on a fee-for-service basis by a federal health care program, provided that such individuals and entities are placed at substantial financial risk for the cost or utilization of items or services furnished to federal health care program beneficiaries.

Again, very specific requirements must be met to fall within the safe harbors, and one should refer to the *Federal Register* for details.

Latest Safe Harbor

On December 4, 2001, the OIG issued the final rule for a safe harbor that applies to certain arrangements under which a hospital might replenish supplies and drugs used while an ambulance transports a patient to the hospital.

Advisory Opinions

As mentioned earlier, HIPAA requires the government to issue advisory opinions on a limited list of issues to help physicians and others determine beforehand whether an arrangement might pose a problem. Usually, one would request an advisory opinion based on complete disclosure of the proposed or current activity—by providing a written explanation of the facts to the OIG.

Often, the government will request additional information and clarifications before rendering an opinion as to whether the proposed activity is legal. Sometimes, the government may simply conclude that there is not enough information to render an opinion.

Technically, the conclusions from advisory opinions apply only to the requesting party. However, the conclusions and facts presented in advisory opinions are relied on by many in the health care industry when analyzing the legality of various arrangements.

The Web site, www.oig.hhs.gov, includes newly issued advisory opinions, recent semiannual reports, press releases, final rules, and other important information with respect to fraud and abuse. This is a good site to monitor recent announcements by the OIG.

Specifically, HIPAA allows advisory opinions for the following matters:

1   What constitutes prohibited remuneration within the meaning of section 1128B(b) of the Social Security Act (SSA), the so-called antikickback statute

2   Whether an arrangement or proposed arrangement satisfies the exemptions set forth in section 1128B(b)(3) for activities that do not result in prohibited remuneration or kickbacks

3   Whether an arrangement or proposed arrangement satisfies the safe harbor criteria that the secretary has established or shall establish by regulation for activities that do not result in prohibited remuneration (ie, kickbacks)

4   What constitutes an inducement to reduce or limit services to individuals entitled to Medicare or Medicaid benefits within the meaning of section 1128B(b)

5   Whether any activity or proposed activity constitutes grounds for the imposition of criminal sanctions, exclusion from participation in Medicare or Medicaid, or civil monetary penalties under sections 1128, 1128A, or 1128B

The Act states that advisory opinions shall *not* address (1) whether the fair market value shall be or was paid or received for any goods, services, or property; and (2) whether an individual is a bona fide employee under the Internal Revenue Code of 1986. The Act states that "each advisory opinion issued by the Secretary shall be binding as to the Secretary and the party or parties requesting the opinion . . . and the failure of a party to seek an advisory opinion may not be introduced into evidence to prove that the party intended to violate the provisions of sections 1128, 1128A, or 1128B." Generally, the Act stipulates that advisory opinions should be issued within 60 days of a request (but delays are possible).[12]

Although seeking an advisory opinion may be appropriate, remember that such opinions are fact specific, and physicians should carefully discuss a request with their attorney. It may take longer than they think to get an opinion, the opinion may be ambiguous, or they may get an opinion explicitly stating that their proposal would not be legal under current law. If physicians decide to request an opinion, they must adequately explain the circumstances so that the advisory opinion will be valid.

Appendix B provides additional information for filing a request for an advisory opinion and a listing of advisory opinions issued through June 2002.

Physician Practice Management Companies' Percentage Fee Arrangements

The following is OIG Advisory Opinion 98-4 regarding what has been a common arrangement when physician practice management companies acquire the assets of a medical practice and charge a percentage of the practice's revenue as a management fee. Even if percentage payments pose a risk, there may be other ways to pay for management services that would not run afoul of antikickback laws (or prohibitions against fee splitting, which Florida's medical board recently cited in an opinion). Physicians should talk with their attorney if they are involved in, or contemplating, a similar arrangement.

OIG Advisory Opinion 98-4 April 1998

[April 15, 1998]
[Name Redacted]
Re: Advisory Opinion No. 98-4

Dear [Name Redacted]:

We are writing in response to your request for an advisory opinion, in which you ask whether a proposed management services contract between a medical practice management company and a physician practice, which provides that the management company will be reimbursed for its costs and paid a percentage of net practice revenues (the "Proposed Arrangement"), would consti-

tute illegal remuneration as defined in the anti-kickback statute, §1128B(b) of the Social Security Act (the "Act").

You have certified that all of the information you provided in your request, including all supplementary letters, is true and correct, and constitutes a complete description of the material facts regarding the Proposed Arrangement. In issuing this opinion, we have relied solely on the facts and information you presented to us. We have not undertaken any independent investigation of such information.

Based on the information provided, we conclude that the Proposed Arrangement may constitute

prohibited remuneration under §1128B(b) of the Act.
[boldface added]

I. Factual Background

A. The Parties

Dr. X is a family practice physician who has incorporated as, and practices under the name of, Company A ("Company A"). Company A is proposing to enter into an agreement to establish a family practice and walk-in clinic with a corporation, Company B ("Company B"). Dr. X is the sole Requestor of this advisory opinion.

B. The Arrangement

Under the Proposed Arrangement, Company A will provide all physician services at the clinic. Company A may hire additional physicians and other medical personnel with the mutual agreement of Company B. Company A will pay all physician compensation and fringe benefits, including but not limited to, licensing fees, continuing education, and malpractice premiums.

Company B will find a suitable location for the clinic and furnish the initial capital for the office, furniture, and operating expenses. Once operational, Company B will provide or arrange for all operating services for the clinic, including accounting, billing, purchasing, direct marketing, and hiring of non-medical personnel and outside vendors.

Company B will also provide Company A with management and marketing services for the clinic, including the negotiation and oversight of health care contracts with various payers, including indemnity plans, managed care plans, and Federal health care programs.

In addition to Company B's activities on behalf of Company A, Company B will set up provider networks. These networks may include Company A and, if required by Company B, Company A has agreed that it will refer its patients to the providers in such networks.

In return for its services, Company B's payment will have three components. Company A will be required to make a capital payment equal to a percentage of the initial cost of each capital asset purchased for Company A per year for six years. Company B will also receive a fair market value payment for the operating services it provides and an at-cost payment for any operating services for which it contracts. Company B will receive a percentage of Company A's monthly net revenues for its management services.

If the percentage payment described above is not permitted by law, then the parties will establish a management fee reflecting the contemplated financial results of the arrangement or, if the parties cannot agree to a fixed amount, the parties will hire an accounting firm to determine an appropriate fixed fee (the "Alternative Proposed Arrangement").

II. Legal Analysis

A. Anti-kickback Statute

The anti-kickback statute, §1128B(b) of the Act, makes it a criminal offense knowingly and willfully to offer, pay, solicit, or receive any remuneration to induce the referral of business covered by a Federal health care program. Specifically, the statute provides that:

> Whoever knowingly and willfully offers or pays [or solicits or receives] any remuneration (including any kickback, bribe, or rebate) directly or indirectly, overtly or covertly, in cash or in kind to any person to induce such person—to refer an individual to a person for the furnishing or arranging for the furnishing of any item or service for which payment may be made in whole or in part under a Federal health care program, or to purchase, lease, order, or arrange for or recommend purchasing, leasing, or ordering any good, facility, service, or item for which payment may be made in whole or in part under a Federal health care program, shall be guilty of a felony.

§1128B(b) of the Act. In other words, the statute prohibits payments made purposefully to induce referrals of business payable by a Federal health care program. The statute ascribes liability to both sides of an impermissible "kickback" transaction. The statute has been interpreted to cover any arrangement where one purpose of the remuneration was to obtain money for the referral of services or to induce further referrals. United States v. Kats, 871 F.2d 105 (9th Cir. 1989); United States v. Greber, 760 F.2d 68 (3d Cir.), cert. denied, 474 U.S. 988 (1985).

Violation of the statute constitutes a felony punishable by a maximum fine of $25,000, imprisonment up to five years or both. Conviction will also lead to automatic exclusion from Federal health care programs, including Medicare and Medicaid. This Office may also initiate administrative proceedings to exclude persons from Federal and State health care programs or to impose civil monetary penalties for fraud, kickbacks, and other prohibited activities. See §1128(b)(7), 1128A(a)(7) of the Act.

Because both the criminal and administrative sanctions related to the anti-kickback implications of the Proposed Arrangement are based on violations of the anti-kickback statute, the analysis for the purposes of this advisory opinion is the same under both. Conviction will also lead to automatic exclusion from Federal health care programs, including Medicare and Medicaid.

[Section deleted]

B. Safe Harbor Regulations

In 1991, the Department of Health and Human Services (the "Department") published safe harbor regulations that define practices that are not subject to the anti-kickback statute because such practices would be unlikely to result in fraud or abuse. Failure to comply with a safe harbor provision does not make an arrangement per se illegal. For this Proposed Arrangement, the only safe harbor regulation potentially available is the personal services and management contracts safe harbor. See 42 C.F.R. §1001.952(d).

The personal services and management contracts safe harbor provides protection for personal services contracts if all of the following six standards are met: (i) the agreement is set out in writing and signed by the parties; (ii) the agreement specifies the services to be performed; (iii) if the services are to be performed on a part-time basis, the schedule for performance is specified in the contract; (iv) the agreement is for not less than one year; (v) the aggregate amount of compensation is fixed in advance, based on fair market value in an arms-length transaction, and not determined in a manner that takes into account the volume or value of any referrals or business otherwise generated between the parties for which payment may be made by Medicare or a State health care program; and (vi) the services performed under the agreement do not involve the promotion of business that violates any Federal or State law.

We conclude that the Proposed Arrangement does not qualify for this safe harbor. In order for an agreement to be protected by this safe harbor, strict compliance with all six standards is necessary. In this case, the compensation is not an aggregate amount, fixed in advance, as the safe harbor requires. Accordingly, the safe harbor standards are not satisfied.

C. Percentage Compensation Arrangement

Because compliance with a safe harbor is not mandatory, the fact that the Proposed Arrangement does not fit within a safe harbor does not mean that the Proposed Arrangement is necessarily unlawful. Rather, we must analyze this Proposed Arrangement on a case-by-case basis.

Percentage compensation arrangements for marketing services may implicate the anti-kickback statute. In our preamble to the 1991 final safe harbor rules, 56 Fed. Reg. 35952 (July 29, 1991), we explained that the anti-kickback statute "on its face prohibits offering or acceptance of remuneration, inter alia, for the purposes of 'arranging for or recommending purchasing, leasing, or ordering any . . . service or item' payable under Medicare or Medicaid. Thus, we believe that many marketing and advertising activities may involve at least technical violations of the statute." 56 Fed. Reg. at 35974.

This Proposed Arrangement is problematic for the following reasons:

- **The Proposed Arrangement may include financial incentives to increase patient referrals.** The compensation that Company B receives for its management services is a percentage of Company A's net revenue, including revenue from business derived from managed care contracts arranged by Company B. Such activities may potentially implicate the anti-kickback statute, because the compensation Company B will receive will be in part for marketing services.

Where such compensation is based on a percentage, there is at least a potential technical violation of the anti-kickback statute. In addition, Company B will be establishing networks of specialist physicians to whom Company A may be required to refer in some circumstances. Further, Company B will presumably receive some compensation for its efforts in connection with the development and operation of these specialist networks. In these circumstances, any evaluation of the Proposed Arrangement requires information about the relevant financial relationships. However, Company B is not a requestor for this advisory opinion, and Company A does not have information regarding Company B's related business arrangements.

Accordingly, we have insufficient information to ascertain the level of risk of fraud or abuse presented by the Proposed Arrangement. (We are also precluded from reaching a conclusion about the Alternative Proposed Arrangement. Such a determination would require us to evaluate whether the agreed upon fee is fixed at fair market value. We are prevented from making that determination by §1128D(b)(3)(A) of the Act, which prohibits our opining on fair market value in an advisory opinion).

- **The Proposed Arrangement contains no safeguards against overutilization.** In light of the proposed establishment of provider networks with required referral arrangements, there is a risk of potential overutilization. Under the Proposed Arrangement, we are unable to determine what, if any, controls will be implemented under managed care contracts negotiated for Company A by Company B. Without such controls, we can not be assured that items and services paid for by Federal health care programs will not be overutilized.

- **The Proposed Arrangement may include financial incentives that increase the risk of abusive billing practices.** Since Company B receives a percentage of Company A's revenue and will arrange for Company A's billing, Company B has an incentive to maximize Company A's revenue. This Office has a longstanding concern that percentage billing arrangements may increase the risk of upcoding and similar abusive billing practices.

III. Conclusion

The advisory opinion process permits the OIG to protect specific arrangements that "contain limitations, requirements, or controls, that give adequate assurances that Federal health care programs cannot be abused." See 62 Fed. Reg. 7350, 7351 (February 19, 1997). Based on the facts we have been presented, the Proposed Arrangement appears to contain no limitations, requirements, or controls that would minimize any fraud or abuse.

Therefore, since we cannot be confident that there is no more than a minimal risk of fraud or abuse, we must conclude that the Proposed Arrangement may involve prohibited remuneration under the anti-kickback statute and thus potentially be subject to sanction under the anti-kickback statute, §1128B(b) of the Act. Any

definitive conclusion regarding the existence of an anti-kickback violation requires a determination of the Page 7 parties' intent, which determination is beyond the scope of the advisory opinion process.

IV. Limitations

The limitations applicable to this opinion include the following:

- This advisory opinion is issued only to Dr. X, who is the Requestor of this opinion. This advisory opinion has no application, and cannot be relied upon, by any other individual or entity.

- This advisory opinion is applicable only to the statutory provision specifically noted above. No opinion is herein expressed or implied with respect to the application of any other Federal, state, or local statute, rule, regulation, ordinance, or other law that may be applicable to the Proposed Arrangement.

- This advisory opinion will not bind or obligate any agency other than the U.S. Department of Health and Human services. This opinion is also subject to any additional limitations set forth at 42 C.F.R. Part 1008.

Sincerely,
/s/
D. McCarty Thornton
Chief Counsel to the Inspector General

(Our conclusion regarding the risk of fraud or abuse in relation to the anti-kickback statute should not be construed to mean that a finding of fraud or abuse is an implied element necessary to establish a violation of the statute.)

Possible Violation of Antikickback
Statutes by Practice Sales and Acquisitions

Some government officials have indicated that practice acquisitions could violate the antikickback statutes if one purpose of the payment is to induce the referral of future Medicare or Medicaid business. Additionally, the safe harbors indicate that, in some circumstances, installment payments lasting longer than 1 year would not be within the safe harbor's protective range (that does not, however, automatically mean a longer period would be illegal).

A letter of opinion (not a formal advisory opinion) written in late 1992 to the Internal Revenue Service (IRS) by an OIG associate general council indicated, among other things, that where a hospital acquires a medical practice, "any amount paid in excess of the fair market value of hard assets of a physician practice would be open to question. Specific items that we believe would raise a question as to whether payment was being made for the value of a referral stream would include, among other things: payment for goodwill; payment for value of ongoing business unit; payment for covenants not to compete; payment for exclusive dealing agreements; payment for patient lists; or payment for patient records."[13]

Since that letter was written, there has been increasing discussion about whether a payment for a reasonable valuation of goodwill would not, of itself, be a violation of Medicare antikickback laws. Further, there is some basis in the law and safe harbors that would appear to allow practice sales or acquisition involving goodwill as long as the transaction is at fair market value. When these arrangements are evaluated, any employment contract associated with the practice sale or acquisition would have to be analyzed as well.

The language in a 1993 letter from the OIG of the Department of Health and Human Services to the American Hospital Association indicates that there is room for payment of amounts in excess of the hard assets, but there may be antikickback implications also. Specifically, the letter states:

> I would like to emphasize that the position I articulated in the December 22, 1992 letter to [the IRS] remains the same. I did not state that payments for intangible assets are illegal per se. Nor have I indicated approval of any particular acquisition practices or valuation methodologies. Since payments for items other than the hard assets of a physician practice could be a payment to induce referrals or could be in return for future referrals, any such payments are subject to scrutiny to determine whether they violate the anti-kickback statute. The fact that the parties may identify the purpose of the payment as something other than a payment for referrals is not determinative.
>
> Similarly, the fact that two different parties may offer to pay the same price for a particular or a comparable physician practice or may use a similar approach in "valuing" the practice does not mean that both will be afforded the same treatment under

the anti-kickback statute. The intent of the parties is the critical element in the determination of a violation under the anti-kickback statute, and different parties may have different purposes and reasons for seeking to acquire a particular physician practice and for paying a particular price. Finally, the facts and circumstances involved in each situation are likely to be different as will be the nature of the relationship between the parties. Consequently, each particular situation must be judged on its own merits and based on its own facts and circumstances.

Turning to the two situations [you presented], . . . either situation could constitute a violation of the anti-kickback statute, depending on the intent of the parties, the nature of the intangible assets, the amounts paid for the intangible assets, and the past and future relationship of the parties, etc. One major factor is where the seller becomes or remains affiliated with the buyer. In such a case, the terms of that continued affiliation as well as the remuneration paid to the seller for services rendered would also need to be taken into account in determining whether a violation exists.

With respect to the second situation involving the purchase of the practice by a hospital, anytime an entity is acquiring a practice where the entity is in a position to benefit from referrals from the practice, there is always a question that a portion of the amount paid for the practice is attributable to the future referrals. As indicated above, it is the intent of the parties and the facts and circumstances of the particular acquisition that are relevant. Accordingly, the fact that a hospital purchases a physician practice for the same amount that another physician might pay does not insulate the hospital from liability under the anti-kickback statute. For example, another physician may offer a high price based on the savings in administrative costs and overhead which could be realized by combining practices. However, a hospital may not have that motivation at all; its offer of the same price could be motivated by a desire to pay for future referrals.[14]

The IRS also has prohibitions against private inurement from tax-exempt organizations. Some officials have argued that it could be viewed as a way of funneling profits to private individuals if the hospital pays an excessive amount for a physician's practice in the community. This could result in revocation of a not-for-profit hospital's tax exemption. Recent IRS rulings seem to indicate that this is not a concern in most cases where a hospital is dealing with physicians and the acquisition is a fair-market-value transaction.

We have seen hospitals use these theories as a rationale in negotiations to offer physicians an inordinately low amount for their practice. At the same time, we have seen other hospitals take a less restrictive view by structuring purchase arrangements to minimize the impact of antikickback and private inurement prohibitions.

Obviously, a physician should thoroughly discuss the situation with his or her attorney before getting too far into negotiations. Some substantial sanctions could be applied against those violating antikickback laws. Alternatively, a hospital might eventually stop making payments by arguing that the purchase agreement is no longer enforceable because it violates federal laws (there is often a clause to this effect in the purchase agreements).

In short, there is considerable confusion over how the law applies. Physicians should work with counsel and advisors to ensure that a practice sale or purchase is structured properly and at a reasonable price.

Conclusion

Before leaving this section, it is important to emphasize that many legitimate arrangements are not addressed in the safe harbors published to date. Safe harbors are generally those identified circumstances that clearly do not violate a law. By nature, however, they are not situations that could or might have some antikickback implications.

The HIPAA requires the government to issue advisory opinions on arrangements with antikickback implications. However, physicians should discuss with their attorney the appropriateness of seeking an advisory opinion, as it is not as simple as it sounds.

Again, the information in this section is a brief summary of antikickback laws and regulations. Physicians who are involved in any arrangement with antikickback implications must carefully analyze—and periodically reanalyze—their situation with their attorney to make sure they fall within the safe harbors or that they have otherwise structured the arrangement to avoid violating antikickback legislation.

Endnotes

1. You do not necessarily have to make or receive an illegal referral to violate the antikickback statutes. Offering a kickback may be enough.

2. 42 USC §1320a-7b.

3. The safe harbors, proposed additional safe harbors, and discussions of the rationale for each are published in several issues of the *Federal Register*, including July 29, 1991; November 5, 1992; September 21, 1993; July 21, 1994; January 25, 1996; and November 19, 1999.

4. Court cases make it clear that one may violate this statute even if there are other reasons for the payments, as long as one of the reasons is to induce referrals. Of course, there are tests as to the significance of the inducement. Realize that an arrangement that has some validity absent the kickback may still violate these statutes if designed to induce referrals. This is another area where your attorney's advice is invaluable.

5. 42 USC §1320a-7b.

6. 42 USC §1320a-7a.

7. A detailed discussion of the safe harbors, proposed additional safe harbors, and discussions of the rationale for each are published in several issues of the *Federal Register*, including July 29, 1991; November 5, 1992; September 21, 1993; July 21, 1994; January 25, 1996; and November 19, 1999.

8. November 19, 1999, *Federal Register*, page 63519.

9. The *term commercially reasonable business purpose* is defined in the November 19, 1999, *Federal Register* as ". . . the test is not merely whether a business purpose is legal or illegal. The 'commercially reasonable business purpose' test is intended to preclude safe harbor protection for health care providers that surreptitiously pay for referrals—whether because of coercion or by their own initiative—by renting more space or equipment or purchasing more services than they actually need from referral sources. By 'commercially reasonable business purpose,' we mean that the purpose must be reasonably calculated to further the business of the lessee or purchaser. In other words, the rental or the purchase must be of space, equipment, or services that the lessee or purchaser needs, intends to utilize, and does utilize in furtherance of its commercially reasonable business objectives. Thus, for example, a space rental contract between a physician and a DME [durable medical equipment] supplier for space in the physician's office that includes extra office space that the DME supplier neither occupies nor uses for its DME business would not be protected by this safe harbor. Nor would the safe harbor protect the lease of more space than would reasonably be rented by a similarly-situated DME supplier negotiating in an arm's-length transaction with a non-referral source lessor. Cost-sharing or risk-sharing arrangements, joint research initiatives, and data collection arrangements may qualify as commercially reasonable business purposes in many circumstances. However, we are aware of abusive arrangements involving contracts with referral sources for data collection services or research projects where the data to be collected or research to be performed have no value to the entity paying for them and are merely pretexts for payments for referrals. Such arrangements do not comply with the safe harbor and are highly suspect under the anti-kickback statute."

10. For example, see the OIG's advisory opinion 99-13, December 7, 1999, regarding certain arrangements for discounted pathology services provided to other physicians (available at Web site www.oig.hhs.gov/fraud/advisoryopinions/opinions.html).

11. The November 19, 1999, *Federal Register* includes the clarification that: "If a seller has done everything that it reasonably could under the circumstances to ensure that the buyer understands its obligation to report the discount accurately, the seller is protected irrespective of the buyer's omissions. **To receive such protection, however, the seller must report the discount to the buyer and inform the buyer of its obligation to report the discount.** To emphasize that the seller's obligations require more than perfunctory compliance with the safe harbor, we proposed adding that the seller must inform the buyer in an effective manner." [boldface added]

12. Government agencies have traditionally opposed issuing advisory opinions, particularly with respect to legislation as complicated as health care fraud and abuse. Consequently, the process may take some time.

13. The letter written by the Associate General Counsel, Inspector General Division, to the IRS is available at Web site www.oig.hhs.gov/fraud/fraudalerts.html.

14. The November, 2, 1993, follow-up letter from Associate General Counsel, Inspector General Division, is available at Web site www.oig.hhs.gov/fraud/fraudalerts.html.

Chapter 5

Stark Self-referral Legislation

Stark I and II—legislation named after US Representative Fortney "Pete" Stark—are aimed at preventing payment for the referral of patients who are Medicare or Medicaid beneficiaries to certain entities providing ancillary services, where the referring physician or an immediate family member has a financial relationship with the entity. Right or wrong, the Stark legislation is based on the presumption that physicians will overutilize such services if they profit from the referrals or orders. In essence, any profit from the related entity providing the service might be a kickback and, therefore, an inducement to refer patients.

Unlike the antikickback statute, the Stark legislation does not take into consideration the intent of the parties, nor is a violator subject to criminal prosecution. A physician may be excluded from the Medicare, Medicaid, and other federal health care programs and face civil monetary penalties. However, it is possible for the government to take criminal action under the antikickback statutes in certain arrangements.

Limits on self-referral were first enacted into a law known as the Stark Amendment as part of the Omnibus Budget Reconciliation Act of 1989. Stark I bars referral of Medicare patients to clinical laboratories by physicians who have, or whose family members have, a financial interest in those laboratories. The Omnibus Budget Reconciliation Act of 1993 expanded the scope of the ban on self-referral to Medicaid and 10 additional designated health services.

Provisions of the Stark Legislation

Referrals of Medicare or Medicaid beneficiaries for the following designated health services may be prohibited under Stark II if the physician has a financial relationship (not just an ownership relationship) with the entity providing the services. Some of these categories are rather broad.

1   Clinical laboratory services

2   Physical therapy services

3   Occupational therapy services

4   Radiology or other diagnostic services

5   Radiation therapy services and supplies

6   Durable medical equipment and supplies

7   Parenteral and enteral nutrients, equipment, and supplies

8   Prosthetics, orthotics, and prosthetic devices and supplies

9   Home health services

10   Outpatient prescription drugs

11   Inpatient and outpatient hospital services

Definitions of these *Designated Health Services* (DHS) are included in the regulations presented in the last section of this chapter.

Stark II provides several exceptions to the general prohibition on referrals. The most common exception occurs when the service is performed within a group or practice (although there may be some consequences for how income is distributed in groups, and some items of service, such as durable medical equipment, may not benefit from this exception). As will be seen, the phrase *within a group* is not quite as straightforward as it appears.

As a general rule, there may be a violation if the service is one of those listed above and there is a financial relationship between the referring or ordering physician and the entity providing the service. If there is a financial relationship, one should then look to see if one of the exceptions to Stark II applies.

Technically, Stark II provisions were effective as of January 1, 1995. To date, however, proposed rules have been published for public comment (in the January 9,

1998, *Federal Register*), but rules have been finalized for only a portion of the law. Until final rules have been published for all aspects, the proposed rules provide some guidance in interpreting the law.[1]

The legislation is extremely complex and confusing. It has essentially taken 10 years for the government to publish a portion of final regulations addressing aspects of the statute. Many hope that additional clarification is forthcoming for some of the legislation's controversial aspects. If physicians find that some of their referrals appear to be in violation of the Stark legislation, they should discuss their situation with an attorney.

The remarks of Kathleen A. Buto, deputy director, Center for Health Plans and Providers, Health Care Financing Administration (HCFA), in May 1999 illustrate the task of writing the final rule and some of the law's significant provisions[2]:

. . . We are evaluating the 12,800 comments we received on these proposed regulations [January 9, 1998], and are open to ideas to further simplify the regulations and the law itself in ways that do not undermine its intent. But we must take care to uphold its intent and prevent arrangements that would increase costs to taxpayers and subject beneficiaries to possible harm from unnecessary tests and procedures.

. . . We have taken steps in our proposed regulations to clarify the law and create appropriate flexibility. One of the most important provisions establishes that referrals to an entity with which a physician has a compensation arrangement are generally permissible as long as the compensation is at "fair market value," furthers a legitimate business purpose, *and is not tied to the volume or value of physician referrals*. This exception goes a long way in simplifying the policy under the law. [italics added]

. . . Adequately defining . . . exceptions and determining whether new exceptions are warranted has proven to be a daunting task. We have spent a great deal of time meeting and talking with industry associations, individual providers, and their attorneys in efforts to deal fairly and proactively with the many issues subject to interpretation. We are continuing these efforts. . . .

. . . The self-referral law works differently from the law against kickbacks, which was enacted as part of the Social Security Amendments of 1972. Enforcement of the anti-kickback law requires proof of "knowing" and "willful" illegal remuneration, such as bribes or rebates,

for patient referrals, and it can result in criminal sanctions. Self-referral laws, on the other hand, are generally self-enforcing.

The simple existence of an improper financial relationship is subject to loss of Medicare payment or a civil fine. This creates a powerful incentive to proactively comply with the law through due diligence efforts to avoid financial arrangements that may unethically lead to substantial increases in use of services. The law's preventive nature makes a highly effective contribution to our increasingly successful efforts to protect Medicare and Medicaid program integrity.

As mentioned above, the law includes many important exceptions. It also gives the Health and Human Services Secretary authority to create new exceptions through regulations as long as they do not create a risk of program or patient abuse. One of the most important exceptions is for most services physicians provide in their own offices or through their group practices. There are more than a dozen additional exceptions, including ones for managed care plans, rural providers, and isolated financial transactions.

Adequately defining these exceptions and determining whether new exceptions are warranted has proven to be a daunting task. We have spent a great deal of time meeting and talking with industry associations, individual providers, and their attorneys in efforts to deal fairly and proactively with the many issues subject to interpretation. We are continuing these efforts.

Regulations

We published proposed regulations for the clinical laboratories referral ban on March 11, 1992, and a final rule with comment period on August 14, 1995. These regulations have been in effect since September 13, 1995.

We published proposed regulations for the other designated services on January 9, 1998. These proposed regulations were generally well received. The American Hospital Association has said they make it easier for physicians and hospitals to work together in integrated systems. The proposed regulations include several clarifications and create new exceptions, providing flexibility for physicians while not compromising the intent of the law. . . .

The Omnibus Reconciliation Act of 1997 instructed the Health Care Financing Administration to issue, upon request, advisory opinions as to whether particular arrangements would violate self-referral policy. We published a final regulation implementing this provision January 9, 1998. To date, we have issued two such advisory opinions and are working on several others.

Reporting and Enforcement

Our proposed regulations also significantly limit the information that physicians are required to report for financial relations related to the 10 new designated services. Also, we are not asking physicians to submit information regarding these financial relationships as we did for clinical laboratory services. Instead, physicians need only keep on file the kind of information that they would normally maintain to meet Internal Revenue Service, Securities Exchange Commission, and other Medicare and Medicaid rules. This would be sufficient to demonstrate compliance in the event of a complaint investigation or spot audit. No other type of enforcement actions will be taken until outstanding questions are resolved and a final rule is published.

Conclusion

While the general response to our proposed regulations was positive, many outstanding issues remain. We extended the public comment period by two months in order to provide more time for interested parties to respond. The public comment period closed on March 10, 1998. We are reviewing the 12,800 comments we received and continuing to evaluate how we should address the many concerns that have been raised in final regulations. Many comments involve issues related to physicians in multi-specialty group practices and to a requirement in the law for direct supervision by physicians of services provided in physician offices. We are considering a wide range of clarifications and other suggestions to determine whether they can be addressed through regulations and would meet the statutory requirement that exceptions not create a risk of program or patient abuse. . . .

Status of Stark Regulations

Discussion in the January 4, 2001, *Federal Register* indicates the long history of Stark legislation and the current status of the regulatory process.

Federal Register: January 4, 2001 (Volume 66, Number 3) Rules and Regulations

From the Federal Register Online via GPO Access [wais.access.gpo.gov]

Part II

Department of Health and Human Services
[Now Centers for Medicare and Medicaid Services]

Health Care Financing Administration

42 CFR Parts 411 and 424

Medicare and Medicaid Programs; Physicians' Referrals to Health Care Entities With Which They Have Financial Relationships; Final Rule

ACTION: Final rule with comment period.

SUMMARY: This final rule with 90-day comment period (Phase I of this rulemaking) incorporates into regulations the provisions in paragraphs (a), (b), and (h) of section 1877 of the Social Security Act (the Act). Under section 1877, if a physician or a member of a physician's immediate family has a financial relationship with a health care entity, the physician may not make referrals to that entity for the furnishing of designated health services (DHS) under the Medicare program, unless an exception applies.

The following services are DHS:

- clinical laboratory services;

- physical therapy services;

- occupational therapy services;

- radiology services, including magnetic resonance imaging, computerized axial tomography scans, and ultrasound services;

- radiation therapy services and supplies;

- durable medical equipment and supplies;

- parenteral and enteral nutrients, equipment, and supplies;

- prosthetics, orthotics, and prosthetic devices and supplies;

- home health services;

- outpatient prescription drugs; and

- inpatient and outpatient hospital services.

In addition, section 1877 of the Act provides that an entity may not present or cause to be presented a Medicare claim or bill to any individual, third party payer, or other entity for DHS furnished under a prohibited referral, nor may we make payment for a designated health service furnished under a prohibited referral.

Paragraph (a) of section 1877 of the Act includes the general prohibition. Paragraph (b) of the Act includes exceptions that pertain to both ownership and compensation relationships, including an in-office ancillary services exception. Paragraph (h) includes definitions that are used throughout section 1877 of the Act, including the group practice definition and the definitions for each of the DHS.

We intend to publish a second final rule with comment period (Phase II of this rulemaking) shortly addressing, to the extent necessary, the remaining sections of the Act. [Emphasis Added] Phase II of this rulemaking will address comments concerning the ownership and investment exceptions in paragraphs (c) and (d) and the compensation exceptions in paragraph (e) of section 1877 of the Act. Phase II of this rulemaking will also address comments concerning the reporting requirements and sanctions provided by paragraphs (f) and (g) of the Act, respectively, and include further consideration of the general exception to the referral prohibition related to both ownership/investment and compensation for services furnished in an ambulatory surgical center (ASC), end-stage renal dialysis facility, or by a hospice in Sec. 411.355(d) of the regulations (this exception presently is in force and effect as to clinical laboratory services). In addition, Phase II of this rulemaking will address section 1903(s) of the Act, which extends aspects of the referral prohibition to the Medicaid Program. Phase II will also address comments received in response to this rulemaking, as appropriate, and certain proposals for new exceptions to section 1877 of the Act not included in the 1998 proposed rulemaking, but suggested in the public comments.

DATES: Effective date: The regulations delineated in Phase I of this rulemaking are effective on January 4, 2002 except for Sec. 424.22(d), which is effective on February 5, 2001. Comment date: We will consider comments if we receive them at the appropriate address, as provided below, no later than 5 p.m. on April 4, 2001. . . .

I. Background

A. *Legislative and Regulatory History*

1. Section 1877 of the Act

Section 6204 of the Omnibus Budget Reconciliation Act of 1989 (Pub. L. 101-239) (OBRA 1989), enacted on December 19, 1989, added section 1877 to the Act. Section 1877 of the Act prohibited a physician from referring a patient to an entity for clinical laboratory services for which Medicare might otherwise pay, if the physician or the physician's immediate family member had a financial relationship with the entity.

The statute defined "financial relationship" as an ownership or investment interest in the entity or a compensation arrangement between the physician (or the physician's immediate family member) and the entity. The statute provided for several exceptions to the prohibition. Some applied to ownership/investment interests and compensation arrangements; others applied only to ownership/investment interests or only to compensation arrangements.

The statute further prohibited an entity from presenting or causing to be presented a Medicare claim or bill to any individual, third party payer, or other entity for clinical laboratory services furnished under a prohibited referral. Additionally, the statute mandated refunding any amount collected under a bill for an item or service furnished under a prohibited referral. Finally, the statute imposed reporting requirements and provided for sanctions, including civil monetary penalty provisions. Section 1877 of the Act became effective on January 1, 1992.

Section 4207(e) of the Omnibus Budget Reconciliation Act of 1990 Pub. L. 101-508) (OBRA 1990), enacted on November 5, 1990, amended certain provisions of section 1877 of the Act to clarify definitions and reporting requirements relating to physician ownership and referral and to provide an additional exception to the prohibition.

Several subsequent laws further changed section 1877 of the Act. Section 13562 of the Omnibus Budget Reconciliation Act of 1993 (Pub. L. 103-66) (OBRA 1993), enacted on August 10, 1993, expanded the referral prohibition to cover 10 "designated health services," in addition to clinical laboratory services, modified some of the existing statutory exceptions, and added new exceptions. Section 152 of the Social Security Act Amendments of 1994 (SSA 1994) (Pub. L. 103-432), enacted on October 31, 1994, amended the list of designated services, effective January 1, 1995, changed the reporting requirements at section 1877(f) of the Act, and modified some of the effective dates established by OBRA 1993. Some provisions relating to referrals for clinical laboratory services were effective retroactively to January 1, 1992, while other provisions became effective on January 1, 1995.

2. Section 1903(s) of the Act

Title XIX of the Act established the Medicaid program to provide medical assistance to individuals who meet certain income and resource requirements. The States operate Medicaid programs in accordance with Federal laws and regulations and with a State plan that we approve. Though States administer the Medicaid programs, the Federal and State governments jointly finance them. We call the Federal government's share of medical assistance expenditures "Federal financial participation" (FFP).

Until OBRA 1993, there were no statutory or regulatory requirements affecting a physician's referrals for services covered under the Medicaid program. Section 13624 of OBRA 1993, entitled "Application of Medicare Rules Limiting Certain Physician Referrals," added a new paragraph (s) to section 1903 of the Act, that extends aspects of the Medicare prohibition on physician referrals to Medicaid. This provision bars FFP in State expenditures for DHS furnished to an individual based on a physician referral that would result in a denial of payment for the services under the Medicare program if Medicare covered the services to the same extent and under the same terms and conditions as under the State Medicaid plan. The statute also made certain reporting requirements in section 1877(f) of the Act and a civil monetary penalty provision in section 1877(g)(5) (related to the reporting requirements) applicable to providers of DHS for which payment may be made under Medicaid in the same manner as they apply to providers of such services for which payment may be made under Medicare. Section 1903(s) of the Act applies to a physician's referrals made on or after December 31, 1994.

B. Regulations History

1. Regulations Published by HCFA [now called CMS] and the Office of the Inspector General (OIG) Relating to Section 1877 of the Act

The following is a summary of the series of regulations we have published in the Federal Register over the past several years to implement the provisions of section 1877 of the Act, as amended, and section 1903(s) of the Act:

On December 3, 1991, we issued an interim final rule with comment period (54 FR 61374) to set forth the reporting requirements under section 1877(f) of the Act.

On March 11, 1992, we issued a proposed rule (57 FR 8588) to implement the self-referral prohibition and exceptions related to referrals for clinical laboratory services established by section 1877 of the Act, and amended by OBRA 1990.

On August 14, 1995, we issued a final rule with comment period (60 FR 41914) incorporating the provisions of OBRA 1993 and SSA 1994 that relate to referrals for clinical laboratory services under section 1877 of the Act, effective January 1, 1992, and revising the March 11, 1992 proposal based on the public comments we received.

On January 9, 1998, we issued a proposed rule (63 FR 1659) to amend the provisions of the August 1995 final rule and to reflect other changes in section 1877 of the Act enacted by OBRA 1993 and SSA 1994 that were effective January 1, 1995. These include, among other changes, the expansion of the referral prohibition to the 10 additional DHS, and the Medicaid expansion.

On January 9, 1998, we published a final rule with comment period (63 FR 1846) incorporating into our regulations the specific procedures we will use to issue advisory opinions, as required under section 1877(g)(6) of the Act. Section 1877(g)(6) of the Act requires that we issue written advisory opinions to outside parties concerning whether the referral of a Medicare patient by a physician for DHS (other than clinical laboratory services) is prohibited under section 1877 of the Act.

We also note that on October 20, 1993, the OIG published a proposed rule (58 FR 54096) to implement the civil money penalty provisions under sections 1877(g)(3) and (g)(4) of the Act. The OIG followed with publication of a final rule with comment period (60 FR 16580) on March 31, 1995.

2. Details About Prior Related Regulations

On August 14, 1995, we published in the Federal Register a final rule with comment period (60 FR 41914) that incorporated into regulations the provisions of section 1877 of the Act prohibiting physician referrals for clinical laboratory services under the Medicare program. That rule incorporated certain expansions and exceptions created by OBRA 1993, and the amendments in SSA 1994. It included only the expansions and other changes that related to prohibited referrals for clinical laboratory services that were retroactively effective to January 1, 1992, and interpreted the new provisions only in a few limited instances in which it was essential to implement the law. That rule also included our responses to the public comments we received on both the December 3, 1991 interim final rule with comment period (56 FR 61374) that established the reporting requirements under section 1877(f) of the Act, and the March 11, 1992 proposed rule (57 FR 8588) that covered section 1877 of the Act, as amended by OBRA 1990, and related to referrals for clinical laboratory services.

Because the August 1995 rule addressed only those changes made by OBRA 1993 and SSA 1994 that had a retroactive effective date of January 1, 1992, we explained our intent to later publish a proposed rule to fully implement the extensive revisions to section 1877 of the Act made by OBRA 1993 and SSA 1994, and to interpret those provisions when necessary. In the later proposed rule, we intended to include the revisions that relate to referrals for the additional DHS (including clinical laboratory services) that became effective January 1, 1995, and to implement the Medicaid expansion in section 1903(s) of the Act that became effective for referrals made on or after December 31, 1994.

As intended, on January 9, 1998, we published the proposed rule (63 FR 1659). The rule was organized as follows: In section I (63 FR 1661 through

1663), we summarized the problems associated with physician self-referrals and the relevant legislative and regulatory background. In section II (63 FR 1663 through 1673), part A, we summarized the provisions of our proposed rule and described how we proposed to alter the final regulation covering referrals for clinical laboratory services to apply it to the additional DHS and to reflect the statutory changes in section 1877 of the Act that were effective on January 1, 1995. In section II, part B, we described the changes we proposed to make to the Medicaid regulations to incorporate section 1903(s) of the Act. In section III (63 FR 1673 through 1705), we discussed in detail how we proposed to interpret any provisions in sections 1877 and 1903(s) of the Act that we believed were ambiguous, incomplete, or that provided us with discretion. We also discussed policy changes or clarifications we proposed to make to the August 1995 rule covering referrals for clinical laboratory services. Section IV (63 FR 1705 through 1715) of the proposed rule included our responses to some of the most common questions concerning physician referrals that we received from physicians, providers, and others in the health care community. We included our interpretations of how the law applies in the situations described to us. Section V (63 FR 1715 through 1719) included a Regulatory Impact Analysis, and section VI (63 FR 1719 through 1720) covered our policy on responding to comments. The proposed regulation text appeared at 63 FR 1720 through 1728.

In the January 1998 proposed rule, we proposed to incorporate the Medicaid expansion in section 1903(s) of the Act into Sec. 435.1012(a) (Limitation to FFP related to prohibited referrals). Section 435.1012(a) stated that no FFP was available for a State's expenditures for certain DHS, as they are defined in proposed Sec. 411.351, furnished to an individual under the State plan. No FFP is available if the services are those furnished on the basis of a physician referral that would, if Medicare provided for coverage of the services to the same extent and under the same terms and conditions as under the State plan, result in the denial of Medicare payment for the services under Secs. 411.351 through 411.360. In Sec. 435.1012(c), we included a cross reference to the procedures we established for individuals or entities to request advisory opinions from us on whether a physician's referrals relating to DHS (other than clinical laboratory services) are prohibited under section 1877 of the Act. Although these advisory opinions

were meant to reflect our interpretation of section 1877 of the Act, they can potentially affect FFP payments to States under the Medicaid program.

Section 1877(b)(3) of the Act excepts from the referral prohibition services furnished to enrollees of certain "prepaid" health plans; however, these exceptions extend only to services furnished to Medicare beneficiaries under Medicare contracts and demonstration projects. As a result, the exception for prepaid arrangements does not apply to physicians who wish to refer in the context of the Medicaid program. In order to give effect to this exception in the Medicaid context, we included, in the January 1998 proposed rule, in Sec. 435.1012(b) an exception for DHS furnished by managed care entities analogous to the Medicare entities excepted under section 1877(b)(3) of the Act. The new exception was meant to cover entities that provide services to Medicaid-eligible enrollees under contract with State Medicaid agencies and under certain demonstration projects. (We discussed these analogous entities in detail in the proposed rule at 63 FR 1697.)

To accommodate the Congress's subsequent creation of the Medicare+Choice (M+C) Program in the Balanced Budget Act of 1997 (Pub. L. 105-33) (BBA 1997), we included an amendment to the physician referral regulations as part of the June 26, 1998 interim final rule with comment period (63 FR 35066) establishing the M+C Program. We amended the final physician self-referral regulations covering referrals for clinical laboratory services by adding an exception in Sec. 411.355(c)(5) for services furnished to prepaid enrollees by a coordinated care plan. We defined a coordinated care plan as such a plan, within the meaning of section 1851(a)(2)(A) of the Act, offered by an organization in accordance with a contract with us under section 1857 of the Act and the M+C regulations. We are reprinting that provision in Phase I of this rulemaking. . . .

II. Development of Phase I of This Final Rulemaking

A. Technical Explanation of Bifurcation of the Regulation

Phase I of this rulemaking implements subsections (a) and (b) of section 1877 of the Act, and related definitions, as applied to the Medicare program. We intend to issue Phase II of this rule-making to cover the remainder of section 1877 of the Act, including its application to the Medicaid program, shortly.

Phase I of This Rulemaking

Given the importance of subsections (a) and (b), and the substantial changes we are making to the January 1998 proposed rule, we are proceeding with the issuance of Phase I of this rulemaking at this time. Further, we are issuing Phase I for comment and delaying its effective date for 1 year to allow individuals and entities engaged in business arrangements affected by Phase I time to restructure those arrangements to comply with the provisions of Phase I, except for Sec. 424.22(d), which is effective February 5, 2001. The statutory provisions interpreted by Phase I remain in effect, as they have been since 1989 for clinical laboratory services and 1993 for all other DHS.

. . . Specifically, section 1877 of the Act imposes a blanket prohibition on the submission of Medicare claims (and payment to the States of FFP under the Medicaid program) for certain DHS when the service provider has a financial relationship with the referring physician, unless the financial relationship fits into one of several relatively specific exceptions. Significantly, no wrongful intent or culpable conduct is required. The primary remedy is simply nonpayment by the program, without penalties. In other words, the basic remedy is recoupment of overpayments by the program. (Of course, wrongful conduct, such as knowingly submitting a claim in violation of the prohibition, can be punished through recoupment of overpayments and imposition of penalties, the False Claims Act, and other Federal statutory and common law remedies.)

The effect of this statutory scheme is that failure to comply with section 1877 of the Act can have a substantial financial result. For example, if a hospital has a $5,000 consulting contract with a surgeon and the contract does not fit in an exception, every claim submitted by the hospital for Medicare beneficiaries admitted or referred by that surgeon is not payable, since all inpatient and outpatient hospital services are DHS.

While the statutory scheme of the physician self-referral prohibition is, in large part, the key to its effectiveness, it obligates us to proceed carefully in determining the scope of activities that are

prohibited. In Phase I of this rulemaking, we have attempted to minimize the impact of the rule on many common physician group governance and compensation arrangements. . . .

With these overall considerations in mind, we have developed several criteria for evaluating our regulatory options. First, we have tried in Phase I of this rulemaking to interpret the prohibitions narrowly and the exceptions broadly, to the extent consistent with the statutory language and intent. As a practical matter, we believe that, while the statute must be implemented to achieve its intent, we should be cautious in interpreting its reach so broadly as to prohibit potentially beneficial financial arrangements. Accordingly, we have tried to focus the regulation on financial relationships that may result in overutilization, which we believe was the main abuse at which the statute was aimed. Some provisions of the January 1998 proposed rule did not appear to address overutilization so much as other potential abuses, such as unfair competition. At the same time, we do not believe the Congress intended us to review every possible designated health service to determine its potential for overutilization. The Congress has already made that determination, and we believe that compliance with the exceptions in Phase I of this rulemaking should not cause undue disruption of the health care delivery system.

Second, a corollary of the above interpretation is that the Congress only intended section 1877 of the Act to establish a minimum threshold for acceptable financial relationships, and that potentially abusive financial relationships that may be permitted under section 1877 of the Act could still be addressed through other statutes that address health care fraud and abuse, including the anti-kickback statute (section 1128B(b) of the Act). In some instances, financial relationships that are permitted by section 1877 of the Act might merit prosecution under section 1128B(b) of the Act. Conversely, conduct that may be proscribed by section 1877 of the Act may not violate the anti-kickback statute.

Third, we have attempted to ensure that Phase I of this rulemaking will not adversely impact the medical care of Federal health care beneficiaries or other patients. In those instances in which we have determined that the provisions of Phase I of this rulemaking may impact current arrangements under which patients are receiving medical care, we have attempted to verify that there are other ways available to structure the arrangement so that patients could continue to receive the care in the same location. In almost all cases, we believe the provisions of Phase I of this rulemaking should not require substantial changes in delivery arrangements, although they may affect the referring physician's or group practice's ability to bill for the care.

In other words, while the provisions of Phase I of this rulemaking may affect a physician's ability to profit financially from the provision of some services, there should be alternative providers available to provide the services in the same setting or alternative business structures that would permit the services to be provided (again, possibly without physician financial interest).

Fourth, we have revised the provisions of our January 1998 proposed rule to conform, as much as possible, to our other policies that affect the same or similar activity. For example, we are dropping the requirement that an in-office ancillary service be supervised under the strict "direct supervision" standards of the "incident to" billing rules in favor of requiring the level of supervision that is mandated under Medicare payment and coverage rules applicable to particular DHS.

Fifth, we have attempted, as much as possible, to establish "bright line" rules so that physicians and health care entities can ensure compliance and minimize administrative costs. We agree with the commenters that as a payment rule, the regulations implementing section 1877 of the Act should establish clear standards, and we have attempted to do so within the constraints of the statutory and regulatory scheme. . . .

. . . Section 1877 of the Act regulates financial relationships; it does not regulate the delivery of services. Section 1877 of the Act does not bar the provision of ancillary services in a physician's office, in a long term care facility, or at nearby, convenient locations. The law only imposes restrictions on a physician who makes a referral for a designated health service if he or she has a financial relationship with the ancillary services provider, such as an employment contract, an office space lease, or an ownership interest. Depending on the structure of the financial relationship, the physician may be able to profit from ordering ancillary services, thereby creating a risk that his or her orders may be motivated, in part,

by personal financial considerations. Statutory and regulatory exceptions are designed to enable physicians to make ancillary services available on-site to their own patients, provided they meet the conditions set forth in the applicable exception. However, nothing in the law prevents physicians from making available convenient ancillary services when the physician has no financial interest in the provision of the services. For example, a physician may arrange for a diagnostic services provider to perform diagnostic tests in the physician's office for which the diagnostic services provider bills, provided that any rental arrangement meets the rental exception in Sec. 411.357(b) and does not violate the anti-kickback statute. Section 1877 of the Act reflects the Congress' unmistakable intent to recognize and accommodate the traditional role played by physicians in the delivery of ancillary services to their patients, while constraining the abuse of the public fisc that results when physician referrals are driven by financial incentives. These regulations reflect that policy balance. . . .

Comment: One commenter stated that we had not informed Medicare beneficiaries about the potential restrictions on their access to care under section 1877 of the Act and its regulations, or informed Medicare providers about the potential restrictions on their ability to provide ancillary services.

Response: Once both Phase I and Phase II of this rulemaking are published, we intend to educate providers further about the new regulations. Providers have been on notice as to section 1877 of the Act since 1989 with respect to clinical laboratory services and 1993 with respect to all other DHS. We intend to provide general information to beneficiaries as well. However, we do not believe beneficiaries will face the restrictions on access that the commenters contemplate.

Indeed, these regulations do not restrict the provision of services to Medicare beneficiaries. If a physician chooses not to make services available to patients if he or she cannot personally benefit financially from services he or she orders, but which are provided by others, the physician is responsible for restricting access. Finally, Phase I of this rulemaking is being, and Phase II of this rulemaking will be, published in the Federal Register and noted on the Department's website, which serves as notice to the affected community.

We believe most providers will also be informed through their trade press, trade associations, and other sources.

. . . Section 1877 of the Act is a civil, not a criminal, statute. A violation of section 1877 of the Act results in nonpayment of claims and monetary sanctions. Criminal penalties or deprivation of liberty are not authorized by section 1877 of the Act.

. . . Because of the significant changes we are making in Phase I of this rulemaking, we are publishing these regulations in final form with a 90-day comment period. We are interested in the industry's views as to the changes we have incorporated into these regulations. Any further changes we deem necessary based on comments will be addressed in Phase II of this rulemaking or shortly thereafter [Note: As of September 3, 2002, Phase II rulemaking has not been promulgated].

. . . [Basic Principle] Section 1877(a) of the Act establishes the basic structure and elements of the statutory prohibition: A physician cannot (1) refer patients to an entity (2) for the furnishing of DHS (3) if there is a financial relationship between the referring physician (or an immediate family member of the referring physician) and the entity, (4) unless the financial relationship fits within one of the specific exceptions in the statute or regulations issued by the Secretary.

. . . Subject to certain exceptions, section 1877(a)(1) of the Act prohibits a physician from making a referral to an entity for the furnishing of DHS for which Medicare would otherwise pay, if the physician (or an immediate family member) has a financial relationship with the DHS entity, and prohibits the DHS entity from billing Medicare or any individual (including, but not limited to, the beneficiary), third party payer, or other entity for those services. A financial relationship is (i) either an ownership or investment interest in the DHS entity (or in another entity that holds an ownership or investment interest in the entity) or (ii) a compensation arrangement with the DHS entity, either directly or indirectly. An ownership or investment interest may exist through equity, debt, or other means.

As defined by section 1877(h)(5) of the Act, a "referral" means a request by a physician for an item or service for which payment may be made under Medicare Part B, including a request for a consultation (including any tests or procedures ordered or performed by the consulting physician or under the supervision of the consulting physician), and the request or establishment of a plan of care by a physician that includes the furnishing of DHS, with certain exceptions for consultations by pathologists, diagnostic radiologists, and radiation oncologists. . . .

[Note: Pages 863–965 of the 01/04/2001 Federal Register are not reproduced here.]

Outline of Phase I of Final Rule

Below is a basic outline of the rulemaking and discussion included in the January 4, 2001, *Federal Register*. Readers must understand that this is a very basic overview of over 100 pages in the January 4, 2001, *Federal Register* and the 1998 proposed rule. There is much more to consider when a physician refers patients for designated health services if the physician has a financial relationship with the entity.

Page number references are those in the January 4, 2001, *Federal Register* (PDF and text file copies are available at the Government Printing Office Web site, www.gpo.gov). The regulations in the final rule are included at the end of this chapter. As of September 3, 2002, Phase II had not been published.

I. Background (Beginning page 857 of the 01/04/2001 *Federal Register*)

Legislative and Regulatory History
Section 1877 of the Act
Section 1903(s) of the Act that Expands Coverage of the Act to Medicaid

Regulations History
Regulations Published by CMS/HCFA and OIG Relating to Section 1877 of the Act

Details about Prior Related Regulations

II. Development of Phase I of this Final Rulemaking (Page 859)

Technical Explanation of Bifurcation of the Regulation

General Comments Regarding the January 1998 Proposed Rule and Responses

III. General Prohibition Under Section 1877 of the Act (Page 863)—A physician cannot (1) refer patients to an entity (2) for the furnishing of Designated Health Services (DHS) (3) if there is a financial relationship between the referring physician (or an immediate family member of the referring physician) and the entity, (4) unless the financial relationship fits within one of the specific exceptions in the statute or regulations issued by the Secretary.

When Is There a Financial Relationship Between the Physician and the Entity? (Page 864)—Basically, any financial relationship between the referring physician and the DHS entity triggers application of the statute, even if the financial relationship is wholly unrelated to a designated health service payable by Medicare or Medicaid.

When Does a Physician Make a Referral? (Page 871)—Under the 01/04/2001 rulemaking, the definition of "referrals that are subject to the general prohibition" do not include services that are *personally performed* by the referring/requesting physician (that is, the referring/requesting physician physically performs the service), and the definition of "entity" is changed to clarify that the referring physician himself or herself is not an entity for purposes of section 1877 of the Act (although the physician's practice is an entity). All other Medicare-covered DHS performed at the request of a referring physician are "referrals" for purposes of section 1877 of the Act. Please note that services performed "incident to" a physician's services may not be excluded because they are not physically performed by the "referring" physician; however, in many cases such services may be excluded from the general prohibition if the in-office ancillary services exception applies (further the 01/04/2002 indicates the government may consider comments regarding this issue when Phase II rules are published).

There are some exceptions to the general prohibition for "referral" of DHS when made by pathologists, diagnostic radiologists or radiation oncologists to the DHS provider.

IV. Physician Compensation Under Section 1877 of the Act: An Overview (Page 875)—Under the 01/04/2001 rulemaking, physicians who personally perform the DHS may be compensated based upon productivity with respect to services they personally perform.

V. "Volume or Value" of Referrals and "Other Business Generated" Standards: An Overview (Page 876)

VI. Exceptions Applicable to Ownership and Compensation Arrangements, Section 1877(b) of the Act (Page 879)—

A. Limited Physician Services (Section 1877(b)(1) of the Act)

B. In-office Ancillary Services (Section 1877(b)(2) of the Act) (Page 880)
Scope of Designated Health Services That Can Be In-office Ancillary Services (Page 881)
Direct Supervision (Page 885)
The Building Requirements (Page 887)
The Billing Requirement (Page 893)

C. Group Practice Definition (Section 1877(h)(4) of the Act) (Page 894)—The definition of a "group practice" is particularly important because exceptions to Stark law prohibitions—such as the *in-office ancillary services exception*—depend upon whether the medical practice will be considered a legitimate "group practice." There are a number of tests, particularly those listed below, that are used to determine if a medical practice is a group practice within the meaning of Section 1877. The intent of the rather lengthy, and at times confusing, discussion in the *Federal Register* is to prevent physicians from taking advantage of acceptable referrals within a group by establishing "a loose confederation of individual physicians bound together primarily to profit from designated health service referrals."

> General Comments (followed by discussion of the tests below)
>
> Two or More Physicians Providing Services Through Single Legal Entity Requirement
>
> Members of the Group Include Only Physician Owners and Full or Part-time Physician Employees
>
> The "Full Range of Services Test"
>
> The "Substantially All Test"
>
> The "Seventy-five Percent Physician-Patient Encounters Test"
>
> Method of Determining Distribution of Income, Expense, Profits Must Be Previously Determined
>
> Unified Business Test
>
> Profit Shares and Productivity Bonuses Are Acceptable If . . . (See 411.352(i))
>
> Group Practice Attestations

D. Prepaid Plans (Section 1877(b)(3) of the Act) (Page 911)

VII. Some Other Regulatory Exceptions (Page 915)

Academic Medical Centers 411.353(e)—The referral/payment prohibitions do apply in academic medical centers that meet a number of requirements, see Section 411.353(e).

Fair Market Value (see §411.357(l))

Non-Monetary Compensation up to $300 and Medical Staff Benefits (Page 920 and see §§411.357(k), (m) and (o))—Discussion of when noncash items such as drug samples, coffee mugs, hospital parking, compliance training, and the like will not be considered a violation of Stark laws. See applicable regulations under Section 411.357. Notice that the $300 limitation does not apply to all subsections, just (k).

VIII. Detailed Definitions of the Designated Health Services (Page 922 and Section 411.351)—

Provides definition of what is included in each of the 11 categories of designated health services (DHS).

General Principles

General Comment: Professional Services as Designated Health Services

Clinical Laboratory Services

Physical Therapy Services

Occupational Therapy Services

Radiology and Certain Other Imaging Services

Radiation Therapy

Durable Medical Equipment (DME)

Parenteral and Enteral Nutrients, Equipment, and Supplies

Prosthetics, Orthotics, and Prosthetic Devices and Supplies

Home Health Services

Outpatient Prescription Drugs

Inpatient and Outpatient Services

Other Definitions (also in Section 411.351)
> Consultation
> Entity
> Fair Market Value
> Group Practic
> Health Professional Shortage Areas
> Employee
> Immediate Family Members
> Referral

Regulations Text (Page 952)

Antikickback vs Self-referral (Stark) Legislation

It is easy to become confused between antikickback legislation discussed in the previous chapter and self-referrals prohibited under the Stark legislation.

The Office of Inspector General (OIG) of the Department of Health and Human Services distinguished the two in the November 19, 1999, *Federal Register* beginning on page 63519:

The Stark Law is a civil statute that generally (i) prohibits physicians from making referrals for clinical laboratory or other designated health services to entities in which the physicians have ownership or other financial interests and (ii) prohibits entities from presenting or causing to be presented claims or bills to any individual, third party payor, or other entity for designated health services furnished pursuant to a prohibited referral. (42 U.S.C. 1395nn(a)(1)).

The anti-kickback statute, on the other hand, is a criminal statute that prohibits the knowing and willful offer, payment, solicitation, or receipt of remuneration to induce Federal health care program business.

. . . Both laws are directed at the problem of inappropriate financial incentives influencing medical decision-making. This similarity notwithstanding, the statutes are different in scope and structural approach. Under the Stark Law, physicians may not refer patients for certain designated health services to entities from which the physicians receive financial benefits, except as allowed in enumerated exceptions. A transaction must fall entirely within an exception to be lawful under the Stark Law.

The anti-kickback statute, on the other hand, establishes an intent-based criminal prohibition with optional statutory and regulatory "safe harbors" that do not purport to define the full range of lawful activity. Rather, safe harbors provide a means of assuring that payment practices are not illegal. Payment practices that do not fully comply with a safe harbor may still be lawful if no purpose of the payment practice is to induce referrals of Federal health care program business.

Because the two statutory schemes are fundamentally different, the conference report for the Stark Law included language clarifying that "any prohibition, exemption, or exception authorized under this provision in no way alters (or reflects on) the scope and application of the anti-kickback provisions in section 1128B of the Social Security Act" (H.R. Conf. Rep. 239, 101st Cong., 1st sess. 856 (1989)).

We are mindful that it may sometimes be burdensome for parties to review their arrangements under two separate statutory schemes. However, it would be inappropriate to adjust our safe harbor provisions in a manner that would prejudice enforcement of the anti-kickback statute merely to conform the safe harbors to an exception or prohibition under section 1877 of the Act.

This is particularly the case in view of the clear legislative intent to keep enforcement under the anti-kickback statute separate from enforcement under section 1877 of the Act. Moreover, variation between the Stark Law exceptions and anti-kickback safe harbors is reasonable in light of the schematic differences between the two statutes.

To the extent the anti-kickback statute and the Stark Law address the same conduct, the Stark Law acts as a structural bar to arrangements that contain a per se conflict of interest. However, even if an arrangement passes muster under the Stark Law, it may still constitute a violation of the anti-kickback statute, if the requisite intent to induce referrals is present.

In-Office Ancillary Services Exception

If designated health services (DHS) are performed in the ordering/requesting physician's office, the Stark law applies. However, there is a very important exception in the law that allows billing the DHS under Medicare and Medicaid. That exception is called the *in-office ancillary services exception.*

The exception for in-office ancillary services, if it applies, allows referrals for designated health services performed within and billed by a group practice. It is common for medical practices to offer diagnostic services such as x-rays and bill for those services under the group provider number. Thus, if these services are provided within the medical group's entity (ie, partnership, professional corporation, or professional association), this exception may apply. However, it is not automatic.

The law implicitly recognizes that solo practitioners will keep all the profits from DHS that fit in the in-office ancillary services exception, whether performed personally or by others.

The definition of a "group practice" is particularly important because exceptions to Stark law prohibitions—such as the *in-office ancillary services exception*—depend upon whether the medical practice will be considered a legitimate "group practice."

There are some important criteria that must be met for the in-office ancillary services exception to apply. Below is the regulation published in the January 4, 2002, *Federal Register* that specifies the in-office ancillary services exception. (Emphasis has been added.)

§411.355 General exceptions to the referral prohibition related to both ownership/investment and compensation.

The prohibition on referrals set forth in §411.353 does not apply to the following types of services:

. . . .

(b) In-office ancillary services. Services (including certain items of durable medical equipment (DME), as defined in paragraph (b)(4) of this section, and infusion pumps that are DME (including external ambulatory infusion pumps), but excluding all other DME and parenteral and enteral nutrients, equipment, and supplies (such as infusion pumps used for PEN), that meet the following conditions:

(1) They are furnished personally by one of the following individuals:
  (i) The referring physician.
  (ii) A physician who is a member of the same group practice as the referring physician.
  (iii) An individual who is supervised by the referring physician or by another physician in the group practice, provided the supervision complies with all other applicable Medicare payment and coverage rules for the services.

(2) They are furnished in one of the following locations:
  (i) **The same building** (as defined in §411.351), but not necessarily in the same space or part of the building, in which—
    (A) The referring physician (or another physician who is a member of the same group practice)

furnishes substantial physician services that are unrelated to the furnishing of DHS payable by Medicare, any other Federal health care payer, or a private payer, even though the unrelated services may lead to the ordering of DHS;

(B) The physician services that are unrelated to the furnishing of DHS in paragraph (b)(2)(i)(A) of this section must represent substantially the full range of physician services unrelated to the furnishing of DHS that the referring physician routinely provides (or, in the case of a referring physician who is a member of a group practice, the full range of physician services that the physician routinely provides for the group practice); and

(C) The receipt of DHS (whether payable by a Federal health care program or a private payer) is not the primary reason the patient comes in contact with the referring physician or his or her group practice.

(ii) A centralized building (as defined in §411.351) that is used by the group practice for the provision of some or all of the group practice's clinical laboratory services.

(iii) A centralized building (as defined in §411.351) that is used by the group practice for the provision of some or all of the group practice's DHS (other than clinical laboratory services).

(3) They must be billed by one of the following:

(i) The physician performing or supervising the service.

(ii) The group practice of which the performing or supervising physician is a member under a billing number assigned to the group practice.

(iii) The group practice if the supervising physician is a "physician in the group" (as defined at §411.351) under a billing number assigned to the group practice.

(iv) An entity that is wholly owned by the performing or supervising physician or by that physician's group practice under the entity's own billing number or under a billing number assigned to the physician or group practice.

(v) An independent third party billing company acting as an agent of the physician, group practice, or entity specified in paragraphs (b)(3)(i) through (b)(3)(iv) of this section under a billing number assigned to the physician, group practice, or entity, provided the billing arrangement meets the requirements of §424.80(b)(6) of this chapter. For purposes of this paragraph (b)(3), a

group practice may have, and bill under, more than one Medicare billing number, subject to any applicable Medicare program restrictions.

(4) For purposes of paragraph (b) of this section, DME covered by the in-office ancillary services exception means canes, crutches, walkers and folding manual wheelchairs, and blood glucose monitors, that meet the following conditions:

(i) The item is one that a patient requires for the purposes of ambulating, uses in order to depart from the physician's office, or is a blood glucose monitor (including one starter set of test strips and lancets, consisting of no more than 100 of each). A blood glucose monitor may be furnished only by a physician or employee of a physician or group practice that also furnishes outpatient diabetes self-management training to the patient.

(ii) The item is furnished in a building that meets the "same building" requirements in the in-office ancillary services exception as part of the treatment for the specific condition for which the patient-physician encounter occurred.

(iii) The item is furnished personally by the physician who ordered the DME, by another physician in the group practice, or by an employee of the physician or the group practice.

(iv) A physician or group practice that furnishes the DME meets all DME supplier standards located in §424.57(c) of this chapter.

(v) The arrangement does not violate the anti-kickback statute, section 1128B(b) of the Act, or any law or regulation governing billing or claims submission.

(vi) All other requirements of the in-office ancillary services exception in paragraph (b) of this section are met.

(5) A designated health service is "furnished" for purposes of paragraph (b) of this section in the location where the service is actually performed upon a patient or where an item is dispensed to a patient in a manner that is sufficient to meet the applicable Medicare payment and coverage rules.

(6) *Special rule for home care physicians.* In the case of a referring physician whose principal medical practice consists of treating patients in their private homes, the "same building" requirements of paragraph (b)(2)(i) of this section are met if the referring physician (or a qualified person accompanying the physician, such as a nurse or technician) provides the DHS contemporaneously with a physician service that is not a designated health service provided by the referring physician to the patient in the patient's private home. For purposes of paragraph (b)(5) of this section, a private home does not include a nursing, long-term care, or other facility or institution.

To qualify for this exception, the 1998 proposed rule would have required "direct supervision" of the performance of DHS. However, the January 4, 2001 rulemaking is somewhat less restrictive requiring that supervision meet existing Medicare and Medicaid coverage rules. Section 411.355(b)(1)(iii) indicates that the exception applies when the service is provided by: "an individual who is supervised by the referring physician or by another physician in the group practice, provided the supervision complies with all other applicable Medicare payment and coverage rules for the services."

To use the in-office exception, a practice must fall within the Stark II definition of a group practice. However, the group practice definition may not be satisfied if members of the group are paid on the basis of the volume or value of referrals or orders for the designated ancillary services, even though performed in the office. For example, if group members are paid by productivity, including the value of designated services they order (but do not personally perform), this exception may not apply (this refers only to Medicare and Medicaid services unless state laws cover other payers). See the next section on compensation arrangements.

Significantly, the in-office ancillary services exception is not available for durable medical equipment (other than infusion pumps, canes, crutches, walkers and folding manual wheelchairs, and blood glucose that meet certain conditions) or for parenteral and enteral nutrients and supplies. Such referrals are strictly prohibited if a financial relationship exists.

Notwithstanding the level of confusion, referrals that do not qualify for the in-office ancillary service exception should be carefully analyzed to ensure compliance with the law. The January 4, 2001 *Federal Register* provides additional clarifying discussion. The page references are provided below:

In-office Ancillary Services (Section 1877(b)(2) of the Act) (Page 880)
Scope of Designated Health Services That Can Be In-office Ancillary Services (Page 881)
Direct Supervision (Page 885)
The Building Requirements (Page 887)
The Billing Requirement (Page 893)

Physician Compensations Formulas in Light of the Stark Laws

The proposed rules issued on January 9, 1998, indicated that it would be a violation of Stark II if a physician in a group receives a direct productivity bonus based on the value of the designated services he or she orders (whether or not he or she performed the test). As written, the proposed rule allowed payment of bonuses to referring physicians "so long as the share or bonus is not determined in any manner that is *directly* related to the volume or value of referrals by the physician."[3] [italics added]

The government takes a different approach in the 01/04/2001 final rulemaking by allowing compensation tied directly to designated health services *personally* performed by the ordering physician as discussed as follows.

January 4, 2001 *Federal Register*

IV. Physician Compensation Under Section 1877 of the Act:

An Overview

Many public comments [to the proposed rule] addressed physician compensation issues. The statute touches on physician compensation in several places: the definition of group practice, the employee exception, and the personal services exception. The interplay of section 1877 of the Act and physician compensation is one of the most significant aspects of the self-referral law.

Obviously, the issue of physician compensation is of critical importance to the physician community. As a starting point, we do not believe that the Congress intended section 1877 of the Act to regulate physician compensation practices, except as necessary to minimize financial incentives to refer DHS to entities with which the physicians have financial relationships.

Having carefully studied the public comments and having reconsidered the statutory provisions, the legislative history, and our January 1998 regulatory proposals, we believe the following general principles govern the application of the statute to the manner in which physicians are paid:

- First, as explained in section III.B of this preamble, for purposes of section 1877 of the Act, the term referral does not include DHS that are personally performed by the physician. As a practical matter, the statutory language and structure indicate Congressional recognition that physicians are commonly compensated based on productivity with respect to services they personally perform.

- Second, with respect to group practices, the Congress intended to confer group practice status on bona fide group practices and not on loose confederations of physicians who come together as a "group" substantially in order to capture the profits of DHS under the in-office ancillary services exception to section 1877 of the Act. To that end, we proposed adding a "unified business" standard to the group practice definition, using the statutory authority the Congress conferred on the Secretary to impose additional standards on group practices. However, in response to comments, we have reconsidered the test for a "unified business"; the final

regulations under Phase I of this rulemaking adopt a considerably more flexible approach to the same end. Under Phase I of this rulemaking, one of several characteristics of a "unified business" is that the group's physician compensation methodologies are established by the centralized management of the group practice. For the limited purposes of establishing that a group practice is a unified business, we think it is appropriate to look at physician compensation derived from all sources, not just from DHS. However, location- and specialty-based compensation practices are expressly permitted with respect to the distribution of revenues derived from services that are not DHS. Such practices may also be allowed for DHS, depending on the circumstances. (See the discussion of the group practice definition in section VI.C of this preamble.)

- Third, except for the limited purpose of determining whether a group practice is a unified business, the physician compensation provisions for group practices under section 1877 of the Act only affect the distribution of revenues derived from DHS. In general, these revenues are likely to comprise a relatively small portion of the total revenues of most group practices. As we indicated in 1998, section 1877 of the Act does not affect the distribution of monies earned from other services. From a practical business standpoint, however, some group practices may find it impractical to segregate DHS revenues. These parties may find it more expedient to allocate compensation in accordance with the methods permitted for DHS revenues under section 1877 of the Act.

- Fourth, the statute implicitly recognizes that solo practitioners will keep all the profits from DHS that fit in the in-office ancillary services exception, whether performed personally or by others.

- **Fifth, section 1877 of the Act contemplates that physicians—whether group practice members, independent contractors, or employees—can be paid in a manner that directly correlates to their own personal labor, including labor in the provision of DHS.** [Emphasis added.] In other words, "productivity," as used in the statute, refers to the quantity and intensity of a physician's own work, but does not include the physician's fruitfulness in generating DHS performed by others (that is, the fruits of passive activity). "Incident to" services are not included in productivity bonuses under the statute unless the services are incident to services personally performed by a referring physician who is in a bona fide group practice. ("Incident to" services must meet the requirements of section 1861(s)(2)(A) of the Act and section 2050, "Services and Supplies," of the Medicare Carriers Manual (HCFA Pub. 14-3), Part 3—Claims Process.) In the case of independent contractors under the personal service arrangements exception and employees under the bona fide employment exception, the amount of compensation for personal productivity is limited to fair market value for the services they personally perform. The fair market value standard in these exceptions acts as an additional check against inappropriate financial incentives. (The personal service arrangements exception, as well as several other exceptions, contains additional restrictions on compensation that varies based on the volume or value of referrals. The volume or value standard is discussed in section V of this preamble.)

- Sixth, the Congress recognized that in the case of group practices, revenues derived from DHS must be distributed to the group practice members in some fashion, even though the members generate the DHS revenue. However, the Congress wished to minimize the economic incentives to generate

unnecessary referrals of DHS. Accordingly, the Congress permitted group practice members (and independent contractors who qualify as "physicians in the group practice") to receive shares of the overall profits of the group, so long as those shares do not directly correlate to the volume or value of referrals generated by the member or "physician in the group practice" for DHS performed by someone else. In addition, the Congress permitted groups to pay their physicians productivity bonuses based directly on personal productivity (including services incident to personally performed services), but precluded groups from paying group practice physicians any productivity bonus based directly on referrals of DHS performed by someone else. As detailed below, we are establishing under Phase I of this rulemaking certain methodologies that describe compensation practices that will be deemed to be indirectly related to the volume or value of DHS referrals for purposes of section 1877(h)(4)(B)(i) of the Act and therefore allowable under section 1877 of the Act. Groups are free to develop their own indirect methodologies, but such methodologies are subject to case-by-case review.

Discussion in the January 4, 2001, *Federal Register* provides insight into profit sharing and productivity bonuses.

Profit Shares and Productivity Bonuses [Page 908]

The Existing Law: In general, the statute provides that a physician who is a member of the group may not be compensated directly or indirectly based on the volume or value of his or her referrals of DHS. In addition, the statute provides that a "physician in a group practice" may receive shares of overall profits of the group or a productivity bonus based on services personally performed or incident to such personally performed services, provided the share or bonus is not determined in a manner that is directly related to the volume or value of referrals by such physician. In other words, group practice compensation formulae that are only indirectly related to the volume or value of referrals of DHS are permissible.

The Proposed Rule: We proposed to interpret the statute to mean that productivity bonuses could only relate to work personally performed by the physician

that results from referrals from other physicians in the group, and could not relate (directly or indirectly) to work that results from self-referrals or DHS referrals to other physicians and other office personnel. Thus, we said that a physician could only receive compensation for his or her own DHS referrals through the aggregation that occurs as part of the overall sharing of group profits. As to the overall sharing of profits, we indicated that profits must be aggregated at the group level and not at a component level.

The Final Rule: In section IV of this preamble, we provide an overview of the physician compensation provisions of section 1877 of the Act. In general, a group practice can segregate its DHS revenues from its other revenues for purposes of compensating physicians; section 1877 of the Act applies only to a practice's DHS revenues. Generally, this income is likely to comprise a relatively small portion of the total revenues of most practices.

Under Phase I of this rulemaking, group practices may pay member physicians and independent contractors who qualify as "physicians in the group" productivity bonuses based directly on the physician's personal productivity (including services incident to such personally performed services that meet the requirements of section 1861(s)(2)(A) of the Act and section 2050 of the Medicare Carriers Manual, Part 3), but may not pay these physicians any bonus based directly on their referrals of DHS that are performed by someone else. The statute also permits group practice members (and independent contractors who qualify as "physicians in the group") to receive shares of the overall profits of the group, so long as those shares do not directly correlate to the volume or value of DHS referrals generated by the physician that are provided by someone else. We are defining "share of overall profits" as meaning a share of the entire profits of the entire group or any component of the group that consists of at least 5 physicians derived from DHS.

Under the statutory scheme, revenues generated by DHS may be distributed to group practice members and physicians in the group in accordance with methods that indirectly take into account DHS referrals. In general, we believe a compensation structure does not directly take into account the volume or value of referrals if there is no direct correlation between the total amount of a physician's compensation and the volume or value of the physician's DHS referrals (regardless of whether the services are personally performed). Phase I of this rulemaking contains specific methodologies that describe compensation methods that are deemed to be indirect. In addition, Phase I of this rulemaking contains additional provisions that allow group practices to devise other reasonable indirect compensation methodologies.

The distribution methods for overall profit shares are as follows:

1. A per capita (that is, per physician) division of the overall profits.

2. A distribution of DHS revenues based on the distribution of the group practice's revenues attributable to services that are not DHS payable by Federal or private payers.

3. Any distribution of DHS revenues if the group practice's DHS revenues are less than 5 percent of the group practice's total revenues and no physician's allocated portion of those revenues is more than 5 percent of the physician's total compensation from the group practice.

The methods for productivity bonuses are as follows:

1. A productivity bonus based on the physician's total patient encounters or RVUs.

2. A productivity bonus based on the allocation of the physician's compensation that is attributable to services that are not DHS payable by Federal or private payers.

3. Any productivity bonus that includes DHS revenues if the group practice's DHS revenues are less than 5 percent of the group practice's total revenues and no physician's allocated portion of those revenues is more than 5 percent of the physician's total compensation from the group.

Comment: Many commenters objected to our proposed interpretation of the statute to mean that productivity bonuses can relate only to work personally performed that results from referrals from other physicians in the group, and cannot relate (directly or indirectly) to work that results from self-referrals. Commenters protested that this interpretation barred any compensation based on a physician's personal productivity for self-referred DHS and was, therefore, contrary to clear statutory intent. Several commenters explained that our interpretation would produce anomalous results in some circumstances. For example, an internist refers a patient with a gastrointestinal complaint to a gastrointestinal specialist, and the specialist evaluates the patient at an initial visit. The specialist subsequently performs an endoscopy on the patient. Under the proposed January 1998 regulations, the endoscopy would be a self-referral by the specialist, and the specialist could not receive a productivity bonus for performing the endoscopy. However, if the specialist referred the patient to another physician in the same group practice for the endoscopy, the specialist could receive compensation indirectly based on that endoscopy. Thus, in the commenter's view, the rule creates a disincentive to perform services and an incentive to refer (which may be contrary to good patient care and not cost effective). The commenter further noted that specialists who perform substantial amounts of DHS are disadvantaged by the proposed interpretation because they cannot be rewarded for personal productivity, while their counterparts, for whom the performance of DHS is a less significant part of their practices, can.

Commenters suggested an interpretation that would permit productivity bonuses for DHS personally performed by the referring physician, but not for DHS referred to others. The commenters generally requested that the final rule allow group practices to compensate members of the group based upon the volume or value of DHS, so long as the services are personally performed by the physician or are incident to the physician's personally performed services. One commenter noted that ancillary services (including ``incident to'' services) performed for one's own patients are more ``personal'' to the ordering or supervising physician than are services he or she performs on colleagues' patients. Commenters also complained that our proposed interpretation would lead to disparate treatment of solo and group practitioners, since solo practitioners could receive the profits from personally performed DHS that they self-refer, whereas group practitioners could not. One commenter thought that this discrepancy would make solo practitioners reluctant to join group practices, thereby discouraging beneficial market integration.

Finally, some commenters noted that many group practices have insufficient information technology systems to track whether a service performed by a physician resulted from a self-referral or a referral from another physician. Commenters asserted that our proposed interpretation would impose a significant additional administrative burden on those groups.

Response: In light of the comments, the changes we have made to our interpretation of the definition of a "referral" and the volume or value standard, and our further review of the statutory language, we are persuaded that our proposed interpretation of the scope of productivity bonuses was unnecessarily restrictive. Accordingly, we have revised the regulation to make clear that group practices may pay member physicians (and independent contractors who qualify as "physicians in the group") productivity bonuses based directly on the physician's personal productivity (including services "incident to" such personally performed services that meet the requirements of section 1861(s)(2)(A) of the Act and section 2050, "Services and Supplies," of the Medicare Carrier's Manual (HCFA Pub. 14-3), Part 3—Claims Process), but may not pay these physicians any bonus based directly on their referrals of DHS that are performed by someone else.

Comment: Commenters sought clarification about the treatment of productivity bonuses for "incident to'" services. One commenter observed that according to longstanding regulatory policies, "incident to" services are services that are an incidental although integral part of a physician's personal, professional service to a patient. Thus, in the commenter's view, there cannot be a referral for "incident to" services in any ordinary sense, since what the ancillary service provider does is part of the physician's service itself. Several commenters expressed

their belief that one purpose of the productivity bonus provision was to allow physicians to receive "credit" for "incident to" services in their compensation. One commenter pointed out that it would be hard to exclude "incident to" services in the calculation of productivity bonuses since claim forms typically do not indicate who performed the "incident to" service (that is, whether the service was performed by the supervising physician or someone else). Other commenters interpreted the statutory reference as equating "incident to" services with "in-office ancillary" services. Under this view, commenters asserted that the statutory language plainly allows productivity bonuses based indirectly on the volume or value of the physician's in-office ancillary services and opposed our proposed interpretation that prohibited any compensation based on referrals for in-office ancillary services.

Response: We agree with the essence of these comments with respect to group practices. Under the final regulation, group practice physicians can receive compensation directly related to the physician's personal productivity and to services incident to the physician's personally performed services, provided the "incident to" services comply with the requirements of section 1861(s)(2)(A) of the Act and section 2050, "Services and Supplies," of the Medicare Carrier's Manual (HCFA Pub. 14-3), Part 3—Claims Process, and any subsequent or additional HHS rules or regulations affecting "incident to" billing. This means that the "incident to" services must be directly supervised by the physician. In other words, the physician (or another clinic physician in the case of a physician-directed clinic) must be present in the office suite and immediately available to provide assistance and direction. Moreover, the person performing the "incident to" services must be an employee of the physician (or the physician-directed clinic). We believe that the heightened supervision requirement imposed by the "incident to" rules provides some assurance that the "incident to" DHS will not be the primary incentive for the self-referral. However, we may revisit the issue of compensation tied to ``incident to'' services if we find that abuses are occurring, especially in the area of physician-directed clinics.

Comment: We received a number of comments seeking clarification related to the methods of paying compensation that are not directly based on the volume or value of referrals. First, commenters urged that we allow pooling of revenues that are not DHS revenues, because such revenues are not governed by the statute. Second, a number of commenters objected to our position in the proposed regulations that overall profits are not profits that "belong only to a particular specialty or subspecialty group" (even if the group is located in several States or has several locations in one State) because "the narrower the pooling, the more likely it will be that a physician will receive compensation for his or her own referrals." Commenters urged that pooling at practice sites with more than a few physicians should not result in any individual's compensation being directly related to the volume or value of his or her referrals, even if DHS revenues are included in the pool. Commenters generally advocated that we allow pooling if at least three physicians are included in the pool and the distribution formula is not related to DHS referrals. Third, commenters offered a variety of suggestions about how to calculate "indirect" compensation. For example, one commenter suggested that compensation be considered "indirect" if the referrals have no mathematical effect on compensation. Others suggested that compensation be considered "indirect" if it is based on per capita calculations, RVUs, patient encounters, hours worked, ownership shares in the practice, or seniority.

Response: First, we are persuaded that we should permit some additional flexibility related to the distribution of shares of overall profits by group practices. Thus, we are defining a "share of overall profits" to mean a share of the entire profits derived from DHS of the entire group practice or any component of the group that consists of at least five physicians. We believe a threshold of at least five physicians is likely to be broad enough to attenuate the ties between compensation and referrals. We are rejecting the suggestion to use a threshold of three physicians because we believe that the lesser threshold would result in pooling that would be too narrow and, therefore, potentially too closely related to DHS referrals. Second, we recognize the need for clear guidance as to appropriate indirect compensation methodologies. For that reason, we are including in Phase I of this rulemaking methodologies that describe compensation distribution systems that we deem to be indirect. In other words, if a group practice wants absolute assurance that its productivity bonuses or profit shares are not directly related to referrals, the group practice may employ one of the regulatory methodologies set forth in Sec. 411.352 of the regulations. Group practices are not required, however, to use these methods. The regulations clarify that other methods (including distributions based on ownership interests or seniority) are acceptable so long as they are reasonable, objectively verifiable, and indirectly related to referrals. These compensation methods should be adequately documented and supporting information must be made available to the Secretary upon request. Under this latter "catch-all" provision, the group practice essentially bears the risk of noncompliance.

Comment: Several commenters sought clarification as to whether an independent contractor could be compensated under the productivity bonus provision of the group practice definition as a "physician in the group," even though independent contractors are not members of the group.

Response: Independent contractors who qualify as "physicians in the group" under the provisions of Sec. 411.351 can receive productivity bonuses under section 1877(h)(4)(B)(i) of the Act.

Comment: One commenter sought clarification as to how providers should treat capitation payments that cover more than one service for purposes of allocating profit shares and productivity bonuses.

Response: In general, we believe that capitation payments are not likely to lead to increased utilization. Parties may use any reasonable allocation method with respect to such payments.

Comment: On page 1691 of the preamble to the January 1998 proposed regulations, we explained our view that "profits should not be pooled and divided between group members so that they relate directly to the number of designated health services for Medicare or Medicaid patients physicians referred to themselves or the value of those self-referrals (such as a value based on complexity of the service)." A commenter objected to the parenthetical statement, asserting that barring consideration of the complexity of the service is contrary to other Medicare payment provisions, which take into consideration the level of training necessary to perform, and difficulty of, certain procedures.

Response: Given our revised interpretation, we believe the parenthetical statement ("such as value based on complexity of the service") is no longer relevant to these regulations. Group practice members can be compensated directly based on their personal productivity (that is, the fruits of their own labors), but not on their productivity in generating referrals. They may only be compensated based indirectly on DHS referrals to other physicians or providers. So long as the compensation is only indirectly related to the volume or value of DHS referrals, we believe it makes little difference if the value of the DHS referrals reflects the complexity of the services.

Comment: A commenter sought clarification that when a physician is a member of a group practice and is also an employee of the group practice, his or her compensation may be determined under the group practice's rules without regard to the employee exception.

Response: We agree that when a physician is a member of a group practice, his or her compensation need only comply with the group practice rules. Meeting the group practice definition allows physicians in the group to refer within the group under the in-office ancillary services exception or the physicians' services exception. However, nothing prevents a physician and group practice from using the employee exception instead. It is important to remember that referrals of DHS are only permitted if an exception, such as the in-office ancillary services exception or employee exception, applies.

Comment: Several commenters were confused by our use of the terms "revenues" and "profits" throughout the preamble to the January 1998 proposed regulations. For example, on page 1691 we stated that "the referring physician can receive a portion of the group's overall pooled revenues from these services as long as the group does not share these profits in a manner that relates directly to who made the referrals for them." Similarly, on the same page we stated that we "regard 'over-all profits of the group' to mean all of the profits or revenues a group can distribute in any form to group members * * *." These commenters requested that the terms "profits" and "revenues" be used in a manner that is consistent with their generally accepted meanings or that definitions of the terms be provided in the regulations.

Response: We agree that the terms "revenues" and "profits" were used inconsistently in the January 1998 proposed regulation. In Phase I of this rulemaking, we have endeavored to use those terms consistent with their generally accepted meanings.

Key Language of the Stark Legislation

This legislation is so important that we have reproduced the key language below. Again, the law is quite confusing, and there have been some indications that certain aspects will be modified. However, as written, many practices may have to change some arrangements—such as how income is distributed for the designated services performed within groups—to comply.

After the legislation, an advisory opinion is provided to illustrate how the government will likely evaluate referrals under Stark.

Stark II

42 USC §1395nn[4]

Limitation on Certain Physician Referrals

TITLE 42—THE PUBLIC HEALTH AND WELFARE

CHAPTER 7—SOCIAL SECURITY

SUBCHAPTER XVIII—HEALTH INSURANCE FOR AGED AND DISABLED

Part C—Miscellaneous Provisions

Sec. 1395nn. Limitation on certain physician referrals

(a) Prohibition of certain referrals
    (1) In general
        Except as provided in subsection (b) of this section, if a physician (or an immediate family member of such physician) has a financial relationship with an entity specified in paragraph (2),then—(A) the physician may not make a referral to the entity for the furnishing of designated health services for which payment otherwise may be made under this subchapter, and (B) the entity may not present or cause to be presented a claim under this subchapter or bill to any individual, third

party payor, or other entity for designated health services furnished pursuant to a referral prohibited under subparagraph (A).[5]

(2) Financial relationship specified

For purposes of this section, a financial relationship of a physician (or an immediate family member of such physician) with an entity specified in this paragraph is—(A) except as provided in subsections (c) and (d) of this section, an ownership or investment interest in the entity, or (B) except as provided in subsection (e) of this section, a compensation arrangement (as defined in subsection (h)(1) of this section) between the physician (or an immediate family member of such physician) and the entity.

An ownership or investment interest described in subparagraph (A) may be through equity, debt, or other means and includes an interest in an entity that holds an ownership or investment interest in any entity providing the designated health service.

(b) General exceptions to both ownership and compensation arrangement prohibitions

[Exceptions] Subsection (a)(1) of this section shall not apply in the following cases:

(1) Physicians' services

In the case of physicians' services (as defined in section 1395x(q) of this title) provided personally by (or under the personal supervision of) another physician in the same group practice (as defined in subsection (h)(4) of this section) as the referring physician.

(2) In-office ancillary services

In the case of services other than durable medical equipment (excluding infusion pumps) and parenteral and enteral nutrients, equipment, and supplies)—(A) that are furnished—

(i) personally by the referring physician, personally by a physician who is a member of the same group practice as the referring physician, or personally by individuals who are directly supervised by the physician or by another physician in the group practice, and

(ii) (I) in a building in which the referring physician (or another physician who is a member of the same group practice) furnishes physicians' services unrelated to the furnishing of designated health services, or (II) in the case of a referring physician who is a member of a group practice,

in another building which is used by the group practice—(aa) for the provision of some or all of the group's clinical laboratory services, or (bb) for the centralized provision of the group's designated health services (other than clinical laboratory services), unless the Secretary determines other terms and conditions under which the provision of such services does not present a risk of program or patient abuse, and (B) that are billed by the physician performing or supervising the services, by a group practice of which such physician is a member under a billing number assigned to the group practice, or by an entity that is wholly owned by such physician or such group practice, if the ownership or investment interest in such services meets such other requirements as the Secretary may impose by regulation as needed to protect against program or patient abuse.

(3) Prepaid plans

in the case of services furnished by an organization—(A) with a contract under section 1395mm of this title to an individual enrolled with the organization, (B) described in section 1395l(a)(1)(A) of this title to an individual enrolled with the organization, (C) receiving payments on a prepaid basis, under a demonstration project under section 1395b-l(a) of this title or under section 222(a) of the Social Security Amendments of 1972, to an individual enrolled with the organization, or (D) that is a qualified health maintenance organization (within the meaning of section 300e-9(d)) . . . to an individual enrolled with the organization.

(4) Other permissible exceptions

In the case of any other financial relationship which the Secretary determines, and specifies in regulations, does not pose a risk of program or patient abuse.

(c) General exception related only to ownership or investment prohibition for ownership in publicly traded securities and mutual funds. Ownership of the following shall not be considered to be an ownership or investment interest described in subsection (a)(2)(A) of this section:

(1) Ownership of investment securities (including shares or bonds, debentures, notes, or other debt instruments) which may be purchased on terms generally available to the public and which are— (A)(i) securities listed on the New York Stock Exchange, the American Stock Exchange, or any

regional exchange in which quotations are published on a daily basis, or foreign securities listed on a recognized foreign, national, or regional exchange in which quotations are published on a daily basis, or (ii) traded under an automated inter-dealer quotation system operated by the National Association of Securities Dealers, and (B) in a corporation that had, at the end of the corporation's most recent fiscal year, or on average during the previous 3 fiscal years, stockholder equity exceeding $75,000,000.

(2) Ownership of shares in a regulated investment company as defined in section 85 1 (a) of the Internal Revenue Code of 1986, if such company had, at the end of the company's most recent fiscal year, or on average during the previous 3 fiscal years, total assets exceeding $75,000,000.

(d) Additional exceptions related only to ownership or investment prohibition

The following, if not otherwise excepted under subsection (b) of this section, shall not be considered to be an ownership or investment interest described in subsection (a)(2)(A) of this section:

(1) Hospitals in Puerto Rico
In the case of designated health services provided by a hospital located in Puerto Rico.

(2) Rural provider
In the case of designated health services furnished in a rural area (as defined in section 1395ww(d)(2)(D) of this title by an entity, if substantially all of the designated health services furnished by such entity are furnished to individuals residing in such a rural area.

(3) Hospital ownership
In the case of designated health services provided by a hospital (other than a hospital described in paragraph (1)) if—(A) the referring physician is authorized to perform services at the hospital and (B) the ownership or investment interest is in the hospital itself (and not merely in a subdivision of the hospital).

(e) Exceptions relating to other compensation arrangements

The following shall not be considered to be a compensation arrangement described in subsection (a)(2)(13) of this section:

(1) Rental of office space; rental of equipment
(A) Office space
Payments made by a lessee to a lessor for the use of premises if—(i) the lease is set out in writing, signed by the parties, and specifies the premises covered by the lease, (ii) the space rented or leased does not exceed that which is reasonable and necessary for the legitimate business purposes of the lease or rental and is used exclusively by the lessee when being used by the lessee, except that the lessee may make payments for the use of space consisting of common areas if such payments do not exceed the lessee's pro rata share of expenses for such space based upon the ratio of the space used exclusively by the lessee to the total amount of space (other than common areas) occupied by all persons using such common areas, (iii) the lease provides for a term of rental or lease for at least 1 year, (iv) the rental charges over the term of the lease are set in advance, are consistent with fair market value, and are not determined in a manner that takes into account the volume or value of any referrals or other business generated between the parties, (v) the lease would be commercially reasonable even if no referrals were made between the parties, and (vi) the lease meets such other requirements as the Secretary may impose by regulation as needed to protect against program or patient abuse.

(B) Equipment
Payments made by a lessee of equipment to the lessor of the equipment for the use of the equipment if—(i) the lease is set out in writing, signed by the parties, and specifies the equipment covered by the lease, (ii) the equipment rented or leased does not exceed that which is reasonable and necessary for the legitimate business purposes of the lease or rental and is used exclusively by the lessee when being used by the lessee, (iii) the lease provides for a term of rental or lease of at least 1 year, (iv) the rental charges over the term of the lease are set in advance, are consistent with fair market value, and are not determined in a manner that takes into account the volume or value of any referrals or other business generated between the parties, (v) the lease would be commercially reasonable even if no referrals were made between the parties, and (vi) the lease meets such other requirements as the Secretary may impose by regulation as needed to protect against program or patient abuse.

(2) Bona fide employment relationships

Any amount paid by an employer to a physician (or an immediate family member of such physician) who has a bona fide employment relationship with the employer for the provision of services if—(A) the employment is for identifiable services, (B) the amount of the remuneration under the employment—(i) is consistent with the fair market value of the services, and (ii) is not determined in a manner that takes into account (directly or indirectly) the volume or value of any referrals by the referring physician, (C) the remuneration is provided pursuant to an agreement which would be commercially reasonable even if no referrals were made to the employer, and (D) the employment meets such other requirements as the Secretary may impose by regulation as needed to protect against program or patient abuse.

Subparagraph (B)(ii) shall not prohibit the payment of remuneration in the form of a productivity bonus based on services performed personally by the physician (or an immediate family member of such physician).

(3) Personal service arrangements

(A) In general Remuneration from an entity under an arrangement (including remuneration for specific physicians' services furnished to a non-profit blood center) if—(i) the arrangement is set out in writing, signed by the parties, and specifies the services covered by the arrangement, (ii) the arrangement covers all of the services to be provided by the physician (or an immediate family member of such physician) to the entity, (iii) the aggregate services contracted for do not exceed those that are reasonable and necessary for the legitimate business purposes of the arrangement, (iv) the term of the arrangement is for at least 1 year, (v) the compensation to be paid over the term of the arrangement is set in advance, does not exceed fair market value, and except in the case of a physician incentive plan described in subparagraph (B), is not determined in a manner that takes into account the volume or value of any referrals or other business generated between the parties, (vi) the services to be performed under the arrangement do not involve the counseling or promotion or a business arrangement or other activity that violates any State or Federal law, and (vii) the arrangement meets such other requirements as the

Secretary may impose by regulation as needed to protect against program or patient abuse.

(B) Physician incentive plan exception

(i) In general in the case of a physician incentive plan (as defined in clause (ii)) between a physician and an entity, the compensation may be determined in a manner (through a withhold, capitation, bonus, or otherwise) that takes into account directly or indirectly the volume or value of any referrals or other business generated between the parties, if the plan meets the following requirements:

(I) No specific payment is made directly or indirectly under the plan to a physician or a physician group as an inducement to reduce or limit medically necessary services provided with respect to a specific individual enrolled with the entity.

(II) In the case of a plan that places a physician or a physician group at substantial financial risk as determined by the Secretary pursuant to section 1395mm(I)(8)(A)(ii) of this title, the plan complies with any requirements the Secretary may impose pursuant to such section.

(III) Upon request by the Secretary, the entity provides the Secretary with access to descriptive information regarding the plan, in order to permit the Secretary to determine whether the plan is in compliance with the requirements of this clause.

(ii) "Physician incentive plan" defined
For purposes of this subparagraph, the term "physician incentive plan" means any compensation arrangement between an entity and a physician or physician group that may directly or indirectly have the effect of reducing or limiting services provided with respect to individuals enrolled with the entity.

(4) Remuneration unrelated to the provision of designated health services

In the case of remuneration which is provided by a hospital to a physician if such remuneration does not relate to the provision of designated health services.

(5) Physician recruitment

In the case of remuneration which is provided by a hospital to a physician to induce the physician to relocate to the geographic area served by the hospital in order to be a member of the medical staff of the hospital, if—(A) the physician is not required to refer patients to the hospital, (B) the amount of the remuneration under the arrangement is not determined in a manner that takes into account (directly or indirectly) the volume or value of any referrals by the referring physician, and (C) the arrangement meets such other requirements as the Secretary may impose by regulation as needed to protect against program or patient abuse.

(6) Isolated transactions [such as one-time sale of practice]

In the case of an isolated financial transaction, such as a one-time sale of property or practice, if (A) the requirements described in subparagraphs (B) and (C) of paragraph (2) are met with respect to the entity in the same manner as they apply to an employer, and (B) the transaction meets such other requirements as the Secretary may impose by regulation as needed to protect against program or patient abuse.

(7) Certain group practice arrangements with a hospital

. . . An arrangement between a hospital and a group under which designated health services are provided by the group but are billed by the hospital if—
(i) with respect to services provided to an inpatient of the hospital, the arrangement is pursuant to the provision of inpatient hospital services under section 1395x(b)(3) of this title, (ii) the arrangement began before December 19, 1989, and has continued in effect without interruption since such date, (iii) with respect to the designated health services covered under the arrangement, substantially all of such services furnished to patients of the hospital are furnished by the group under the arrangement, (iv) the arrangement is pursuant to an agreement that is set out in writing and that specifies the services to be provided by the parties and the compensation for services provided under the agreement, (v) the compensation paid over the term of the agreement is consistent with fair market value and the compensation per unit of services is fixed in

advance and is not determined in a manner that takes into account the volume or value of any referrals or other business generated between the parties, (vi) the compensation is provided pursuant to an agreement which would be commercially reasonable even if no referrals were made to the entity, and (vii) the arrangement between the parties meets such other requirements as the Secretary may impose by regulation as needed to protect against program or patient abuse.

(8) Payments by a physician for items and services
Payments made by a physician—(A) to a laboratory in exchange for the provision of clinical laboratory services, or (B) to an entity as compensation for other items or services if the items or services are furnished at a price that is consistent with fair market value.

(f) Reporting requirements
Each entity providing covered items or services for which payment may be made under this subchapter shall provide the Secretary with the information concerning the entity's ownership, investment, and compensation arrangements, including—

(1) the covered items and services provided by the entity, and (2) the names and unique physician identification numbers of all physicians with an ownership or investment interest (as described in subsection (a)(2)(A) of this section), or with a compensation arrangement (as described in subsection (a)(2)(B) of this section), in the entity, or whose immediate relatives have such an ownership or investment interest or who have such a compensation relationship with the entity.

Such information shall be provided in such form, manner, and at such times as the Secretary shall specify. The requirement of this subsection shall not apply to designated health services provided outside the United States or to entities which the Secretary determines provides services for which payment may be made under this subchapter very infrequently.

(g) Sanctions

(1) Denial of payment
No payment may be made under this subchapter for a designated health service which is provided in violation of subsection (a)(1) of this section.

(2) Requiring refunds for certain claims

If a person collects any amounts that were billed in violation of subsection (a)(1) of this section, the person shall be liable to the individual for, and shall refund on a timely basis to the individual, any amounts so collected.

(3) Civil money penalty and exclusion for improper claims

Any person that presents or causes to be presented a bill or a claim for a service that such person knows or should know is for a service for which payment may not be made under paragraph (1) or for which a refund has not been made under paragraph (2) shall be subject to a civil money penalty of not more than $15,000 for each such service. The provisions of section 1320a-7a of this title (other than the first sentence of subsection (a) and other than subsection (b)) shall apply to a civil money penalty under the previous sentence in the same manner as such provisions apply to a penalty or proceeding under section 1320a-7a(a) of this title.

(4) Civil money penalty and exclusion for circumvention schemes

Any physician or other entity that enters into in arrangement or scheme (such as a cross-referral arrangement) which the physician or entity knows or should know has a principal purpose of assuring referrals by the physician to a particular entity which, if the physician directly made referrals to such entity, would be in violation of this section, shall be subject to a civil money penalty of not more than $100,000 for each such arrangement or scheme. The provisions of section 1320a-7a of this title (other than the first sentence of subsection (a) and other than subsection (b)) shall apply to a civil money penalty under the previous sentence in the same manner as such provisions apply to a penalty or proceeding under section 1320a-7a(a) of this title.

(5) Failure to report information

Any person who is required, but fails, to meet a reporting requirement of subsection (f) of this section is subject to a civil money penalty of not more than $10,000 for each day for which reporting is required to have been made. The provisions of section 1320a-7a of this title (other than the first sentence of subsection (a) and other than subsection (b)) shall apply to a civil money penalty under the previous sentence in the same manner as

such provisions apply to a penalty or proceeding under section 1320a-7a(a) of this title.

(h) Definitions and special rules

For purposes of this section:

(1) Compensation arrangement; remuneration

(A) The term "compensation arrangement" means any arrangement involving any remuneration between a physician (or an immediate family member of such physician) and an entity other than an arrangement involving only remuneration described in subparagraph (C).

(B) The term "remuneration" includes any remuneration, directly or indirectly, overtly or covertly, in cash or in kind.

(i) Remuneration described in this subparagraph is any remuneration consisting of any of the following: (i) The forgiveness of amounts owed for inaccurate tests or procedures, mistakenly performed tests or procedures, or the correction of minor billing errors. (ii) The provision of items, devices, or supplies that are used solely to—

(ii) collect, transport, process, or store specimens for the entity providing the item, device, or supply, or (II) order or communicate the results of tests or procedures for such entity. (iii) A payment made by an insurer or a self-insured plan to a physician to satisfy a claim, submitted on a fee for service basis, for the furnishing of health services by that physician to an individual who is covered by a policy with the insurer or by the self-insured plan, if (I) the health services are not furnished, and the payment is not made, pursuant to a contract or other arrangement between the insurer or the plan and the physician, (II) the payment is made to the physician on behalf of the covered individual and would otherwise be made directly to such individual, (III) the amount of the payment is set in advance, does not exceed fair market value, and is not determined in a manner that takes into account directly or indirectly the volume or value of any referrals, and (IV) the payment meets such other requirements as the Secretary may impose by regulation as needed to protect against program or patient abuse.

(2) Employee

An individual is considered to be "employed by" or an "employee" of an entity if the individual would be considered to be an employee of the entity under the usual common law rules applicable in determining the employer-employee relationship (as applied for purposes of section 3121(d)(2) of the Internal Revenue Code of 1986).

(3) Fair market value

The term "fair market value" means the value in arms length transactions, consistent with the general market value, and, with respect to rentals or leases, the value of rental property for general commercial purposes (not taking into account its intended use) and, in the case of a lease of space, not adjusted to reflect the additional value the prospective lessee or lessor would attribute to the proximity or convenience to the lessor where the lessor is a potential source of patient referrals to the lessee.

(4) Group practice

(A) Definition of group practice

The term "group practice" means a group of 2 or more physicians legally organized as a partnership, professional corporation, foundation, not-for-profit corporation, faculty practice plan, or similar association—(i) in which each physician who is a member of the group provides substantially the full range of services which the physician routinely provides, including medical care, consultation, diagnosis, or treatment, through the joint use of shared office space, facilities, equipment and personnel (ii) for which substantially all of the services of the physicians who are members of the group are provided through the group and are billed under a billing number assigned to the group and amounts so received are treated as receipts of the group, (iii) in which the overhead expenses of and the income from the practice are distributed in accordance with methods previously determined, (iv) except as provided in subparagraph (B)(i), in which no physician who is a member of the group directly or indirectly receives compensation based on the volume or value of referrals by the physician, (v) in which members of the group personally conduct no less than 75 percent of the physician-patient encounters of the group practice, and (vi) which meets such other standards as the Secretary may impose by regulation.

(B) Special rules

(i) Profits and productivity bonuses

A physician in a group practice may be paid a share of overall profits of the group, or a productivity bonus based on services personally performed or services incident to such personally performed services, so long as the share or bonus is not determined in any manner which is directly related to the volume or value of referrals by such physician.

(ii) Faculty practice plans

In the case of a faculty practice plan associated with a hospital, institution of higher education, or medical school with an approved medical residency training program in which physician members may provide a variety of different specialty services and provide professional services both within and outside the group, as well as perform other tasks such as research, subparagraph (A) shall be applied only with respect to the services provided within the faculty practice plan.

(5) Referral; referring physician

(A) Physicians' services

Except as provided in subparagraph (C), in the case of an item or service for which payment may be made under part B of this subchapter, the request by a physician for the item or service, including the request by a physician for a consultation with another physician (and any test or procedure ordered by, or to be performed by (or under the supervision of) that other physician), constitutes a 'referral' by a 'referring physician'.

(B) Other items

Except as provided in subparagraph (C), the request or establishment of a plan of care by a physician which includes the provision of the designated health service constitutes a 'referral' by a 'referring physician'.

(C) Clarification respecting certain services integral to a consultation by certain specialists

A request by a pathologist for clinical diagnostic laboratory tests and pathological examination services, a request by a radiologist for diagnostic radiology services, and a request by a radiation oncologist for radiation therapy, if such services are furnished by (or under the supervision of) such pathologist, radiologist, or radiation oncologist pursuant to a consultation requested by another physician does not constitute a 'referral' by a 'referring physician'.

(6) Designated health services
The term "designated health services" means any of the following items or services:
(A) Clinical laboratory services.
(B) Physical therapy services.

(C) Occupational therapy services.
(D) Radiology or other diagnostic services.
(E) Radiation therapy services.
(F) Durable medical equipment.
(G) Parenteral/enteral nutrients, equipment, and supplies.
(H) Prosthetics, orthotics, and prosthetic devices.
(I) Home health services.
(J) Outpatient prescription drugs.
(K) Inpatient and outpatient hospital services.

Many observers expect publication of final regulations during 2000 or early 2001. Notwithstanding the absence of final regulations, Stark II is law. Physicians need to begin thinking about how this act may impact their practice. Some medical practices will need to make changes to ensure compliance with the law. Some groups may need to modify physician compensation arrangements to comply with the law and proposed regulations. Finally, some states have adopted similar legislation that complicates matters as well.

Advisory Opinions

CMS issues advisory opinions that discuss whether a physician's referrals relating to certain designated health services (other than clinical laboratory services) are prohibited under the Medicare program by section 1877 of the Social Security Act. To date, there are only a couple of advisory opinions that have been issued. CMS's Stark Advisory Opinion Web site, www.cms.gov/physicians/aop/default.asp, includes two advisory opinions related to physician self-referrals (these opinions should not be confused with OIG advisory opinions).

Advisory opinion 98-002 is instructive as to the analysis the government would use in looking at potential prohibited referrals. Readers should note that these advisory opinions were written before publication of the Phase I final rule.

Re: Advisory Opinion No. HCFA-AO-98-002

Dear [Redacted]:

We are writing in response to your request for an advisory opinion (AO), in which you pose the following question: Whether the partners and physician employees of a proposed partnership may, under the "in-office ancillary services" exception defined in section 1877(b)(2) of the Social Security Act (the Act), refer Medicare and/or Medicaid patients to the partnership for eyeglass prescriptions filled subsequent to cataract surgery with the insertion of an intraocular lens.

You have certified that all of the information you have provided in your request, including all supplementary materials and letters, is true and correct, and constitutes a complete description of the parties, relationships and facts regarding the proposed arrangement. In issuing this opinion we have relied solely on the facts and information you have presented to us. We have not undertaken an independent investigation of this information. If material facts have not been disclosed or have changed since we accepted your request, these differences could nullify the validity of this AO.

Based on the information provided, we conclude that the partners and employees of the proposed partnership would qualify for the in-office ancillary services exception.

Factual Background

The two Requestors propose to form a partnership, "Partnership," for the purpose of providing ophthalmology services for patients, and eyeglasses and contact lenses for patients and non-patients. We are using the term non-patient to mean a person who gets a prescription for eyeglasses or contact lenses from someplace other than the partnership, but comes to Partnership to have that prescription filled.

Each Requestor has one ophthalmologist shareholder and several physician employees; each Requestor currently leases its own office space, and proposes an additional site for the partnership, so Partnership would operate at three locations. Requestors have proposed to assign all leases and employment contracts to Partnership, for those employees who have agreed to work for the partnership. (One of the employees of one of the Requestors has refused to assign his contract to the partnership. Requestors have since submitted that

this physician has not renewed his contract, and will no longer be a factor in the proposed arrangement.) Each Requestor will contribute 50 percent of the assets of the partnership and will receive 50 percent of the revenues left after expenses are met and each employee has been paid. Each physician owner and physician employee is paid a salary that is unrelated to referrals.

Legal Analysis

A. The Referral Prohibition

Section 1877 of the Act prohibits a physician from referring a Medicare patient to an entity for certain designated health services if the physician has a financial relationship with the entity, unless an exception applies. A financial relationship exists if the physician has an ownership or investment interest in the furnishing entity, or a compensation arrangement with the entity. In the proposed arrangement, it appears that the physician partners will have an ownership interest in an entity that will furnish eyeglasses and contact lenses to patients following cataract surgery with the insertion of an intraocular lens. The partners will also have a compensation arrangement with the entity in the form of salary payments, as will other physician employees who will be paid a salary.

The list of designated health services that appears in section 1877 (h)(6) of the Act includes "prosthetic devices," which are defined in the Medicare statute in section 1861 (s)(8) as including one pair of conventional eyeglasses or contact lenses furnished subsequent to each cataract surgery with insertion of an intraocular lens. (This is the only circumstance under which Medicare covers prescription eyeglasses or contact lenses.) We have stated in a proposed rule covering a physician's referrals for designated health services that we are proposing to define the term "prosthetic devices" for the purposes of the referral prohibition in the same manner as it is defined in the Medicare statute. (See 63 FR 1678 (January 9, 1998).) Although the proposed rule has not been promulgated in final form, it reflects our current interpretation of the law.

Section 1903(s) of the Act applies some of the referral rules to the Medicaid program.

In the Medicaid context, eyeglasses are generally covered under a category separate from prosthetic devices under the authority of section 1905 (a)(12) of the Act. As we have explained in the proposed rule mentioned above, when the definition of a designated health service differs under a State's Medicaid plan (which lists the services a State covers) from the definition under Medicare, we propose to assume that the services included under the State's plan take precedence. (See 63 FR 1673-74.) In Requestors' state, eyeglasses are not considered to be a prosthetic device. As long as a State does not classify eyeglasses as a prosthetic device or otherwise as a designated health service, there are no physician referral implications for any Medicaid referrals for them.

Since it appears that the proposed arrangement would be a financial relationship for purposes of Medicare referrals under section 1877, the physicians involved can only refer to Partnership if an exception applies. The Requestors have specifically asked whether the in-office ancillary services exception would make the referrals of the partners and physician employees acceptable.

B. Group Practice

Requestors have stated that they wish their partnership to be considered a group practice, and that they want this group practice to qualify for the in-office ancillary services exception.

To qualify for the in-office ancillary services exception, Requestors must first meet the definition of a group practice as set forth in section 1877(h)(4)(A)of the Act: "The term 'group practice' means a group of 2 or more physicians legally organized as a partnership . . . or similar association—(i) in which each physician who is a member of the group provides substantially the full range of services which the physician routinely provides . . . through the joint use of shared office space, facilities, equipment and personnel, (ii) for which substantially all of the services of the physicians who are members of the group are provided through the group and are billed under a billing number assigned to the group and amounts so received are treated as receipts of the group, (iii) in which the overhead expenses of and the income from the practice are distributed in accordance with methods previously determined, (iv) except as provided in subparagraph (B)(i) [which relates to profits and productivity bonuses], in which no physician who is a member of the group directly or indirectly receives compensation based on the volume or value of referrals by the physician, and (v) in which members of the group personally conduct no less than 75 percent of the physician-patient encounters of the group practice. . . ."

1. Substantially the full range of services

Section 1877(h)(4)(A)(i) requires that each member of the group provide "substantially the full range of services

which the physician routinely provides . . . through the joint use of shared office space, facilities, equipment and personnel." Requestors have certified that each physician who is a member of Partnership will practice the same range of ophthalmology services as the physician currently does. Further, since all leases have been assigned to the partnership, it appears that all facilities and office space will be shared, as well as the personnel who will be employed by the partnership.

2. Substantially all of the members' services are provided through the group and are billed by the group

Section 1877(h)(4)(A)(ii) requires that "substantially all of the services of the physicians who are members of the group are provided through the group and are billed under a billing number assigned to the group and amounts so received are treated as receipts of the group. . . ." In our final regulation governing referrals for clinical laboratory services in 42 CFR 411.351, we defined a group practice by stating that at least 75 percent of the total patient care services of the group practice members must be furnished through the group and be billed in the name of the group. We measured "patient care services" by the total patient care time each member spends on these services. In our proposed rule covering referrals for other designated health services, we proposed to clarify certain aspects of the "substantially all" test. In the discussion at 63 FR 1688, we stated that we expect a group to look at a physician's total patient care time during a week, furnished both inside and outside of the group practice, to determine what percent of this time is furnished through the one group. Requestors have indicated to us that member physicians will be performing 100 percent of their patient care services through Partnership. Provided that this is accurate, we conclude that they will meet this part of the test.

Requestors have certified in a letter to HCFA that billing will be done under one billing number assigned to the partnership, all receipts from billing done on behalf of the partners and the employees of the partnership will be treated as receipts of the group, and expenses will be paid as expenses of the group. We therefore believe that this part of the test will be satisfied.

3. Overhead expenses and income from the practice shall be distributed in accordance with previously determined methods

HCFA believes that this provision is ambiguous and has proposed to interpret it to mean that a group must have in place methods for distribution prior to the time period the group has earned the income or incurred the costs. (See 63 FR 1690.)

The Partnership Agreement details that expenses of the practice such as rent, utilities, and salaries will be paid out of the income to the practice before any profits are distributed, and the employment contracts detail the precise amounts of each member's annual salary. Profits over and above salaries and expenses will be distributed on a 50 percent basis between the partners, as detailed in the Partnership Agreement. We therefore believe that the arrangement satisfies our interpretation of this part of the test.

4. No physician member will be compensated, directly or indirectly, based on the volume or value of referrals

Under section 1877(h)(4)(A)(iv), no physician member of the group may receive compensation based on the volume or value of that physician's own referrals. However, section 1877(h)(4)(B)(I) qualifies this statement by allowing that "a physician in a group practice may be paid a share of overall profits of the group, or a productivity bonus based on services personally performed or services incident to such personally performed services, so long as the share or bonus is not determined in any manner which is directly related to the volume or value of referrals by such physician."

Partnership's employment contracts indicate that physician employees will be compensated on a straight salary basis. These salaries are based on the number of hours worked, multiplied by a pre-determined amount that varies slightly among the employees. This variance reflects differences in education and experience among the members, and is not based on the volume or value of past or projected future referrals. In addition to salary, employees also receive a health benefit package. While there is no fair market value test for the compensation that a group practice can pay a physician member under section 1877(h) (4) (A), if a physician appears to be paid an inordinately high salary for his or her work, we would assume that the group is compensating the physician for referrals by including the payments as part of a set salary. Because we are not in a position to determine whether the wages and benefits under the arrangement are fair, we condition this advisory opinion on the requirement that the salaries and benefits are in line with what similarly situated ophthalmologists in the geographical area receive for comparable work, without the value of any referrals included in the development of the salary package.

The Partnership Agreement states that physician owners will each be paid both an annual salary and a 50 percent share of the profits, which will be based solely on the percentage of the ownership interest of each owner.

The employees are to be paid on a pre-determined hourly salary, without receiving a bonus related to the volume or value of referrals for designated health services. Partnership has not proposed any other forms of compensation or incentives for owners or employees. It therefore appears that this part of the test will be satisfied.

5. Members of the group provide at least 75 percent of the physician-patient encounters

HCFA has proposed to interpret "member of the group" to include physician owners and employees of the group. (See 63 FR 1687.) Since Partnership has indicated in correspondence with HCFA that all physician-patient encounters will be performed by members of the group, Partnership's proposal will meet this part of the test.

B. In-office Ancillary Services Exception

In order to qualify for the in-office ancillary services exception, Partnership must not only meet the definition of a group practice but also demonstrate that it meets the criteria set forth in section 1877(b)(2)(A) of the Act, which exempts services that are furnished "(i) personally by the referring physician, personally by a physician who is a member of the same group practice as the referring physician, or personally by individuals who are directly supervised by the physician or another physician in the group practice, and (ii)(I) in a building in which the referring physician (or another physician who is a member of the same group practice) furnishes physicians' services unrelated to the furnishing of designated health services, or (II) in the case of a referring physician who is a member of a group practice, in another building which is used by the group practice for the centralized provision of the group's designated health services (other than clinical laboratory services). . . ." In addition, under (b)(2)(B), the services must be billed by the physician performing or supervising the services or the group practice of which such physician is a member under a billing number assigned to the group practice, or by an entity that is wholly owned by the physician or the group practice.

1. Services furnished or supervised by the referring physician or by a member of the same group practice

Requestors would meet this part of the test if a member of the group personally furnishes or directly supervises a non-member in the furnishing of the designated health service. By regulation in 42 CFR 411.351, in terms of referrals involving only clinical laboratory services, we have interpreted "direct supervision" to mean "supervision by a physician who is present in the office suite and immediately available to provide assistance and direction throughout the time services are being performed." The January 9, 1998 proposed rule further defines "present in the office suite" as meaning that the physician must be present in the suite in which the services are being furnished, at the time they are being furnished, except that the definition does allow certain unexpected absences and certain routine absences of short duration. (See 63 FR 1684.)

Requestors can meet this requirement by assuring that at least one of the four physician members of the group is present at each of the three locations at any given time. Requestors have not specifically addressed this management issue in their communication with us, but have stated verbally that they intend to comply with HCFA's opinion on how to meet each prong of each test. The direct supervision requirement applies only to Medicare covered designated health services. Thus, as long as at least one physician member is in the office suite performing or directly supervising a non-member employee in the furnishing of eyeglasses or contact lenses that qualify as designated health services that are covered under Medicare, this part of the test will be met.

2. Services furnished in an appropriate location

Except as described below, designated health services must be furnished in a building in which the referring physician or another physician member of the group practice is furnishing physicians' services unrelated to the furnishing of designated health services. We have proposed to interpret "unrelated to designated health services" as any services that are not listed as designated health services in section 1877 (h) (6), even if these services lead to a physician requesting a designated health service (see 63 FR 1695). Since the partnership proposes to offer a broader range of ophthalmology services than those considered to be designated health services at each of its locations, we believe that this requirement will be met.

Alternatively, a group practice can meet the location test if the designated health services are furnished in another building that is used by the group for the centralized provision of designated health services. Partnership could arrange its locations such that no additional physicians' services are furnished where the eyeglasses are furnished, provided that a physician is on the premises to either furnish the eyeglasses or to directly supervise non-member employees who are furnishing the eyeglasses.

3. Services billed under the billing number assigned to the group practice

Requestors have certified that partners and physician employees of Partnership would bill under a common billing number assigned to the partnership. Provided that

they obtain and use a billing number assigned to the group practice, this provision will be met.

Conclusion

We find that the proposed partnership arrangement is a group practice and that the designated health services performed or supervised by members of the group will meet the in-office ancillary services exception, provided that all of the above-mentioned criteria are met.

Limitations of This Opinion

The limitations that apply to this Advisory Opinion include the following:

This AO and the validity of conclusions reached in it are based entirely on the accuracy of the information that you have presented to us.

This AO is relevant only to the specific question(s) posed at the beginning of this opinion. This AO is limited in scope to the specific arrangement described in this letter and has no application to other arrangements, even those which appear to be similar in nature or scope.

This AO does not apply to, nor can it be relied upon, by any individual or entity other than the Requestor. This AO may not be introduced in any matter involving an entity or individual that is not a Requestor to this opinion.

Our Advisory Opinion authority originates from Section 1877 of the Social Security Act, which specifically contains a prohibition against certain physician referrals. This AO may not be construed as permission to avoid compliance with any other Federal, State or local laws which may apply to the arrangement.

This AO will not bind or obligate any agency other than the U.S. Department of Health and Human Services. Under 42 CFR 411.382, HCFA reserves the right to reconsider the issues posed in this AO and, where public interest requires, rescind or revoke this opinion.

This opinion is also subject to any additional limitations set forth at 42 CFR 411.370 et seq.

Sincerely,
/S/
Robert A. Berenson, M.D.
Director
Center for Health Plans and Providers

There is another advisory opinion that evaluates a proposed ambulatory surgery center in a rural area with nonsurgeon physician investors. CMS has indicated they are currently working on other opinions.

Identifying Potential Kickbacks and Physician Self-referral Problems

Identifying instances that may violate the antikickback and physician self-referral statutes is a matter of looking at contractual and informal arrangements between physicians and ancillary health care entities.

Typically, any contractual relationships among physicians and other providers, payments for medical directorships, joint venture arrangements, ownership interests in a health care service provider, physician compensation arrangements within a group, and the like should be reviewed. Interviews with managers and physicians may be required. Some informal arrangements among physicians and others may need to be reviewed as well.

Do not, however, assume that such arrangements are necessarily illegal. There are many legitimate arrangements that contribute to the delivery of quality medical care.

Regulations Published in the January 4, 2001, Federal Register

The regulations included in this section were published in the January 4, 2001, *Federal Register*, which provides the final rulemaking for Phase I of "Physicians' Referrals to Health Care Entities With Which They Have Financial Relationships." The 97 pages of discussion in the *Federal Register* preceding the regulations below are not included here. These pages provide important clarifications and examples and should be reviewed if a physician makes "referrals" for Designated Health Services to an entity in which they have a financial relationship.

Federal Register: January 4, 2001 (Volume 66, Number 3)
Rules and Regulations

From the Federal Register Online via GPO Access [wais.access.gpo.gov]

Part II

Department of Health and Human Services
[Now Centers for Medicare and Medicaid Services]

Health Care Financing Administration
42 CFR Parts 411

Medicare and Medicaid Programs; Physicians' Referrals to Health Care Entities With Which They Have Financial Relationships; Final Rule

ACTION: Final rule with comment period.

[Note: The 97 pages preceding the regulations below are not included in this excerpt, but they provide important clarifications and interpretations.]

For the reasons set forth in the preamble, HCFA amends 42 CFR chapter IV as set forth below:

PART 411—EXCLUSIONS FROM MEDICARE AND LIMITATIONS ON MEDICARE PAYMENT

A. Part 411 is amended as follows:
  1. The authority citation for part 411 continues to read as follows:

  Authority: Secs. 1102 and 1871 of the Social Security Act (42 U.S.C. 1302 and 1395hh).

Subpart A—General Exclusions and Exclusions of Particular Services

  2. In §411.1, paragraph (a) is revised to read as follows:

§411.1 Basis and scope.
  (a) *Statutory basis.* Sections 1814(a) and 1835(a) of the Act require that a physician certify or recertify a patient's need for home health services but, in general, prohibit a physician from certifying or recertifying the need for services if the services will be furnished by an HHA in which the physician has a significant ownership interest, or with which the physician has a significant financial or contractual relationship. Sections 1814(c), 1835(d), and 1862 of the Act exclude from Medicare payment certain specified services. The Act provides

special rules for payment of services furnished by the following: Federal providers or agencies (sections 1814(c) and 1835(d)); hospitals and physicians outside of the U.S. (sections 1814(f) and 1862(a)(4)); and hospitals and SNFs of the Indian Health Service (section 1880 of the Act). Section 1877 of the Act sets forth limitations on referrals and payment for designated health services furnished by entities with which the referring physician (or an immediate family member of the referring physician) has a financial relationship.

Subpart J—Physician Ownership of, and Referral of Patients or Laboratory Specimens to, Entities Furnishing Clinical Laboratory or Other Health Services

  3. Section 411.350 is revised to read as follows:

§411.350 Scope of subpart.
  (a) This subpart implements section 1877 of the Act, which generally prohibits a physician from making a referral under Medicare for designated health services to an entity with which the physician or a member of the physician's immediate family has a financial relationship.

  (b) This subpart does not provide for exceptions or immunity from civil or criminal prosecution or other sanctions applicable under any State laws or under Federal law other than section 1877 of the Act. For example, although a particular arrangement involving a physician's financial relationship with an entity may not prohibit the physician from making referrals to the entity under this subpart, the arrangement may nevertheless violate another provision of the Act or other laws administered by HHS, the Federal Trade Commission, the Securities and Exchange Commission, the Internal Revenue Service, or any other Federal or State agency.

  (c) This subpart requires, with some exceptions, that certain entities furnishing covered services under

Medicare Part A or Part B report information concerning their ownership, investment, or compensation arrangements in the form, manner, and at the times specified by HCFA.

4. Section 411.351 is revised to read as follows:

§411.351 Definitions.

As used in this subpart, unless the context indicates otherwise:

Centralized building means all or part of a building, including, for purposes of this definition only, a mobile vehicle, van, or trailer that is owned or leased on a full-time basis (that is, 24 hours per day, 7 days per week, for a term of not less than 6 months) by a group practice and that is used exclusively by the group practice. Space in a building or a mobile vehicle, van, or trailer that is shared by more than one group practice, by a group practice and one or more solo practitioners, or by a group practice and another provider (for example, a diagnostic imaging facility) is not a centralized building for purposes of this rule. This provision does not preclude a group practice from providing services to other providers (for example, purchased diagnostic tests) in the group practice's centralized building. A group practice may have more than one centralized building.

Clinical laboratory services means the biological, microbiological, serological, chemical, immunohematological, hematological, biophysical, cytological, pathological, or other examination of materials derived from the human body for the purpose of providing information for the diagnosis, prevention, or treatment of any disease or impairment of, or the assessment of the health of, human beings, including procedures to determine, measure, or otherwise describe the presence or absence of various substances or organisms in the body, as specifically identified by the CPT and HCPCS codes posted on the HCFA web site, http://www.hcfa.gov, (and in annual updates published in the *Federal Register* and posted on the HCFA web site), except as specifically excluded on the HCFA web site and in annual updates. All services identified on the HCFA web site and in annual updates are clinical laboratory services for purposes of these regulations. Any service not specifically identified on the HCFA web site, as amended from time to time and published in the *Federal Register*, is not a clinical laboratory service for purposes of these regulations.

Consultation means a professional service furnished to a patient by a physician if the following conditions are satisfied:

(1) The physician's opinion or advice regarding evaluation and/or management of a specific medical problem is requested by another physician.

(2) The request and need for the consultation are documented in the patient's medical record.

(3) After the consultation is provided, the physician prepares a written report of his or her findings, which is provided to the physician who requested the consultation.

(4) With respect to radiation therapy services provided by a radiation oncologist, a course of radiation treatments over a period of time will be considered to be pursuant to a consultation, provided the radiation oncologist communicates with the referring physician on a regular basis about the patient's course of treatment and progress.

Designated health services (DHS) means any of the following services (other than those provided as emergency physician services furnished outside of the U.S.), as they are defined in this section:

(1) Clinical laboratory services.

(2) Physical therapy, occupational therapy, and speech-language pathology services.

(3) Radiology and certain other imaging services.

(4) Radiation therapy services and supplies.

(5) Durable medical equipment and supplies.

(6) Parenteral and enteral nutrients, equipment, and supplies.

(7) Prosthetics, orthotics, and prosthetic devices and supplies.

(8) Home health services.

(9) Outpatient prescription drugs

(10) Inpatient and outpatient hospital services.

Except as otherwise noted in these regulations, the term "designated health services (DHS)" means only DHS payable, in whole or in part, by Medicare. DHS do not include services that are reimbursed by Medicare as part of a composite rate (for example, ambulatory surgical center services or SNF Part A payments), except to the extent the services listed in paragraphs (1) through (10) of this definition are themselves payable through a composite rate (that is, all services provided as home health services or inpatient and outpatient hospital services are DHS).

Durable medical equipment (DME) and supplies has the meaning given in section 1861(n) of the Act and §414.202 of this chapter.

Employee means any individual who, under the common law rules that apply in determining the employer-employee relationship (as applied for purposes of section

3121(d)(2) of the Internal Revenue Code of 1986), is considered to be employed by, or an employee of, an entity. (Application of these common law rules is discussed in 20 CFR 404.1007 and 26 CFR 31.3121(d)-1(c).)

Entity means a physician's sole practice or a practice of multiple physicians or any other person, sole proprietorship, public or private agency or trust, corporation, partnership, limited liability company, foundation, not-for-profit corporation, or unincorporated association that furnishes DHS. For purposes of this definition, an entity does not include the referring physician himself or herself, but does include his or her medical practice. A person or entity is considered to be furnishing DHS if it is the person or entity to which HCFA makes payment for the DHS, directly or upon assignment on the patient's behalf, except that if the person or entity has reassigned its right to payment to an employer pursuant to §424.80(b)(1) of this chapter; a facility pursuant to §424.80(b)(2) of this chapter; or a health care delivery system, including clinics, pursuant to §424.80(b)(3) of this chapter (other than a health care delivery system that is a health plan (as defined in §1000.952(l) of this title), and other than any managed care organization (MCO), provider-sponsored organization (PSO), or independent practice association (IPA) with which a health plan contracts for services provided to plan enrollees), the person or entity furnishing DHS is the person or entity to which payment has been reassigned. Provided further, that a health plan, MCO, PSO, or IPA that employs a supplier or operates a facility that could accept reassignment from a supplier pursuant to §§424.80(b)(1) and (b)(2) of this chapter is the entity furnishing DHS for any services provided by such supplier.

Fair market value means the value in arm's-length transactions, consistent with the general market value. "General market value" means the price that an asset would bring, as the result of *bona fide* bargaining between well-informed buyers and sellers who are not otherwise in a position to generate business for the other party; or the compensation that would be included in a service agreement, as the result of bona fide bargaining between well-informed parties to the agreement who are not otherwise in a position to generate business for the other party, on the date of acquisition of the asset or at the time of the service agreement. Usually, the fair market price is the price at which bona fide sales have been consummated for assets of like type, quality, and quantity in a particular market at the time of acquisition, or the compensation that has been included in bona fide service agreements with comparable terms at the time of the agreement. With respect to the rentals and leases

described in §411.357(a) and (b), "fair market value" means the value of rental property for general commercial purposes (not taking into account its intended use). In the case of a lease of space, this value may not be adjusted to reflect the additional value the prospective lessee or lessor would attribute to the proximity or convenience to the lessor when the lessor is a potential source of patient referrals to the lessee. For purposes of this section, a rental payment does not take into account intended use if it takes into account costs incurred by the lessor in developing or upgrading the property or maintaining the property or its improvements.

Home health services means the services described in section 1861(m) of the Act and part 409, subpart E of this chapter.

Hospital means any entity that qualifies as a "hospital" under section 1861(e) of the Act, as a "psychiatric hospital" under section 1861(f) of the Act, or as a "rural primary care hospital" under section 1861(mm)(1) of the Act, and refers to any separate legally organized operating entity plus any subsidiary, related entity, or other entities that perform services for the hospital's patients and for which the hospital bills. However, a "hospital" does not include entities that perform services for hospital patients "under arrangements" with the hospital.

HPSA means, for purposes of this subpart, an area designated as a health professional shortage area under section 332(a)(1)(A) of the Public Health Service Act for primary medical care professionals (in accordance with the criteria specified in part 5 of this title).

Immediate family member or member of a physician's immediate family means husband or wife; birth or adoptive parent, child, or sibling; stepparent, stepchild, stepbrother, or stepsister; father-in-law, mother-in-law, son-in-law, daughter-in-law, brother-in-law, or sister-in-law; grandparent or grandchild; and spouse of a grandparent or grandchild.

"Incident to" services means those services that meet the requirements of section 1861(s)(2)(A) of the Act and section 2050 of the Medicare Carriers Manual (HCFA Pub. 14-3), Part 3—Claims Process. (Those wishing to subscribe to program manuals should contact either the Government Printing Office (GPO) or the National Technical Information Service (NTIS) at the following addresses: Superintendent of Documents, Government Printing Office, ATTN: New Orders, P.O. Box 371954, Pittsburgh, PA 15250-7954, Telephone (202) 512-1800, Fax number (202) 512-2250 (for credit card orders); or

National Technical Information Service, Department of Commerce, 5825 Port Royal Road, Springfield, VA 22161, Telephone (703) 487-4630. In addition, individual manual transmittals and Program Memoranda can be purchased from NTIS. Interested parties should identify the transmittal(s) they want. GPO or NTIS can give complete details on how to obtain the publications they sell. Additionally, all manuals are available at the following Internet address: http://www.hcfa.gov/pubforms/progman.htm.)

Inpatient hospital services means those services as defined in section 1861(b) of the Act and §409.10(a) and (b) of this chapter and includes inpatient psychiatric hospital services listed in section 1861(c) of the Act and inpatient rural primary care hospital services, as defined in section 1861(mm)(2) of the Act. "Inpatient hospital services" do not include emergency inpatient services provided by a hospital located outside of the U.S. and covered under the authority in section 1814(f)(2) of the Act and part 424, subpart H of this chapter, or emergency inpatient services provided by a nonparticipating hospital within the U.S., as authorized by section 1814(d) of the Act and described in part 424, subpart G of this chapter. These services also do not include dialysis furnished by a hospital that is not certified to provide end-stage renal dialysis (ESRD) services under subpart U of part 405 of this chapter. Inpatient hospital services include services that a hospital provides for its patients that are furnished either by the hospital or by others under arrangements with the hospital. "Inpatient hospital services" do not include professional services performed by physicians, physician assistants, nurse practitioners, clinical nurse specialists, certified nurse midwives, and certified registered nurse anesthetists and qualified psychologists if Medicare reimburses the services independently and not as part of the inpatient hospital service (even if they are billed by a hospital under an assignment or reassignment).

Laboratory means an entity furnishing biological, microbiological, serological, chemical, immunohematological, hematological, biophysical, cytological, pathological, or other examination of materials derived from the human body for the purpose of providing information for the diagnosis, prevention, or treatment of any disease or impairment of, or the assessment of the health of, human beings. These examinations also include procedures to determine, measure, or otherwise describe the presence or absence of various substances or organisms in the body. Entities only collecting or preparing specimens (or both) or only serving as a mailing service and not performing testing are not considered laboratories.

List of CPT/HCPCS Codes Used to Describe Certain Designated Health Services Under the Physician Referral Provisions (Section 1877 of the Social Security Act) means the list of certain designated health services under section 1877 of the Act initially posted on the HCFA web site and updated annually thereafter in an addendum to the physician fee schedule final rule and on the HCFA web site.

Member of the group means, for purposes of this rule, a direct or indirect physician owner of a group practice (including a physician whose interest is held by his or her individual professional corporation or by another entity), a physician employee of the group practice (including a physician employed by his or her individual professional corporation that has an equity interest in the group practice), a locum tenens physician (as defined in this section), or an on-call physician while the physician is providing on-call services for members of the group practice. A physician is a member of the group during the time he or she furnishes "patient care services" to the group as defined in this section. An independent contractor or a leased employee is not a member of the group. "Locum tenens physician" means a physician who substitutes (that is, "stands in the shoes") in exigent circumstances for a regular physician who is a member of the group, in accordance with applicable reassignment rules and regulations, including section 3060 of the Medicare Carriers Manual (HCFA Pub. 14-3), Part 3—Claims Process.

Outpatient hospital services means the therapeutic, diagnostic, and partial hospitalization services listed under sections 1861(s)(2)(B) and (C) of the Act; outpatient services furnished by a psychiatric hospital, as defined in section 1861(f) of the Act; and outpatient rural primary care hospital services, as defined in section 1861(mm)(3) of the Act. Emergency services covered in nonparticipating hospitals are excluded under the conditions described in section 1835(b) of the Act and subpart G of part 424 of this chapter. "Outpatient hospital services" includes services that a hospital provides for its patients that are furnished either by the hospital or by others under arrangements with the hospital. "Outpatient hospital services" do not include professional services performed by physicians, physician assistants, nurse practitioners, clinical nurse specialists, certified nurse midwives, certified registered nurse anesthetists, and qualified psychologists if Medicare reimburses the services independently and not as part of the outpatient hospital service (even if they are billed by a hospital under an assignment or reassignment).

Outpatient prescription drugs means all prescription drugs covered by Medicare Part B.

Parenteral and enteral nutrients, equipment, and supplies means the following services (including all HCPCS level 2 codes for these services):

(1) *Parenteral nutrients, equipment, and supplies*, meaning those items and supplies needed to provide nutriment to a patient with permanent, severe pathology of the alimentary tract that does not allow absorption of sufficient nutrients to maintain strength commensurate with the patient's general condition, as described in section 65-10 of the Medicare Coverage Issues Manual (HCFA Pub. 6); and

(2) *Enteral nutrients, equipment, and supplies*, meaning items and supplies needed to provide enteral nutrition to a patient with a functioning gastrointestinal tract who, due to pathology to or nonfunction of the structures that normally permit food to reach the digestive tract, cannot maintain weight and strength commensurate with his or her general condition, as described in section 65-10 of the Medicare Coverage Issues Manual (HCFA Pub. 6).

Patient care services means any tasks performed by a physician in the group practice that—

Address the medical needs of specific patients or patients in general, regardless of whether they involve direct patient encounters; or

Generally benefit a particular practice.

Patient care services can include, for example, the services of physicians who do not directly treat patients, such as time spent by a physician consulting with other physicians or reviewing laboratory tests, or time spent training staff members, arranging for equipment, or performing administrative or management tasks.

Physical therapy, occupational therapy, and speech-language pathology services means those particular services identified by the CPT and HCPCS codes on the HCFA web site (and in annual updates published in the *Federal Register*). All services identified on the HCFA web site and in annual updates are physical therapy, occupational therapy, and speech-language pathology services for purposes of these regulations. Any service not specifically identified on the HCFA web site, as amended from time to time and published in the *Federal Register*, is not a physical therapy, occupational therapy, or speech-language pathology service for purposes of these regulations.

The list of codes identifying physical therapy, occupational therapy, and speech-language pathology services for purposes of these regulations includes the following:

(1) *Physical therapy services*, meaning those outpatient physical therapy services (including speech-language pathology services) described at section 1861(p) of the Act that are covered under Medicare Part A or Part B, regardless of who provides them, if the services include—

(i) Assessments, function tests and measurements of strength, balance, endurance, range of motion, and activities of daily living;

(ii) Therapeutic exercises, massage, and use of physical medicine modalities, assistive devices, and adaptive equipment;

(iii) Establishment of a maintenance therapy program for an individual whose restoration potential has been reached; however, maintenance therapy itself is not covered as part of these services; or

(iv) Speech-language pathology services that are for the diagnosis and treatment of speech, language, and cognitive disorders that include swallowing and other oral-motor dysfunctions.

(2) *Occupational therapy services*, meaning those services described at section 1861(g) of the Act that are covered under Medicare Part A or Part B, regardless of who provides them, if the services include—

(i) Teaching of compensatory techniques to permit an individual with a physical or cognitive impairment or limitation to engage in daily activities;

(ii) Evaluation of an individual's level of independent functioning;

(iii) Selection and teaching of task-oriented therapeutic activities to restore sensory-integrative function; or

(iv) Assessment of an individual's vocational potential, except when the assessment is related solely to vocational rehabilitation.

Physician means a doctor of medicine or osteopathy, a doctor of dental surgery or dental medicine, a doctor of podiatric medicine, a doctor of optometry, or a chiropractor, as defined in section 1861(r) of the Act.

Physician in the group practice means a member of the group practice, as well as an independent contractor physician, during the time the independent contractor is furnishing patient care services (as defined in this section) to the group practice under a contractual arrangement with the group practice to provide services to the group practice's patients in the group practice's facilities. The contract must contain the same restrictions on compensation that apply to members of the group practice under §411.352(g) (or the contract fits in the personal services exception in §411.357(d)), and the independent contractor's arrangement with the group practice must comply with the reassignment rules at §424.80(b)(3) of this chapter (see also section 3060.3 of the Medicare Carriers Manual (HCFA Pub. 14-3), Part 3—Claims Process). Referrals from an independent contractor who is a physician in the group are subject to the prohibition on referrals in §411.353(a), and the group practice is subject to the limitation on billing for those referrals in §411.353(b).

Physician incentive plan means any compensation arrangement between an entity and a physician or physician group that may directly or indirectly have the effect of reducing or limiting services furnished with respect to individuals enrolled with the entity.

Plan of care means the establishment by a physician of a course of diagnosis or treatment (or both) for a particular patient, including the ordering of services.

Prosthetics, Orthotics, and Prosthetic Devices and Supplies means the following services (including all HCPCS level 2 codes for these services that are covered by Medicare):

(1) *Orthotics*, meaning leg, arm, back, and neck braces, as listed in section 1861(s)(9) of the Act.

(2) *Prosthetics*, meaning artificial legs, arms, and eyes, as described in section 1861(s)(9) of the Act.

(3) *Prosthetic devices*, meaning devices (other than a dental device) listed in section 1861(s)(8) of the Act that replace all or part of an internal body organ, including colostomy bags, and one pair of conventional eyeglasses or contact lenses furnished subsequent to each cataract surgery with insertion of an intraocular lens.

(4) *Prosthetic supplies*, meaning supplies that are necessary for the effective use of a prosthetic device (including supplies directly related to colostomy care).

Radiation therapy services and supplies means those particular services and supplies identified by the CPT and HCPCS codes on the HCFA web site and in annual updates published in the *Federal Register*. All services identified on the HCFA web site and in annual updates are *radiation therapy services and supplies* for purposes of these regulations. Any service not specifically identified on the HCFA web site, as amended from time to time and published in the *Federal Register*, is not a *radiation therapy service or supply* for purposes of these regulations. The list of codes for radiation therapy services and supplies identified on the HCFA web site and in annual updates is based on section 861(s)(4) of the Act and §410.35 of this chapter but does not include nuclear medicine procedures.

Radiology and certain other imaging services means those particular services identified by the CPT and HCPCS codes on the HCFA web site and in annual updates published in the *Federal Register* (except as otherwise specifically excluded on the HCFA web site and in annual updates). All services identified on the HCFA web site and in annual updates are *radiology and certain other imaging services* for purposes of these regulations. Any service not specifically identified on the HCFA web site, as amended from time to time and published in the *Federal Register*, is not a *radiology or certain other imaging service* for purposes of these regulations. The list of *radiology and certain other imaging services* set forth on the HCFA web site and in annual updates includes the professional and technical components of any diagnostic test or procedure using x-rays, ultrasound, or other imaging services, computerized axial tomography, or magnetic resonance imaging, as covered under section 1861(s)(3) of the Act and §§410.32 and 410.34 of this chapter but does not include—

(1) X-ray, fluoroscopy, or ultrasonic procedures that require the insertion of a needle, catheter, tube, or probe through the skin or into a body orifice;

(2) Radiology procedures that are integral to the performance of, and performed during, nonradiological medical procedures; and

(3) Nuclear medicine procedures.

Referral—

(1) Means either of the following:

(i) Except as provided in paragraph (2) of this definition, the request by a physician for, or ordering of, or the certifying or recertifying of the need for, any designated health service for which payment may be made under Medicare Part B, including a request for a consultation with another physician and any test or procedure ordered by or to be performed by (or under the supervision of) that other physician, but not including any designated health service *personally* performed or provided by the referring physician. A designated health service is not personally performed or provided by the referring physician if it is performed or provided by any other person, including, but not limited to, the referring physician's employees, independent contractors, or group practice members.

(ii) Except as provided in paragraph (2) of this definition, a request by a physician that includes the provision of any designated health service for which payment may be made under Medicare, the establishment of a plan of care by a physician that includes the provision of such a designated health service, or the certifying or recertifying of the need for such a designated health service, but not including any designated health service *personally* performed or provided by the referring physician. A designated health service is not personally performed or provided by the referring physician if it is performed or provided by any other person including, but not limited to, the referring physician's employees, independent contractors, or group practice members.

(2) Does not include a request by a pathologist for clinical diagnostic laboratory tests and pathological examination services, by a radiologist for diagnostic radiology services, and by a radiation oncologist for radiation therapy, if—

(i) The request results from a consultation initiated by another physician (whether the request for a consultation was made to a particular physician or to an entity with which the physician is affiliated); and

(ii) The tests or services are furnished by or under the supervision of the pathologist, radiologist, or radiation oncologist.

(3) Can be in any form, including, but not limited to, written, oral, or electronic.

Referring physician means a physician who makes a referral as defined in this section or who directs another person or entity to make a referral or who controls referrals made by another person or entity.

Remuneration means any payment or other benefit made directly or indirectly, overtly or covertly, in cash or in kind, except that the following are not considered remuneration for purposes of this section:

(1) The forgiveness of amounts owed for inaccurate tests or procedures, mistakenly performed tests or procedures, or the correction of minor billing errors.

(2) The furnishing of items, devices, or supplies (not including surgical items, devices, or supplies) that are used solely to collect, transport, process, or store specimens for the entity furnishing the items, devices, or supplies or are used solely to order or communicate the results of tests or procedures for the entity.

(3) A payment made by an insurer or a self-insured plan to a physician to satisfy a claim, submitted on a fee-for-service basis, for the furnishing of health services by that physician to an individual who is covered by a policy with the insurer or by the self-insured plan, if—

(i) The health services are not furnished, and the payment is not made, under a contract or other arrangement between the insurer or the plan and the physician;

(ii) The payment is made to the physician on behalf of the covered individual and would otherwise be made directly to the individual; and

(iii) The amount of the payment is set in advance, does not exceed fair market value, and is not determined in a manner that takes into account directly or indirectly the volume or value of any referrals.

Same building means a structure with, or combination of structures that share, a single street address as assigned by the U.S. Postal Service, excluding all exterior spaces (for example, lawns, courtyards, driveways, parking lots) and interior parking garages. For purposes of this rule, the "same building" does not include a mobile vehicle, van, or trailer.

5. Section 411.352 is added to read as follows:

§411.352 Group practice.

For purposes of this subpart, a group practice is a physician practice that meets the following conditions:

(a) *Single legal entity.* The group practice must consist of a single legal entity formed primarily for the purpose of being a physician group practice in any organizational form recognized by the State in which the group practice achieves its legal status, including, but not limited to, a partnership, professional corporation, limited liability company, foundation, not-for-profit corporation, faculty practice plan, or similar association. The single legal entity may be organized by any party or parties, including, but not limited to, physicians, health care facilities, or other persons or entities (including, but not limited to, physicians individually incorporated as professional corporations). The single legal entity may not be organized or owned (in whole or in part) by another medical practice that is an operating physician practice (regardless of whether the medical practice meets the conditions for a group practice under this section). For purposes of this rule, a single legal entity does not include informal affiliations of physicians formed substantially to share profits from referrals, or separate group practices under common ownership or control through a physician practice management company, hospital, health system, or other entity or organization. A group practice that is otherwise a single legal entity may itself own subsidiary entities.

(b) *Physicians.* The group practice must have at least two physicians who are members of the group (whether employees or direct or indirect owners), as defined in this section.

(c) *Range of care.* Each physician who is a <u>member of the group</u>, as defined in §411.351, must furnish substantially the full range of patient care services that the physician routinely furnishes, including medical care, consultation, diagnosis, and treatment, through the joint use of shared office space, facilities, equipment, and personnel.

(d) *Services furnished by group practice members.*

(1) Except as provided in paragraphs (d)(2) and (d)(3) of this section, substantially all of the patient care services of the physicians who are <u>members of the group</u> (that is, at least 75 percent of the total patient care services of the group practice members) must be furnished through the group and billed under a billing number assigned to the group, and the amounts received must be treated as receipts of the group. "Patient care services" must be measured by one of the following:

(i) The total time each member spends on patient care services documented by any reasonable means (including, but not limited to, time cards, appointment schedules, or personal diaries). (For example, if a physician practices 40 hours a week and spends 30 hours on patient care services for a group practice, the physician has spent 75 percent of his or her time providing patient care services for the group.)

(ii) Any alternative measure that is reasonable, fixed in advance of the performance of the services being measured, uniformly applied over time, verifiable, and documented.

(2) The data used to calculate compliance with this "substantially all test" and related supportive documentation must be made available to the Secretary upon request.

(3) The "substantially all test" does not apply to any group practice that is located solely in an HPSA, as defined in §411.351.

(4) For a group practice located outside of an HPSA (as defined in §411.351), any time spent by a group practice member providing services in an HPSA should not be used to calculate whether the group practice has met the "substantially all test," regardless of whether the member's time in the HPSA is spent in a group practice, clinic, or office setting.

(5) During the "start up" period (not to exceed 12 months) that begins on the date of the initial formation of a new group practice, a group practice must make a reasonable, good faith effort to ensure that the group practice complies with the requirement set forth in paragraph (d)(1) of this section as soon as practicable, but no later than 12 months from the date of the initial formation of the group practice. This paragraph (d)(5) does not apply when an existing group practice admits a new member or when an existing group practice reorganizes.

(e) *Distribution of expenses and income.* The overhead expenses of, and income from, the practice must be distributed according to methods that are determined before the receipt of payment for the services giving rise to the overhead expense or producing the income. Nothing in this rule prevents a group practice from adjusting its compensation methodology prospectively, subject to restrictions on the distribution of revenue from DHS under paragraph (i) of this section.

(f) *Unified business.*

(1) The group practice must be a unified business having at least the following features:

(i) Centralized decision-making by a body representative of the group practice that maintains effective control over the group's assets and liabilities (including, but not limited to, budgets, compensation, and salaries).

(ii) Consolidated billing, accounting, and financial reporting.

(iii) Centralized utilization review.

(2) Location and specialty-based compensation practices are permitted with respect to revenues derived from services that are not DHS and may be permitted with respect to revenues derived from DHS under paragraph (i) of this section.

(g) *Volume or value of referrals.* No physician who is a member of the group practice directly or indirectly receives compensation based on the volume or value of referrals by the physician, except as provided in paragraph (i) of this section.

(h) *Physician-patient encounters.* Members of the group must personally conduct no less than 75 percent of the physician-patient encounters of the group practice.

(i) *Special rule for productivity bonuses and profit shares.*

(1) A physician in a group practice may be paid a share of overall profits of the group, or a productivity bonus based on services that he or she has personally performed (including services "incident to" those personally performed services as defined in §411.351), provided that the share or bonus is not determined in any manner that is directly related to the volume or value of referrals of DHS by the physician.

(2) "Overall profits" means the group's entire profits derived from DHS payable by Medicare or Medicaid or the profits derived from DHS payable by Medicare or Medicaid of any component of the group practice that consists of at least five physicians. The share of overall profits will be

deemed <u>not</u> to relate directly to the volume or value of referrals if <u>one</u> of the following conditions is met:

(i) The group's profits are divided per capita (for example, per member of the group or per physician in the group).

(ii) Revenues derived from DHS are distributed based on the distribution of the group practice's revenues attributed to services that are not DHS payable by any Federal health care program or private payer.

(iii) Revenues derived from DHS constitute less than 5 percent of the group practice's total revenues, and the allocated portion of those revenues to each physician in the group practice constitutes 5 percent or less of his or her total compensation from the group.

(iv) Overall profits are divided in a reasonable and verifiable manner that is not directly related to the volume or value of the physician's referrals of DHS.

(3) A productivity bonus for personally performed services (including services "incident to" those personally performed services as defined in §411.351) will be deemed <u>not</u> to relate directly to the volume or value of referrals of DHS if <u>one</u> of the following conditions is met:

(i) The bonus is based on the physician's total patient encounters or relative value units (RVUs). The methodology for establishing RVUs is set forth in §414.22 of this chapter.

(ii) The bonus is based on the allocation of the physician's compensation attributable to services that are not DHS payable by any Federal health care program or private payer.

(iii) Revenues derived from DHS are less than 5 percent of the group practice's total revenues, and the allocated portion of those revenues to each physician in the group practice constitutes 5 percent or less of his or her total compensation from the group practice.

(iv) The bonus is calculated in a reasonable and verifiable manner that is not directly related to the volume or value of the physician's referrals of DHS.

(4) Supporting documentation verifying the method used to calculate the profit shares or productivity bonus under paragraphs (i)(2) and (i)(3) of this section, and the resulting amount of compensation, must be made available to the Secretary upon request.

6. Section 411.353 is revised to read as follows:

§411.353 Prohibition on certain referrals by physicians and limitations on billing.

(a) *Prohibition on referrals.* Except as provided in this subpart, a physician who has a direct or indirect financial relationship with an entity, or who has an immediate family member who has a direct or indirect financial relationship with the entity, may not make a referral to that entity for the furnishing of DHS for which payment otherwise may be made under Medicare. A physician's prohibited financial relationship with an entity that furnishes DHS is not imputed to his or her group practice or its members or its staff; however, a referral made by a physician's group practice, its members, or its staff may be imputed to the physician, if the physician directs the group practice, its members, or its staff to make the referral or if the physician controls referrals made by his or her group practice, its members, or its staff.

(b) *Limitations on billing.* An entity that furnishes DHS pursuant to a referral that is prohibited by paragraph (a) of this section may not present or cause to be presented a claim or bill to the Medicare program or to any individual, third party payer, or other entity for the DHS performed pursuant to the prohibited referral.

(c) *Denial of payment.* Except as provided in paragraph (e) of this section, no Medicare payment may be made for a designated health service that is furnished pursuant to a prohibited referral.

(d) *Refunds.* An entity that collects payment for a designated health service that was performed under a prohibited referral must refund all collected amounts on a timely basis, as defined in §1003.101 of this title.

(e) *Exception for certain entities.* Payment may be made to an entity that submits a claim for a designated health service if—

(1) The entity did not have actual knowledge of, and did not act in reckless disregard or deliberate ignorance of, the identity of the physician who made the referral of the designated health service to the entity; and

(2) The claim otherwise complies with all applicable Federal laws, rules, and regulations.

7. Section 411.354 is added to read as follows:

§411.354 Financial relationship, compensation, and ownership or investment interest.

(a) *Financial relationships.*

(1) *Financial relationship means—*

(i) A direct or indirect ownership or investment interest (as defined in paragraph (b) of this section) in any entity that furnishes DHS; or

(ii) A direct or indirect compensation arrangement (as defined in paragraph (c) of this section) with an entity that furnishes DHS.

(2) A direct financial relationship exists if remuneration passes between the referring physician (or a member of his or her immediate family) and the entity furnishing DHS without any intervening persons or entities (not including an agent of the physician, the immediate family member, or the entity furnishing DHS).

(3) An indirect financial relationship exists under the conditions described in paragraphs (b)(5) and (c)(2) of this section.

(b) *Ownership or investment interest.* An ownership or investment interest may be through equity, debt, or other means, and includes an interest in an entity that holds an ownership or investment interest in any entity that furnishes DHS.

(1) An ownership or investment interest includes, but is not limited to, stock, partnership shares, limited liability company memberships, as well as loans, bonds, or other financial instruments that are secured with an entity's property or revenue or a portion of that property or revenue.

(2) An ownership or investment interest in a subsidiary company is neither an ownership or investment interest in the parent company, nor in any other subsidiary of the parent, unless the subsidiary company itself has an ownership or investment interest in the parent or such other subsidiaries. It may, however, be part of an indirect financial relationship.

(3) Ownership and investment interests do not include, among other things—

    (i) An interest in a retirement plan;

    (ii) Stock options and convertible securities until the stock options are exercised or the convertible securities are converted to equity (before this time they are compensation arrangements as defined in paragraph (c) of this section);

    (iii) An unsecured loan subordinated to a credit facility (which is a compensation arrangement as defined in paragraph (c) of this section); or

    (iv) An "under arrangements" contract between a hospital and an entity owned by one or more physicians (or a group of physicians) providing DHS "under arrangements" to the hospital.

(4) An ownership or investment interest that meets an exception set forth in §§411.355 or 411.356 need not also meet an exception for compensation arrangements set forth in §411.357 with respect to profit distributions, dividends, interest payments on secured obligations, or the like.

(5) *Indirect ownership or investment interest.*

    (i) An indirect ownership or investment interest exists if—

        (A) Between the referring physician (or immediate family member) and the entity furnishing DHS there exists an unbroken chain of any number (but no fewer than one) of persons or entities having ownership or investment interests between them; and

        (B) The entity furnishing DHS has actual knowledge of, or acts in reckless disregard or deliberate ignorance of, the fact that the referring physician (or immediate family member) has some ownership or investment interest (through any number of intermediary ownership or investment interests) in the entity furnishing the DHS.

    (ii) The entity furnishing DHS need not know, or act in reckless disregard or deliberate ignorance of, the precise composition of the unbroken chain or the specific terms of the ownership or investment interests that form the links in the chain.

(c) *Compensation arrangement.* A compensation arrangement can be any arrangement involving remuneration, direct or indirect, between a physician (or a member of a physician's immediate family) and an entity. An "under arrangements" contract between a hospital and an entity providing DHS "under arrangements" to the hospital creates a compensation arrangement for purposes of these regulations.

    (1) A compensation arrangement does not include any of the following:

        (i) The portion of any business arrangement that consists solely of the remuneration described in section 1877(h)(1)(C) of the Act and in paragraphs (1) through (3) of the definition of the term "remuneration" in §411.351. (However, any other portion of the arrangement may still constitute a compensation arrangement.)

        (ii) Payments made by a consultant to a referring physician under §414.65(e) of this chapter.

    (2) *Indirect compensation arrangement.* An <u>indirect</u> compensation arrangement exists if—

        (i) Between the referring physician (or a member of his or her immediate family) and the entity furnishing DHS there exists an unbroken chain of any number (but not fewer than one) of persons or entities that have financial relationships (as defined in paragraph (a) of this section) between them (that is, each link in the chain has either an ownership or investment interest or a compensation arrangement with the preceding link);

        (ii) The referring physician (or immediate family member) receives aggregate compensation from the person or entity in the chain with which the physician (or immediate family member) has a *direct* financial relationship that varies with, or otherwise reflects, the volume or value of referrals or other business generated by the referring physician for the entity furnishing the DHS. If the financial relationship between the physician (or immediate family member) and the person or entity in the chain with which the referring physician (or immediate family member) has a direct financial relationship is an ownership or investment interest, the determination whether the aggregate compensation varies with, or otherwise reflects, the volume or value of referrals or other business generated by the referring physician for the entity furnishing the DHS will be measured by the nonownership or noninvestment interest closest to the referring physician (or immediate family member). (For example, if a referring physician has an ownership interest in company A, which owns company B, which has a compensation arrangement with company C, which has a compensation arrangement with entity D that furnishes DHS, we would look to the aggregate compensation between company B and company C for purposes of this paragraph (c)(2)(ii)); and

(iii) The entity furnishing DHS has actual knowledge of, or acts in reckless disregard or deliberate ignorance of, the fact that the referring physician (or immediate family member) receives aggregate compensation that varies with, or otherwise reflects, the value or volume of referrals or other business generated by the referring physician for the entity furnishing the DHS.

(d) *Special rules on compensation.* The following special rules apply only to compensation under section 1877 of the Act and these regulations in subpart J of this part.

(1) Compensation will be considered "set in advance" if the aggregate compensation or a time-based or per unit of service-based (whether per-use or per-service) amount is set in advance in the initial agreement between the parties in sufficient detail so that it can be objectively verified. The payment amount must be fair market value compensation for services or items actually provided, not taking into account the volume or value of referrals or other business generated by the referring physician at the time of the initial agreement or during the term of the agreement. Percentage compensation arrangements do not constitute compensation that is "set in advance" in which the percentage compensation is based on fluctuating or indeterminate measures or in which the arrangement results in the seller receiving different payment amounts for the same service from the same purchaser.

[Note: A notice in the *Federal Register,* December 3, 2001 provides a partial delay in the last sentence above: " . . . A 1-year delay in the effective date of the last sentence in Sec. 411.354(d)(1) will give Department officials the opportunity to reconsider

the definition of compensation that is 'set in advance' as it relates to percentage compensation methodologies in order to avoid unnecessarily disrupting existing contractual arrangements for physician services. Accordingly, the last sentence of Sec. 411.354(d)(1), which would have become effective January 4, 2002, will not become effective until January 6, 2003. DATES: Effective date: The effective date of the last sentence in Sec. 411.354(d)(1) of the final rule published in the Federal Register on January 4, 2001 (66 FR 856), is delayed for 1 year, from January 4, 2002 until January 6, 2003."]

(2) Compensation (including time-based or per unit of service-based compensation) will be deemed not to take into account "*the volume or value of referrals*" if the compensation is fair market value for services or items actually provided and does not vary during the course of the compensation agreement in any manner that takes into account referrals of DHS.

(3) Compensation (including time-based or per unit of service-based compensation) will be deemed to not take into account "*other business generated between the parties*" so long as the compensation is fair market value and does not vary during the term of the agreement in any manner that takes into account referrals or other business generated by the referring physician, including private pay health care business.

(4) A physician's compensation may be conditioned on the physician's referrals to a particular provider, practitioner, or supplier, so long as the compensation arrangement—

(i) Is fixed in advance for the term of the agreement;

(ii) Is consistent with fair market value for services performed (that is, the payment does not take into account the volume or value of anticipated or required referrals);

(iii) Complies with an applicable exception under §§411.355 or 411.357; and

(iv) Complies with the following conditions:

(A) The requirement to make referrals to a particular provider, practitioner, or supplier is set forth in a written agreement signed by the parties.

(B) The requirement to make referrals to a particular provider, practitioner, or supplier does not apply if the patient expresses a preference for a different provider, practitioner, or supplier; the patient's insurer determines the provider, practitioner, or supplier; or the referral is not in the patient's best medical interests in the physician's judgement.

8. Section 411.355 is revised to read as follows:

§411.355 General exceptions to the referral prohibition related to both ownership/investment and compensation.

The prohibition on referrals set forth in §411.353 does not apply to the following types of services:

(a) *Physician services.*

(1) Physician services as defined in §410.20(a) of this chapter that are furnished—

(i) Personally by another physician who is a member of the referring physician's group practice or is a physician in the same group practice (as defined in §411.351) as the referring physician; or

(ii) Under the supervision of another physician who is a member of the referring physician's group practice or is a physician in the same group practice (as defined at §411.351) as the referring physician, provided that the supervision complies with all other applicable Medicare payment and coverage rules for the physician services.

(2) For purposes of paragraph (a) of this section, "physician services" includes only those "incident to" services (as defined in §411.351) that are physician services under §410.20(a) of this chapter.

(3) All other "incident to" services (for example, diagnostic tests, physical therapy) are outside the scope of paragraph (a) of this section.

(b) *In-office ancillary services.* Services (including certain items of durable medical equipment (DME), as defined in paragraph (b)(4) of this section, and infusion pumps that are DME (including external ambulatory infusion pumps), but excluding all other DME and parenteral and enteral nutrients, equipment, and supplies (such as infusion pumps used for PEN), that meet the following conditions:

(1) They are furnished personally by one of the following individuals:

(i) The referring physician.

(ii) A physician who is a member of the same group practice as the referring physician.

(iii) An individual who is supervised by the referring physician or by another physician in the group practice, provided the supervision complies with all other applicable Medicare payment and coverage rules for the services.

(2) They are furnished in one of the following locations:

(i) The same building (as defined in §411.351), but not necessarily in the same space or part of the building, in which—

(A) The referring physician (or another physician who is a member of the same group practice) furnishes substantial physician services that are unrelated to the furnishing of DHS payable by Medicare, any other Federal health care payer, or a private payer, even though the unrelated services may lead to the ordering of DHS;

(B) The physician services that are unrelated to the furnishing of DHS in paragraph (b)(2)(i)(A) of this section must represent substantially the full range of physician services unrelated to the furnishing of DHS that the referring physician routinely provides (or, in the case of a referring physician who is a member of a group practice, the full range of physician services that the physician routinely provides for the group practice); and

(C) The receipt of DHS (whether payable by a Federal health care program or a private payer) is not the primary reason the patient comes in contact with the referring physician or his or her group practice.

(ii) A centralized building (as defined in §411.351) that is used by the group practice for the provision of some or all of the group practice's clinical laboratory services.

(iii) A centralized building (as defined in §411.351) that is used by the group practice for the provision of some or all of the group practice's DHS (other than clinical laboratory services).

(3) They must be billed by one of the following:

(i) The physician performing or supervising the service.

(ii) The group practice of which the performing or supervising physician is a member under a billing number assigned to the group practice.

(iii) The group practice if the supervising physician is a "physician in the group" (as defined at §411.351) under a billing number assigned to the group practice.

(iv) An entity that is wholly owned by the performing or supervising physician or by that physician's group practice under the entity's own billing number or under a billing number assigned to the physician or group practice.

(v) An independent third party billing company acting as an agent of the physician, group practice, or entity specified in paragraphs (b)(3)(i) through (b)(3)(iv) of this section under a billing number assigned to the physician, group practice, or entity, provided the billing arrangement meets the requirements of §424.80(b)(6) of this chapter. For purposes of this paragraph (b)(3), a group practice may have, and bill under, more than one Medicare billing number, subject to any applicable Medicare program restrictions.

(4) For purposes of paragraph (b) of this section, DME covered by the in-office ancillary services exception means canes, crutches, walkers and folding manual wheelchairs, and blood glucose monitors, that meet the following conditions:

(i) The item is one that a patient requires for the purposes of ambulating, uses in order to depart from the physician's office, or is a blood glucose monitor (including one starter set of test strips and lancets, consisting of no more than 100 of each). A blood glucose monitor may be furnished only by a physician or employee of a physician or group practice that also furnishes outpatient diabetes self-management training to the patient.

(ii) The item is furnished in a building that meets the "same building" requirements in the in-office ancillary services exception as part of the treatment for the specific condition for which the patient-physician encounter occurred.

(iii) The item is furnished personally by the physician who ordered the DME, by another physician in the group practice, or by an employee of the physician or the group practice.

(iv) A physician or group practice that furnishes the DME meets all DME supplier standards located in §424.57(c) of this chapter.

(v) The arrangement does not violate the anti-kickback statute, section 1128B(b) of the Act, or any law or regulation governing billing or claims submission.

(vi) All other requirements of the in-office ancillary services exception in paragraph (b) of this section are met.

(5) A designated health service is "furnished" for purposes of paragraph (b) of this section in the location where the service is actually performed upon a patient or where an item is dispensed to a patient in a manner that is sufficient to meet the applicable Medicare payment and coverage rules.

(6) *Special rule for home care physicians.* In the case of a referring physician whose principal medical practice consists of treating patients in their private homes, the "same building" requirements of paragraph (b)(2)(i) of this section are met if the referring physician (or a qualified person accompanying the physician, such as a nurse or technician) provides the DHS contemporaneously with a physician service that is not a designated health service provided by the referring physician to the patient in the patient's private home. For purposes of paragraph (b)(5) of this section, a private home does not include a nursing, long-term care, or other facility or institution.

(c) *Services furnished by an organization (or its contractors or subcontractors) to enrollees.* Services furnished by an organization (or its contractors or subcontractors) to enrollees of one of the following prepaid health plans (not including services provided to enrollees in any other plan or line of business offered or administered by the same organization):

(1) An HMO or a CMP in accordance with a contract with HCFA under section 1876 of the Act and part 417, subparts J through M of this chapter, which set forth qualifying conditions for Medicare contracts; enrollment, entitlement, and disenrollment under Medicare contracts; Medicare contract requirements; and change of ownership and leasing of facilities: effect on Medicare contracts.

(2) A health care prepayment plan in accordance with an agreement with HCFA under section 1833(a)(1)(A) of the Act and part 417, subpart U of this chapter.

(3) An organization that is receiving payments on a prepaid basis for Medicare enrollees through a demonstration project under section 402(a) of the Social Security Amendments of 1967 (42 U.S.C. 1395b-1) or under section 222(a) of the Social Security Amendments of 1972 (42 U.S.C. 1395b-1 note).

(4) A qualified HMO (within the meaning of section 1310(d) of the Public Health Service Act).

(5) A coordinated care plan (within the meaning of section 1851(a)(2)(A) of the Act) offered by an organization in accordance with a contract with HCFA under section 1857 of the Act and part 422 of this chapter.

(d) *Clinical laboratory services furnished in an ambulatory surgical center (ASC) or end-stage renal disease (ESRD) facility, or by a hospice* if payment for those services is included in the ASC rate, the ESRD composite rate, or as part of the per diem hospice charge, respectively.

(e) *Academic medical centers.*

(1) Services provided by an academic medical center if all of the following conditions are met:

(i) The referring physician—

(A) Is a <u>bona fide</u> employee of a component of the academic medical center on a full-time or substantial part-time basis. ("Components" of an academic medical center means an affiliated medical school, faculty practice plan, hospital, teaching facility, institution of higher education, or departmental professional corporation.);

(B) Is licensed to practice medicine in the State;

(C) Has a <u>bona fide</u> faculty appointment at the affiliated medical school; and

(D) Provides either substantial academic or substantial clinical teaching services for which the faculty member receives compensation as part of his or her employment relationship with the academic medical center.

(ii) The total compensation paid for the previous 12-month period (or fiscal year or calendar year) from all academic medical center components to the referring physician is set in advance and, in the aggregate, does not exceed fair market value for the services provided, and is not determined in a manner that takes into account the volume or value of any referrals or other business generated by the referring physician within the academic medical center.

(iii) The academic medical center must meet all of the following conditions:

(A) All transfers of money between components of the academic medical center must directly or indirectly support the missions of teaching, indigent care, research, or community service.

(B) The relationship of the components of the academic medical center must be set forth in a written agreement that has been adopted by the governing body of each component.

(C) All money paid to a referring physician for research must be used solely to support bona fide research.

(iv) The referring physician's compensation arrangement does not violate the anti-kickback statute, section 1128B(b) of the Act.

(2) The "academic medical center" for purposes of this section consists of—

(i) An accredited medical school (including a university, when appropriate);

(ii) An affiliated faculty practice plan that is a 501(c)(3) or (c)(4) of the Internal Revenue Code nonprofit, tax-exempt organization under IRS regulations (or is a part of such an organization under an umbrella designation); and

   (iii) One or more affiliated hospital(s) in which a majority of the hospital medical staff consists of physicians who are faculty members and a majority of all hospital admissions are made by physicians who are faculty members.

(f) *Implants in an ASC.* Implants, including, but not limited to, cochlear implants, intraocular lenses, and other implanted prosthetics, implanted prosthetic devices and implanted DME that meet the following conditions:

   (1) The implant is furnished by the referring physician or a member of the referring physician's group practice in a Medicare-certified ASC (under part 416 of this chapter) with which the referring physician has a financial relationship.

   (2) The implant is implanted in the patient during a surgical procedure performed in the same ASC where the implant is furnished.

   (3) The arrangement for the furnishing of the implant does not violate the Federal anti-kickback statute, section 1128B(b) of the Act.

   (4) Billing and claims submission for the implants complies with all Federal and State laws and regulations.

   (5) The exception set forth in this paragraph (f) does not apply to any financial relationships between the referring physician and any entity other than the ASC in which the implant is furnished to and implanted in the patient.

(g) *EPO and other dialysis-related outpatient prescription drugs furnished in or by an ESRD facility.* EPO and other dialysis-related outpatient prescription drugs that are identified by the CPT and HCPCS codes on the HCFA web site, http://www.hcfa.gov, and in annual updates published in the Federal Register and that meet the following conditions:

   (1) The EPO and other dialysis-related drugs are furnished in or by an ESRD facility. For purposes of this paragraph, "furnished" means that the EPO or drugs are either administered or dispensed to a patient in or by the ESRD facility, even if the EPO or drugs are furnished to the patient at home.

"Dialysis-related drugs" means certain drugs required for the efficacy of dialysis, as identified on the HCFA web site and in annual updates.

   (2) The arrangement for the furnishing of the EPO and other dialysis-related drugs does not violate the Federal anti-kickback statute, section 1128B(b) of the Act.

   (3) Billing and claims submission for the EPO and other dialysis related drugs complies with all Federal and State laws and regulations.

   (4) The exception set forth in this paragraph (g) does not apply to any financial relationships between the referring physician and any entity other than the ESRD facility that furnishes the EPO and other dialysis-related drugs to the patient.

(h) *Preventive screening tests, immunizations, and vaccines.* Preventive screening tests, immunizations, and vaccines that are covered by Medicare and identified by the CPT® and HCPCS codes included on the HCFA web site and in annual updates published in the Federal Register and that meet the following conditions:

   (1) The preventive screening tests, immunizations, and vaccines are subject to HCFA-mandated frequency limits.

   (2) The preventive screening tests, immunizations, and vaccines are reimbursed by Medicare based on a fee schedule.

   (3) The arrangement for the provision of the preventive screening tests, immunizations, and vaccines does not violate the Federal anti-kickback statute, section 1128B(b) of the Act.

   (4) Billing and claims submission for the preventive screening tests, immunizations, and vaccines complies with all Federal and State laws and regulations.

   (5) To qualify under this exception, the preventive screening tests, immunizations, and vaccines must be covered by Medicare and must be listed on the HCFA web site and in annual updates.

(i) *Eyeglasses and contact lenses following cataract surgery.* Eyeglasses and contact lenses that are covered by Medicare when furnished to patients following cataract surgery that meet the following conditions:

(1) The eyeglasses or contact lenses are provided in accordance with the coverage and payment provisions set forth in §410.36(a)(2)(ii) and §414.228 of this chapter, respectively.

(2) The arrangement for the furnishing of the eyeglasses or contact lenses does not violate the Federal anti-kickback statute, section 1128B(b) of the Act.

(3) Billing and claims submission for the eyeglasses or contact lenses complies with all Federal and State laws and regulations.

9. In §411.357, paragraph (j) is added and reserved, and paragraphs (k), (l), (m), (n), (o), and (p) are added to read as follows:

§411.357 Exceptions to the referral prohibition related to compensation arrangements.

(j) [Reserved]

(k) *Non-monetary compensation up to $300.* Compensation from an entity in the form of items or services (not including cash or cash equivalents) that does not exceed an aggregate of $300 per year, if all of the following conditions are satisfied:

(1) The compensation is not determined in any manner that takes into account the volume or value of referrals or other business generated by the referring physician.

(2) The compensation may not be solicited by the physician or the physician's practice (including employees and staff members).

(3) The compensation arrangement does not violate the Federal anti-kickback statute, section 1128B(b) of the Act.

(l) *Fair market value compensation.* Compensation resulting from an arrangement between an entity and a physician (or an immediate family member) or any group of physicians (regardless of whether the group meets the definition of a group practice set forth in §411.351) for the provision of items or services by the physician (or an immediate family member) or group practice to the entity, if the arrangement is set forth in an agreement that meets the following conditions:

(1) It is in writing, signed by the parties, and covers only identifiable items or services, all of which are specified in the agreement.

(2) It specifies the timeframe for the arrangement, which can be for any period of time and contain a termination clause, provided the parties enter into only one arrangement for the same items or services during the course of a year. An arrangement made for less than 1 year may be renewed any number of times if the terms of the arrangement and the compensation for the same items or services do not change.

(3) It specifies the compensation that will be provided under the arrangement. The compensation must be set in advance, be consistent with fair market value, and not be determined in a manner that takes into account the volume or value of any referrals or any other business generated by the referring physician.

(4) It involves a transaction that is commercially reasonable (taking into account the nature and scope of the transaction) and furthers the legitimate business purposes of the parties.

(5) It meets a safe harbor under the anti-kickback statute in §1001.952 of this title, has been approved by the OIG under a favorable advisory opinion issued in accordance with part 1008 of this title, or does not violate the anti-kickback provisions in section 1128B(b) of the Act.

(6) The services to be performed under the arrangement do not involve the counseling or promotion of a business arrangement or other activity that violates a State or Federal law.

(m) *Medical staff incidental benefits.* Compensation in the form of items or services (not including cash or cash equivalents) from a hospital to a member of its medical staff when the item or service is used on the hospital's campus, if all of the following conditions are met:

(1) The compensation is offered to all members of the medical staff without regard to the volume or value of referrals or other business generated between the parties.

(2) The compensation is offered only during periods when the medical staff members are making

rounds or performing other duties that benefit the hospital or its patients.

(3) The compensation is provided by the hospital and used by the medical staff members only on the hospital's campus.

(4) The compensation is reasonably related to the provision of, or designed to facilitate directly or indirectly the delivery of, medical services at the hospital.

(5) The compensation is consistent with the types of benefits offered to medical staff members—

 (i) By other hospitals within the same local region; or

 (ii) If no such hospitals exist within the same local region, by comparable hospitals in comparable regions.

(6) The compensation is of low value (that is, less than $25) with respect to each occurrence of the benefit (for example, each meal given to a physician while he or she is serving patients who are hospitalized must be of low value).

(7) The compensation is not determined in any manner that takes into account the volume or value of referrals or other business generated between the parties.

(8) The compensation arrangement does not violate the Federal anti-kickback provisions in section 1128B(b) of the Act.

(n) *Risk sharing arrangements.* Compensation pursuant to a risk-sharing arrangement (including, but not limited to, withholds, bonuses, and risk pools) between a managed care organization or an independent physicians association and a physician (either directly or indirectly through a subcontractor) for services provided to enrollees of a health plan, provided that the arrangement does not violate the Federal anti-kickback statute, section 1128B(b) of the Act, or any law or regulation governing billing or claims submission. For purposes of this paragraph (n), "health plan" and

"enrollees" have the meanings ascribed to those terms in §1001.952(l) of this title.

(o) *Compliance training.* Compliance training provided by a hospital to a physician (or the physician's immediate family member) who practices in the hospital's local community or service area, provided the training is held in the local community or service area. For purposes of this paragraph (o), "compliance training" means training regarding the basic elements of a compliance program (for example, establishing policies and procedures, training of staff, internal monitoring, reporting) or specific training regarding the requirements of Federal health care programs (for example, billing, coding, reasonable and necessary services, documentation, unlawful referral arrangements).

(p) *Indirect compensation arrangements.* Indirect compensation arrangements, as defined in §411.354(c)(2), if all of the following conditions are satisfied:

(1) The compensation received by the referring physician (or immediate family member) described in §411.354(c)(2)(ii) is fair market value for services and items actually provided not taking into account the value or volume of referrals or other business generated by the referring physician for the entity furnishing DHS.

(2) The compensation arrangement described in §411.354(c)(2)(ii) is set out in writing, signed by the parties, and specifies the services covered by the arrangement, except in the case of a bona fide employment relationship between an employer and an employee, in which case the arrangement need not be set out in a written contract, but must be for identifiable services and be commercially reasonable even if no referrals are made to the employer.

(3) The compensation arrangement does not violate the anti-kickback statute or any laws or regulations governing billing or claims submission.

[Note: Additional regulations will be issued when Phase II is published. Phase II has not been published as of September 3, 2002.]

Endnotes

1. There is a comment in the final rule for Stark I legislation that says: "Even though we will [cover services listed in Stark II] under a separate proposed rule, this final rule . . . will affect how we review referrals involving any of the designated health services [under Stark II]" (August 14, 1995, *Federal Register*, page 41916).

2. May 13, 1999, Kathleen A. Buto, deputy director, Center for Health Plans and Providers, HCFA, Physician Self-referral Regulations Before the Committee on Ways and Means, Subcommittee on Health.

3. Specifically, the proposed rule originally stated: "Thus, we believe a physician's compensation can reflect a bonus for designated health services the physician personally performs or 'incident to' services the physician directly supervises, provided the services result from the referral of a physician other than the one performing or supervising the service. A physician in this situation is not being compensated based on the volume or value of his or her own referrals. A physician can receive compensation for *his or her own referrals* for designated health services only through the aggregation that occurs as part of over-all sharing of profits." [italics added] The 01/04/2001 final rulemaking takes a different approach.

4. Section 1877 of the Social Security Act.

5. Under the final rule, "immediate family member or member of a physician's immediate family" means husband or wife; birth or adoptive parent, child, or sibling; stepparent, stepchild, stepbrother, or stepsister; father-in-law, mother-in-law, son-in-law, daughter-in-law, brother-in-law, or sister-in-law; grandparent or grandchild; and spouse of a grandparent or grandchild.

Chapter 6

Entities Involved in Fraud and Abuse Investigations

The following entities and organizations may be involved in a fraud or abuse investigation.

- The Department of Justice (DOJ)

- United States Attorney General

- Federal Bureau of Investigation

- State agency for health care administration

- State licensing board

- Medicare/Medicaid carriers and intermediaries

- Office of Inspector General, Department of Health and Human Services (HHS)
  - Office of Audit Services
  - Office of Investigations

- Drug Enforcement Administration

- Internal Revenue Service (IRS)

- United States Postal Service

- Health Care Financing Administration (HCFA)

- Utilization and quality control peer review organizations (PROs)

- State attorneys general

- State Medicaid fraud units

- State bureau of investigation

- Private payers

- Self-insured companies

- Beneficiaries

- Competitors

- Present and previous employees

The HCFA administers the Medicare program. The HCFA oversees the payment of claims by local carriers and intermediaries, conducts fiscal audits, and sets policy to prevent and to recover overpayments. Within HCFA's Bureau of Program Operations is the Office of Benefits Integrity, which oversees each carrier's operations related to fraud, audit, medical review, the collection of overpayments, and the imposition of civil monetary penalties for certain violations of Medicare law.

Medicare Carriers and Intermediaries

The HCFA contracts with local carriers (ie, usually private insurance companies) to pay Part B claims for the Medicare program and intermediaries to pay Part A benefits.[1] The carrier's primary role regarding fraud and abuse is to identify cases of suspected fraud and abuse, develop them thoroughly, and, in a timely manner, take immediate action to ensure that monies are not inappropriately paid out and any mistaken payments are recouped.

The success of any carrier or intermediary in detecting fraud and abuse depends on how closely its medical review (MR) unit and its fraud unit work together. Each carrier requires personnel within the MR unit, whether they be in claims adjudication, payment utilization review, or a professional relations function, to take responsibility for identifying fraud and abuse and to be familiar with internal procedures for forwarding potential fraud cases to its fraud unit.

Carrier's Medical Review Unit

Each MR unit has the responsibility to ensure that services for which claims are submitted are medically necessary and appropriate. This includes the responsibility to detect and take action to correct program abuses. The term *abuse* includes incidents or actions of providers, physicians, or suppliers of services that are inconsistent with accepted sound medical practices, directly or indirectly resulting in (1) unnecessary costs to the program, (2) improper payment, or (3) program payment for services that fail to meet professionally recognized standards of care or are medically unnecessary.

As discussed in Chapter 1, the distinction between "abuse" and "fraud" is not always clear. The degree of intent possessed by the provider or supplier to abuse the Medicare program is often the measurement used. The MR units usually work closely with the fraud unit to resolve these types of occurrences, especially in situations where a provider has repeatedly submitted bills for which payment has been denied. Similarly, when the fraud unit has determined that a situation is not fraudulent, but rather abusive in nature, it usually refers those situations back to the MR unit for disposition.

This is a pivotal point in determining whether a physician's case is handled by the carrier or proceeds along a path that could ultimately result in criminal or civil monetary penalties. Cases handled by the MR unit will normally end in an overpayment request and/or an educational effort to improve compliance in the future (assuming that noncompliance is demonstrated in an audit or after completion of appeals). An overpayment request would include an assessment for any monies the carrier believes were received in error plus interest applied during the period the overpayments occurred.

Carrier's Fraud Unit

In general, a fraud unit is responsible for preventing, detecting, and deterring fraud and abuse within its service area. It determines the factual bases for leads and allegations of fraud made by beneficiaries, providers, HCFA, the Office of Inspector General (OIG), and others.

When appropriate, the fraud unit refers cases to the OIG for coordination of civil and criminal prosecution and/or application of administrative sanctions, including exclusion. Dissemination of information about fraud and abuse, both internally and externally, often originates from the fraud unit. Physicians may have seen fraud alert-type newsletters coming from their carriers. If and when a matter is referred to the OIG, the investigation will be intensified.

The Office of Inspector General

The OIG of the Department of HHS[2] performs audits and inspections of the Medicare program and other HHS programs as well as pursues investigations of suspected instances of fraud and abuse. In carrying out its responsibilities, the OIG may request information or assistance from HCFA and its contractors, including PROs.

The OIG has access to HCFA's files, records, and data as well as those of HCFA's contractors. The OIG investigates fraud, develops cases, and has the authority to take civil action in the form of civil monetary penalties and program exclusion, and to refer cases to the DOJ for further criminal or civil action.

The OIG has three divisions that might become involved in fraud and abuse cases.

1   Office of Civil Fraud and Administrative Adjudication: This office is responsible for coordinating activities that result in the negotiation and imposition of civil monetary penalties, assessments, and program exclusions. It works with the Office of Investigations, Office of Audit Services, HCFA, and other organizations in the development of health care fraud and exclusion cases.

2   Office of Investigations: The Office of Investigations, within OIG, is staffed with professional criminal investigators and is responsible for all HHS criminal investigations, including Medicare fraud. The Office of Investigations investigates allegations of fraud or abuse whether committed by contractors, grantees, beneficiaries, or providers of service (eg, fraud allegations involving physicians and other providers, contract fraud, and cost report fraud claimed by hospitals).

The Office of Investigations presents cases to the US Attorney's Office within the Department of Justice for civil or criminal prosecution.

When a physician or other person is determined to have failed to comply with his or her obligations in a substantial number of cases or to have grossly and flagrantly violated any obligation in one or more instances, the Office of Investigations may refer the case to the Office of Civil Fraud and Administrative Adjudication for consideration of one or both of the following sanctions:

- An exclusion from participation in the federal health care programs or any state health care programs as defined under 1128(h) of the Social Security Act

- The imposition of a corporate integrity agreement, including a monetary penalty, as a condition to continued participation in the Medicare program and state health care programs.

These two sanctions have been used extensively when the Department of Justice refuses to prosecute.

3   Office of Audit Services: This office conducts comprehensive audits to promote economy and efficiency and to prevent waste in operations and programs. The Office of Audit Services may request data for use in auditing aspects of Medicare and other HHS programs and is often involved in assisting the Office of Investigations in its role in investigations and prosecutions.

Occasionally, the OIG will get investigative help from the Federal Bureau of Investigation (FBI), which has allocated a significant number of its agents to help combat health care fraud. Under a special memorandum of understanding between the DOJ, OIG, and HCFA, the FBI has direct access to carrier data and other records to the same extent as the OIG.

Department of Justice

The OIG presents cases to the US Attorney's Office within the DOJ for civil or criminal prosecution. The FBI may also get involved in investigations of alleged health care fraud and abuse.

The DOJ may begin investigations as a result of private citizens' bringing *qui tam* actions against a physician or other health care professionals or entities. Under the Federal False Claims Act (FCA), in certain circumstances private individuals can file an action on behalf of the United States and obtain part of any recovery by the government in the action. The *qui tam* statute provides financial incentives to expose fraudulent activities. More than half of the $480 million the DOJ was awarded in health care fraud cases in fiscal year 1998 involved judgments or settlements related partially or completely to allegations in *qui tam* cases. More than one half of all *qui tam* suits involve allegations of fraud against HHS (ie, Medicare and Medicaid).[3] (Also, see Chapter 3 for a discussion of *qui tam* actions.)

The following excerpts from a joint report by HHS and DOJ illustrate activities related to fraud and abuse.[4]

The Department of Health and Human Services and the Department of Justice Health Care Fraud and Abuse Control Program
Annual Report for FY 1998
February 1999

United States Attorneys

Health care fraud involves many different types of schemes that defraud Medicare, Medicaid, the Department of Veterans Affairs, or other insurers or providers. The fraudulent activity may include double billing schemes, kickbacks, billing for unnecessary or unperformed tests, or may be related to the quality of the medical care provided.

United States Attorneys' offices (USAOs) criminally and civilly prosecute health care professionals, providers, and other specialized business entities who engage in health care fraud, and work with the Department's Civil and Criminal Divisions, and the FBI.

USAOs continue to cooperate closely with numerous federal, state and local law enforcement agencies who are involved in the prevention, evaluation, detection, and investigation of health care fraud. In addition to the HHS/OIG and HCFA, these agencies include the State Medicaid Fraud Control Units; Inspectors General Offices of other federal agencies; the Drug Enforcement Administration; Department of Defense, Defense Criminal Investigative Service; and the TRICARE Support Office in the Department of Defense.

To assist in coordination and communication at national, state, and local levels, each USAO has appointed both a criminal and civil health care fraud coordinator. Prior to the enactment of HIPAA, USAOs dedicated substantial resources to combating health care fraud, HIPAA allocations have supplemented these efforts.

Training

The Executive Office for the United States Attorneys' Office of Legal Education (OLE) is tasked with the responsibility for providing health care fraud training for USAO, and DOJ attorneys, investigators, and auditors.

. . . While the primary student body at each of these courses were DOJ employees, personnel from HHS/OIG and other agencies were also invited to participate as presenters and students. Additionally, USAO attorneys, investigators and auditors participated in a number of non-OLE sponsored, multi-agency health care fraud training courses over the last year.

Accomplishments—Criminal Prosecutions

The primary objective of criminal prosecution efforts is to ensure the integrity of our Nation's health care programs and to punish and deter those who, through their fraudulent activities, abuse the health care system and the taxpayers.

Each time a criminal case is referred to a USAO from the FBI, HHS/OIG, or other law enforcement agency, it is opened as a matter pending in the district. A case remains a matter until an indictment or information is filed or the case is declined for prosecution. In 1998, the USAOs had 1,866 criminal matters pending involving 2,986 defendants, a 23 percent increase over 1997. 322 cases were filed with 439 defendants. This represents a 14 percent increase over cases filed in 1997. Health care fraud convictions include both guilty pleas and guilty verdicts. During 1998, there were 219 criminal health care fraud convictions, involving 326 defendants.

Accomplishments—Civil Cases

Civil health care fraud efforts constitute a major focus of Affirmative Civil Enforcement (ACE) activities. The ACE Program is a powerful legal tool used to help ensure that federal laws are obeyed, and that violators provide compensation to the government for losses and damages they cause as a result of fraud, waste, and abuse. Civil health care fraud matters ordinarily involve the United States utilizing the False Claims Act, as well as the common law of fraud, payment by mistake, unjust enrichment and conversion, to recover damages from those who have knowingly submitted false or fraudulent claims. Additionally, in conjunction with a defendant committing a criminal health care fraud offense, the United States may file a civil proceeding using the Fraud Injunction Statute, to ensure assets traceable to such violation are available to repay those victims the defendant has defrauded.

Each time a civil matter is referred to a USAO it is opened as a matter pending in the district. Civil health care fraud matters are referred directly from federal or state investigative agencies, or result from filings by private persons known as "relators," who file suits on behalf of the Federal Government under the 1986 qui tam amendments to the False Claims Act and may be entitled to share in the recoveries resulting from these lawsuits.

At the end of 1998, the USAOs had 3,471 civil health care fraud matters pending. A matter becomes a case when the United States files a civil complaint, or intervenes in a qui tam complaint, in United States District Court. A large majority of civil health care fraud cases and matters are settled without a complaint ever being filed. In 1998, civil health care fraud cases filed increased 20 percent over 1997, from 89 to 107.

Civil Division

Civil Division attorneys vigorously pursue civil remedies in health care fraud matters, working closely with the USAOs, the FBI, the Inspectors General of HHS and Defense, as well as other federal and state law enforcement agencies. A total of 161 new health care fraud matters were initiated in 1998. In addition to pursuing more health care fraud allegations, the Civil Division is pursuing an increasing number of health care fraud cases in which the apparent single damages are particularly high.

Criminal Division

The Fraud Section of the Criminal Division develops and implements white collar crime policy and provides support to the Criminal Division, the Department and other federal agencies on white collar crime issues. The Fraud Section supports the USAOs with legal and investigative guidance and, in certain instances, provides trial attorneys to prosecute criminal fraud cases. For several years, a major focus of Fraud Section personnel and resources has been to investigate and prosecute fraud involving federal health care programs.

The Fraud Section has provided guidance to FBI agents, AUSAs and Criminal Division attorneys on criminal, civil and administrative tools to combat health care fraud, and worked on an inter-agency level through:

- updates on criminal, civil, administrative and regulatory efforts to combat health care fraud.

- updates on significant appellate decisions concerning health care fraud prosecutions.

- participation in the negotiated rulemaking committee which sought to develop standards for the shared risk exception to liability under the anti-kickback statute. The committee met several times and developed a committee report which is presently being worked by HHS into its final form.

- development of guidance on suspension of Medicare payments to ensure program integrity. The memorandum provides information to Department attorneys and AUSAs concerning the standards and process for suspension of Medicare payments. It also encourages the attorneys to engage in effective and timely communication with representatives of HCFA to discuss all significant issues which may impact the government's decision whether to employ the suspension remedy in a particular instance.

- development of a Statement of Principles for the Sharing of Health Care Fraud Information Between the DOJ and Private Health Plans. This is a general statement of principles governing the Department's exchange of health care fraud information with private health insurance plans as required by the HCFAC Program Guidelines issued by the Attorney General and the Secretary.

- providing frequent advice and written materials to AUSAs, and investigative agents, on confidentiality and disclosure issues regarding medical records which arise in the course of investigations and legal proceedings.

- reviewing and commenting on numerous requests for advisory opinions submitted by health care providers to the HHS/OIG and consulting with the HHS/OIG on draft advisory opinions per the requirements of HIPAA.

Justice Management Division

The Justice Management Division, Debt Collection Management Staff continues to perform various administrative and coordination duties. The duties of this office include: budget formulation, oversight and coordinating with the Office of Management and Budget and HCFA; development and data collection for the internal program evaluation; coordinating with HHS/OIG and the Department of the Treasury on the tracking of collections; coordinating with the GAO on required audits; and preparation and coordination of the annual report.

Federal Bureau of Investigation

Successful health care fraud enforcement cannot be achieved by any one agency alone. Investigations must be a cooperative effort if they are to be successful in combating the increasing problems of health care fraud. The FBI is involved in this cooperative effort. The FBI works many health care fraud cases on a joint basis with other federal agencies, including the HHS/OIG. These two federal agencies collaborate through attendance at health care fraud working groups, attend each others training conferences, and have a liaison program between the two organizations.

In addition, the Health Care Fraud task forces represent the coordinated efforts of the FBI, state and local law enforcement, investigative agencies such as Inspectors General, and private industry. The FBI and HHS/OIG share a common commitment to ending fragmented health care fraud enforcement.

In addition to providing new statutory tools to combat health care fraud, HIPAA specified mandatory funding to the FBI for health care fraud enforcement. In 1998, $56 million was provided by HIPAA for 569 positions (340 agents). The FBI used this funding, in large part, to fund an additional 44 agents and 28 support positions for health care fraud and to create several new dedicated Health Care Fraud Squads. This increase in personnel resources along with the direct FBI funding increased the number of FBI agents addressing health care fraud in the fourth quarter of 1998 to approximately 460 agents as compared to 112 in 1992.

As the FBI has increased the number of agents assigned to health care fraud investigations, the caseload has increased dramatically from 591 cases in 1992, to 2,700 cases through 1998. The FBI caseload is divided between those health plans receiving government funds and those that are privately funded. Criminal health care fraud convictions resulting from FBI investigations have risen from 116 in 1992, to 352 through the third quarter in 1998.

Health care fraud investigations are among those investigations having the highest priority within the FBI. The investigations are generally complex and require specific knowledge, skills and abilities to successfully investigate.

Often sophisticated, innovative and creative ideas are needed to combat and eventually prosecute the perpetrators of these crimes. As the complexity and long-term nature of health care fraud investigations increase, the FBI anticipates that the number of FBI investigations and convictions will begin to level off.

A considerable portion of the increased funding was utilized to support major health care fraud investigations. In addition, operational support has been provided for FBI national initiatives focusing on pharmaceutical diversion, chiropractic fraud, and medical clinics. Further, the Health Care Fraud Unit, FBI Headquarters, supported individual field offices with equipment and supplies to assist in numerous individual investigations.

Utilization and Quality Control Peer Review Organizations

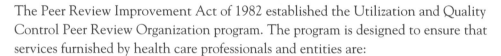

The Peer Review Improvement Act of 1982 established the Utilization and Quality Control Peer Review Organization program. The program is designed to ensure that services furnished by health care professionals and entities are:

1   Provided economically

2   Medically necessary

3   Of a quality that meets professionally recognized standards of health care

4   Supported by the appropriate evidence of medical necessity and quality in the form and fashion that the reviewing PRO may reasonably require (including copies of the necessary documentation) to ensure that the practitioner or other individual is meeting these obligations

State Medicaid Fraud Control Units

The Medicaid fraud control units (MFCUs) are responsible for investigating fraud. At present, 47 states have MFCUs and are receiving funds and technical assistance from OIG. Three states—Nebraska, North Dakota, and Idaho—have received waivers from establishing MFCUs as required by the Omnibus Budget Reconciliation Act of 1993.

The MFCUs conduct investigations and bring to prosecution persons charged with defrauding the Medicaid program or with patient abuse and neglect. During fiscal year 1999, OIG administered approximately $89.7 million in grants to the MFCUs to facilitate their mission.[5]

Although most Medicaid fraud cases are investigated by the MFCUs, OIG occasionally works with them and/or other law enforcement agencies on such cases.

The OIG's April to September 1999 *Semiannual Report* discusses some new joint audits of Medicaid.

Federal and State Partnership: Joint Audits of Medicaid

One of OIG's major initiatives has been to work more closely with State auditors in reviewing the Medicaid program. To foster the creation of these joint review efforts and to provide broader coverage of the Medicaid program, the Partnership Plan was developed. The partnership approach has been an overwhelming success in ensuring more effective use of scarce audit resources by both the Federal and the State audit sectors.

To date, partnerships have been developed in 22 States. Extensive sharing of audit ideas, approaches and objectives has taken place between Federal and State auditors. Completed reports have resulted in identifying potential program savings of $145 million and over $39 million in overpayment recoveries of Federal and State government funds.

Conclusion

Generally, one can conclude that as long as a resolving Medicare issue stays at the carrier level and is not referred to the OIG or DOJ, the matter (eg, an overpayment request) remains characterized as abusive activity.

If it requires the attention of the OIG or DOJ (ie, has been referred by the carrier fraud unit), these agencies explore ways to establish the existence of willful intent that would constitute fraud. At this point, there is little question but that the physician needs to contact an attorney.

Most audits are initiated by your Medicare carrier. A very small percentage of these will be turned over to the OIG to pursue fraud. You should do everything you can to supply your carrier with information in your medical records that indicate the services performed and medical necessity for those services. If you have any concern about a carrier-initiated audit, it is time to talk to your attorney.

Endnotes

1. The Medicare program is divided into two parts: (1) hospital insurance (Part A) and (2) medical insurance (Part B). Part A covers inpatient hospital services, limited stays in skilled nursing homes, hospice care, and some home health care. Part A coverage is responsible for hospital reimbursement under diagnosis-related groups. Entities known as *intermediaries* handle Part A services.

    Part B Medicare covers physician services, durable medical equipment, outpatient hospital services, x-rays, laboratory tests, home health, ambulance services, and the like. Entities known as Medicare *carriers* handle most Part B services. This publication focuses on physician services under Part B.

2. Actually, there are a number of Offices of Inspector General in addition to that of the Department of Health and Human Services that may become involved with health care fraud investigations: Department of Defense, Department of Labor, Office of Personnel Management, and Railroad Retirement Board.

3. Health Care Fraud Report, Department of Justice, fiscal year 1998. The full report is available at Web site www.usdoj.gov/dag/pubdoc/health98.htm.

4. The full report is available at Web site www.usdoj.gov/ag/98hipaa_ar.htm.

5. *Semiannual Report*, OIG, April-September 1999.

Chapter 7

Medicare Claims Review and Audits

When a Medicare claim is submitted, it is reviewed on several levels before it is paid. Today, these *prepayment* reviews are handled by computers in most cases. Postpayment review may also occur months, or even years, after payout is made.

Prepayment Review

Entitlement/Processing Issues

Before a claim is paid, certain factors, such as beneficiary eligibility, possibility of duplicate claim submissions, services excluded from coverage, and presence of other insurance coverage that may be primary to Medicare, must be checked. These factors are usually handled automatically by computer claims processing systems. If a problem arises with a particular claim, it will usually be returned as unprocessable.

Prepayment Review Edits

Medicare's computer—and occasionally staff—compare CPT® and ICD-9 codes and other information placed on claim forms against a number of prepayment edits before a claim is approved for payment. The edits may vary by physician specialty or provider category.[1] The general categories of prepayment edits are presented below.

- Procedure to procedure
  - Relationship between procedures
  - Example: office visit during surgical-postoperative period or procedures failing "correct coding" edits

- Procedure to provider
  - Specific procedures used by specific providers
  - Example: vascular surgery billed by an internist

- Procedure to sex
  - Services that may only be provided to a specific sex
  - Example: hysterectomy on a male patient

- Frequency to time
  - Specific procedures screened within certain time guidelines
  - One of the more complex edit categories

- Diagnosis to procedure
  - Specific procedures screened against a specific range of diagnosis codes
  - Example: level 5 office visit for a sore throat

- Procedure to provider certification
  - Specific procedures screened against the coverage guidelines for specific types of providers or suppliers
  - Example: podiatrists may bill Medicare only for certain procedures

A Medicare carrier's computer system automatically rejects claims with a high probability of being incorrect or medically unnecessary based on computer edits. In the past, some carriers used seemingly arbitrary edits, such as more than one custodial nursing home visit in a month; more than 31 subsequent hospital visits during a hospital stay; more than four electrocardiograms per year for a patient with a diagnosis of angina; automatic referral of certain types of services to medical review before payment; etc.[2] Today's screens are supposedly based on actual data that indicate potential aberrant billing.

For many common CPT® codes, Medicare Carrier's and others maintain computer files with "acceptable" ICD-9 diagnoses codes that supposedly justify the service billed. If a claim is submitted with a given CPT® code, the computer will check to see if the claim includes an "acceptable" diagnosis code. If not, the claim will be rejected, perhaps with a notice requesting additional information. These CPT® and

ICD-9 code pairings are computer edits. (See Chapter 8 for additional information on prepayment edits and medical necessity denials.)

Medicare's Correct Coding Initiative

A number of prepayment edits in Medicare's claims processing system are a result of a project started in 1996, which led to development of a massive database that identified inappropriate CPT® coding combinations and established certain coding policies. These policies and prepayment edits were developed by AdminaStar Federal, Inc, and incorporated into the *National Correct Coding Policy Manual for Part B Medicare Carriers*.

In addition to containing various coding guidelines and policy statements, the *Correct Coding Policy Manual* includes extensive coding edits that Medicare carriers use to approve or deny payment when two or more CPT® codes are billed for the same date of service by the same physician. These edits are revised quarterly. The *Correct Coding Policy Manual* is a useful tool in dealing with Medicare and even other payers when trying to determine if it is appropriate to bill one code with another code.[3]

A number of the correct coding policies clarify or add valuable insight into coding issues. Please keep in mind that a few of the Correct Coding Initiative policies appear to be in conflict with previous Medicare guidelines. Therefore, physicians should watch for carrier announcements before necessarily assuming there has been a change. In fact, AdminaStar prefaces its policy manuals with the statement: "These Correct Coding Policies do not supersede any specific Medicare coding, coverage, or payment policies."

Surprisingly, very few correct coding policies are currently aimed at evaluation and management services. However, a number of policies appear in these sections: Anesthesia, Surgery, Radiology, Laboratory, and Medicine.

Recently, the government began considering the use of other private contractors to develop better screens and enhanced audit programs. Consequently, we may see implementation of dramatically new prepayment edits.

Postpayment Review

The previous sections looked at *prepayment* edits that prevent payment from being made for claims that may have inaccurate beneficiary information, incorrect physician information, or CPT® or ICD-9 codes that may be inappropriate. Thus, payment is not made until the claim is corrected or documentation is submitted that supports the services and diagnoses billed.

Postpayment review and audits occur months, perhaps several years, after a claim is paid. Usually, the period from the date of service to the date of a postpayment audit is somewhere between 1 and 3 years, but it could be longer. Using these audits, Medicare carriers could recoup previous payments (plus interest) by asserting that the physician billed the wrong CPT® code or that the physician's medical records do not support medical necessity.

One medical director for a Medicare carrier made the following statement, which summarizes the postpayment review process:

> When reviewing claims, we **look first at *documentation* to see if the physician actually performed the service billed**. That is, did he/she perform each of the components of say a Level 5 Office Visit. In surgical cases we may look to see if a "Reduction with Manipulation" was billed when the service was really the lower paying "Reduction <u>without</u> Manipulation."

> If we are convinced the service billed was actually performed and that it meets Medicare coverage and billing guidelines, **then we look to see if it was medically necessary for the patient's condition** as reported using ICD-9 codes and/or documentation in the medical records. That is, was a Level 5 Office Visit necessary for a patient with a cold?

> **If the review fails either test, the claim is denied or down-coded to a lower-paying service.** Of course, we also look at any other special coverage or billing guidelines that may apply to the services performed. [boldface added]

Some of these postpayment audits are almost routine in that there is little suspicion that the physician or others are involved in a fraudulent activity. Many of the audits for evaluation and management codes were of this nature because carriers looked at the process as an educational effort during the first few years.

Of course, even "routine" audits could be elevated to the fraud category if a pattern of gross upcoding or billing for services not performed were identified. Some government officials are proposing that carriers perform more random audits, rather than relying as much on picking outliers or focused audits.

In many cases, Medicare carriers will select physicians for audits by comparing their utilization rate for certain CPT® codes to those of their peers (in the same locality and specialty). There are many legitimate reasons why physicians might appear on these reports: Medicare does not have their correct specialty[4]; they saw a higher number of severely ill patients during the period under review than their peers did (one who specializes in certain complicated problems might utilize higher levels or certain services more often than others); or peers are actually undercoding their claims. However, simply seeing more Medicare patients than others would not have an impact because utilization rates are calculated per beneficiary.

Actually, Medicare carriers audit a very small percentage of physicians annually. However, the odds certainly increase if a physician continues to fall at the upper end of utilization profiles. If a physician provides higher levels of service, it is extremely important to review medical record documentation to ensure that it passes muster in relation to CPT® requirements. Similarly, it is important to ensure that documentation supports the medical necessity of diagnostic tests.

Determination of Overpayments From an Audit

Audits are usually made on a small number of Medicare patient encounters. When an audit determines that an overpayment occurred, a carrier can request repayment of the actual dollars represented by the charts reviewed. For example, if billings for 24 of 25 encounters reviewed were considered correct, a carrier could ask for repayment of the amount at issue from the one remaining patient encounter. Usually this would be a relatively small amount. (Appealing audit determinations is discussed later.)

Unfortunately, carriers often use a small sample to calculate a larger repayment request. Assume that a sample of 25 patient encounters resulted in a carrier issuing an overpayment request for $1,000 and during the past 3 years the audited physician has billed the codes in the sample a total of 500 times. While it is a little more complicated than this, essentially Medicare carriers may issue an overpayment request for $20,000 (500/25 X $1,000), plus interest, through a process of extrapolation.

Extrapolation can result in some very large overpayment requests. Consultants report overpayment determinations in the hundreds of thousands of dollars for physicians with a large Medicare patient base.[5]

Statistically Valid Random Samples and Consent Settlements

Medicare carriers can assess these extrapolated overpayment requests by conducting a *Statistically Valid Random Sample* (SVRS), or they may reach a *Consent Settlement* based on a much smaller sample size than necessary for a SVRS. A statistically valid random sample would likely require audit of many more patient encounters than the 25 in the example above in most medical practices.

But a carrier could look at 25 encounters and notify the physician or other health care professional that they believe a larger sampling would produce an overpayment request of at least $20,000. At that point, the carrier could offer to settle without conducting the more complex and timely SVRS.

We have elected not to reproduce the statistical formulae and calculations required to conduct an SVRS. Readers may access the instructions by reviewing the *Medicare Program Integrity Manual* available at www.cms.hhs.gov/manuals/108_pim/pim83c03.asp (select Chapter 8 of the manual for discussion of sampling and consent settlements) and the *Medicare Carriers Manual* at www.cms.hhs.gov/manuals/14_car/3b7000.asp (select Sections 7151–7170). The discussion in the *Medicare Carriers Manual* also includes information on compromise settlements (talk with your attorney), possibility of installment payments over a few months (not years) in hardship cases, and the like.

Section 8.3.3 of the *Medicare Integrity Program Manual* includes the following comments about consent settlements:

> The consent settlement process is an appropriate tool to modify a provider's billing practice while limiting contractor costs in monitoring provider practice patterns. Consent settlement documents carefully explain, in a neutral tone, what rights a provider waives by accepting a consent settlement. Also, the documents must explain in a neutral tone the consequences of not accepting a consent settlement. A key feature of a consent settlement is a binding statement that the provider agrees to waive any rights to appeal the decision regarding the potential overpayment.
>
> The consent settlement agreement must carefully explain this to ensure that the provider is knowingly and intentionally agreeing to a waiver of rights. A consent settlement correspondence must contain:
>
> - A complete explanation of the review and the review findings;
>
> - A thorough discussion of Sections 1879 and 1870 determinations where applicable; and
>
> - The consequences of deciding to accept or decline a consent settlement.
>
> When offering a provider a consent settlement, contractors may choose to present the consent settlement letter to the provider in a face-to-face meeting. The consent settlement correspondence describes the three options available to the provider.
>
> - Option 2—Acceptance of Potential Projected Overpayment
>
> Providers selecting Option 2 agree to refund the entire limited projected overpayment amount without submitting additional documentation. These providers forfeit their right to appeal the adjudication determinations made on the sampled cases and the potential projected overpayment that resulted from extrapolating to the universe. For providers who elect Option 1, do not audit any additional claims for the service under review within the time period audited. (If desired, waive Option 2.)
>
> - Option 1—Acceptance of Capped Potential Projected Overpayment
>
> Providers selecting Option 1 agree to submit additional pre-existing documentation. Review this additional documentation and adjust the potential projected overpayment amount accordingly. Do not audit any additional claims for the service under review within the time period audited for providers who elect Option 1.

- Option 3—Election to Proceed to SVRS

If a provider fails to respond, this option is selected by default. For providers who select this option knowingly or by default, thereby rejecting the consent settlement offer and retaining their full appeal rights, contractors shall:

Notify the provider of the actual overpayment and refer to overpayment recoupment staff. (See PIM Section 8); and Initiate an expanded review of a SVRS of the provider's claims for the service under review. (See PIM Section 8.3.2)

If the review results in a decision to recoup overpayment through the consent settlement process, the consent settlement must have been initiated within 12 months of the selection process. . . .

Readers should realize that a request from a Medicare carrier or other payer for documentation from a relatively small number of patient encounters can expand rapidly to a large overpayment request. And there is always the possibility that the audit results will be forwarded to the OIG and Department of Justice for determination of whether charges of fraudulent billing are warranted.[6]

Later we provide some tips for surviving an audit. If subjected to an audit, one will obviously want to present legitimate documentation and arguments that minimize the amounts the carrier determines were overpaid. Any improvement in the results of the small sample will minimize potential overpayment assessments in a consent settlement situation. Further, in subsequent appeals, those subject to an audit will want to rebut as many adverse findings as possible. But readers should understand that it is much easier to withstand an audit when adequate documentation is written or dictated at the time of service.

Outline of Postpayment Medicare Audit Process

Most physicians who have had to return money to Medicare or Medicaid have done so on the basis of an overpayment request following a postpayment audit by a Medicare carrier. As discussed above, postpayment audits usually result when a physician's utilization pattern for a specific service is markedly different from the pattern of peers. For example, a physician's frequency distribution of established patient office visits may indicate that usage of CPT® code 99215 is significantly greater than that of others in his or her specialty. Similarly, a physician may have a significantly higher utilization rate for diagnostic tests than peers do.

In these cases, a Medicare carrier might decide to review documentation for a small number of patient encounters to determine if there is justification for the higher utilization rates. On the basis of the audit findings, the carrier could decide to issue an overpayment request to the audited physician. The letter requesting repayment will provide details on how the overpayment was calculated, the physician's options for repayment, and appeals rights. Recipients of such letters should carefully comply with dates and options to ensure availability of appeal and other rights.

Below is a detailed outline of the postpayment audit process and the physician's appeal rights. While this is the audit process most physicians would experience, there are variations, such as investigations that include demands for immediate access to records, search warrants, and suspension of payments while an investigation is made. In these more aggressive situations, law enforcement agencies are usually involved.

I. Initial notification is provided by carrier, usually by a letter requesting copies of medical record documentation for specified patients and dates of service.[7]
    A. Letter describes random sample.[8]
    B. Letter may include indication of reason for audit.
    C. Copy of physician profile may be included if pertinent to audit.
    D. Thirty days are given to submit records or other support for services as billed (time period may be extended when justified).
    E. Sometimes carrier will go directly to a hospital, nursing home, or other facility and review records without physician's knowledge.
    F. If records are not submitted, carrier will usually deny services and issue an overpayment request.

II. Audit of records is usually conducted by a registered nurse from the medical review department or carrier medical director. Usually, the review will compare services billed to documentation in medical record to determine if billing was correct and services were medically necessary.

III. Physician may be contacted for additional information or clarification.

IV. Services of outside physician consultants of audited physician's specialty may be used in some instances.

V. File is reviewed with medical review committee and Medicare carrier medical director.

VI. Overpayment letter is sent to physician (assuming adverse findings), including following information[9]:
    A. Overpayment amount
    B. Individual audit findings report for each selected beneficiary
    C. Detailed findings from review
    D. Information from related publications
        1. Medicare Part B publications such as newsletters
        2. AMA CPT® book
        3. Medicare Carrier Manual guidelines or other such governmental publications
    E. Determination of "at fault" section 1870 of the Social Security Act and "liability" section 1879 of the Social Security Act

  F. Repayment options
    1. Full payment within 30 days
    2. Monthly installment, promissory (dependent on amount at issue)
    3. Financial alternate plan
    4. Automatic withhold from future claims payments
    5. Interest rate, approximately 13% to 15%
  G. Discussion of appeal rights (be sure to comply with time tables outlined in letter)

(Also see "Consent Settlements" in item IX.)

VII. CMS-mandated letters are sent to sample beneficiaries informing them to seek refunds for any amount paid out of their pocket for the denied services (these letters can create total confusion—beneficiaries are told they can appeal).[10]
  A. Letter usually states services were paid in error.
  B. Letter may state: "If there is a pattern of improper billing, we will refer this file for special handling."

VIII. Medicare hearing and appeal rights
  A. Amounts must exceed $100.00 for fair hearing.
  B. Request must be made within 180 days of the letter (the overpayment letter should include instructions).
    1. Send request in writing, certified mail, receipt requested.
  C. Hearing officer is usually a Medicare employee.
    1. Hearing officers are supposed to be unbiased and fair.
    2. They must be thoroughly familiar with Medicare regulations.
    3. Some carriers use attorneys as hearing officers.
    4. They must have general understanding of medical matters and terminology.
    5. Hearing officers must not be involved with initial decision.
    6. Hearing can be in person, on the record, or by telephone (overpayment letter will include details).
    7. All hearings are tape recorded (except for on the record).
    8. Physicians are entitled to transcripts or copy of tapes.
  D. According to Medicare Carrier Manual section 12016, a hearing must be scheduled within 120 days of request (although experience indicates there are often delays).
  E. Fair hearing decision should be rendered in 30 days according to Medicare (but it often takes longer).
  F. If physician is unhappy with fair hearing decision, he or she may appeal.
    1. Administrative law judge (ALJ) hearing must be requested within 60 days of fair hearing decision.
      a. Request in writing, certified mail, receipt requested.
      b. Be prepared to wait at least 1 year for hearing.
    2. Outstanding amount must be at least $500.
    3. Administrative law judge is an employee of the Social Security Administration.

    a. Most ALJ hearings are in person.

    b. They are much more formal than fair hearing.

    c. All testimony is under oath.

    d. Proceedings are tape recorded.

    e. Decisions are either unfavorable, partially favorable, or fully favorable.

    f. Hearing does not require representation by an attorney (but attorney's presence is often a good idea, especially if amounts are large).

    g. Preparation is key to obtaining desired result; flexibility is essential.

    h. Use of outside physician consultant is possible.

    i. Content of decision is at judge's discretion.

G. If physician is not satisfied with the ALJ decision, he or she may request a hearing by the Appeals Counsel.

    1. Hearing must be requested within 60 days of ALJ hearing decision.

    2. Appeals counsel can decide on its own to review any case.

    3. Hearing is not in person.

    4. Appeals counsel will review entire record.

    5. Additional information can be submitted by physician.

H. Next level of appeal would be through federal district courts.

IX. Consent settlements in overutilization cases

A. A consent settlement may be offered in the event the carrier convinces the physician he or she was at fault for the overpayment. Three options are offered at the time of a consent settlement.

    1. Acceptance of potential projected overpayment

        a. Physician agrees to refund entire limited projected overpayment without submitting additional documentation.

        b. Physician waives right to appeal adjudication determinations made on sampled cases and potential projected overpayment.

    2. Acceptance of capped potential projected overpayment

        a. Physician agrees to submit additional preexisting documentation.

        b. Physician agrees to overpayment as calculated after review of additional documentation.

        c. Physician waives right to appeal.

    3. Election to proceed to a statistically valid random sample

        a. Refer to step I of the Medicare audit process.

The audit process can be quite disconcerting for any physician. Physicians often feel singled out, and the carrier's letters can be threatening, particularly an overpayment request. Consultants report overpayment requests for a single physician in excess of $250,000 based on extrapolation from a random sample of 25 to 50 records.

Tips for Surviving an Audit

The recommendations below apply to the type of carrier audits just discussed. There are other concerns when it is likely that enforcers are looking into more serious offenses that could include criminal charges as well as civil penalties.

1   Cooperate with the carrier and supply information that is specifically requested. Do not send any additional information, such as records for other beneficiaries. Furnish only the portions of the record that are specifically requested. If the carrier needs additional documentation, it will request it.

While consultants generally advise limiting the information submitted to carriers to copies of medical records for the specific dates of service requested, it may be necessary to provide additional information if those records do not adequately describe the encounter.

Physicians should review all documentation before it is submitted to a Medicare carrier to make sure it clearly supports the services provided and the medical necessity for those services. While records should not be changed under any circumstances, an addendum can be added to include all pertinent aspects of the encounter and the patient's condition and treatment.

Too often, consultants report offices merely copying inadequate notes and sending them in without proper review. This is another reason to make sure original documentation is up to par. If it is, it will include all the information needed by an auditor. If documentation is inadequate, physicians could find themselves facing a large overpayment request or even more serious criminal charges.

Admittedly, even the best records may not prevent an auditor from denying services, but complete documentation improves the odds and will help when a physician appeals a carrier's decision.

2   Submit all records requested in a timely manner.

3   When copies of x-rays or other diagnostic tests are sent, be sure the lesion or pathology in question can be identified. Be sure to keep originals.

4   Make sure all records are legible; however, do not alter them. Altering records could turn a routine carrier audit into something more serious. If the records cannot be read, print or type an interpretation on another sheet and attach it to the medical record in question. When handwritten documentation is difficult to read, some practices send typewritten transcriptions attached to the original handwritten documentation, clearly marked as follows:

TRANSCRIPTION OF ORIGINAL RECORD
Mrs Gene Clark
Date of Service 12/31/99

5   If reference in a note is made to other records, the other records should also be provided.

6   Send all requested information by *certified mail, receipt requested*. Make and retain copies of all records you send. Make sure that you do not misplace the originals.

7   Exercise caution when talking to representatives of the carrier or any persons who may be involved in the review. Statements you make may be documented and used as potential evidence against you.

8   Communicate effectively with office staff to prevent any misunderstanding or misstatements. If you are being reviewed by Medicare, appoint only one person in your office to handle inquiries relative to the audit. The designated representative should be well informed as to the seriousness of the process and advised to keep you informed of all inquiries from Medicare personnel.

Designated office staff can coordinate responses if they are experienced in dealing with carrier audits and medical records. The physician still bears the responsibility, and he or she should review any information sent to the carrier before it is transmitted to ensure that the response adequately describes services performed and the medical necessity for those services.

Again, if there is any concern that this is anything more than a routine carrier audit, have an attorney review the response (it may be a good idea even if you are not concerned). Remember, if things escalate from a routine carrier audit to one involving fraudulent activity, *intent* will play an important part in the investigation and ultimate outcome.

9   If the carrier contacts you for an explanation of a complaint, make every effort to provide an accurate answer.

10   When preparing to exercise appeal rights, organize thoughts and materials. You are attempting to convince another medical professional that your actions were appropriate and that the bill for the services rendered was correct or that the codes used were reasonable in view of published guidelines and other information generally available to physicians. Remember that the final results of the audit may be extrapolated to reflect a representation of the overpayment for all services rendered during the review period. Any adverse findings that are overturned—no matter how small—will minimize ultimate recoupments.

11   In preparation for appeal, review all relevant Medicare Part B publications and portions of the AMA CPT® book that relate to the issues pertinent to your case. You will be better prepared if you know the arguments that will be presented by the carrier. Also, you want to make sure that you have been audited on the basis of the guidelines in place when the service was provided (consultants report cases where auditors used guidelines implemented after services were rendered).

12   Do not make any attempts to contact the beneficiaries or other potential persons who may be called in by the carrier. If the carrier determines this to be the case, it may be used against you at a later time. Potentially, you could be charged with obstructing an investigation.

13   Remain under control at all times when dealing with the carrier or any other persons or entities involved in hearing an appeal. Any statements made in anger could be used against you when subjective decisions are to be made.

Too often, physicians respond to these requests by writing a tersely worded letter to the carrier because they feel their professional decisions are being questioned. You are better off directing this energy into a response that clearly indicates the services performed and the medical necessity for services under review—this is what we did, and why we did it.

Keep in Mind

In conducting these types of postpayment audits, carriers usually look to see if documentation supports the services performed, the medical necessity for the services, and whether services and claim forms indicate compliance with any special Medicare coverage and billing guidelines existing at that time. If the review fails any of these tests, the claim is denied or downcoded to a lower-paying service.

Preparing for a Hearing: Fair Hearings and Administrative Law Judge

The following outline provides guidelines on preparing for a fair hearing or a hearing before an ALJ.

    I.   Request copy of complete record from carrier:
        A.   Stratified random sample claim listing
        B.   All carrier internal memorandums
        C.   Copies of any correspondence or communications
        D.   Complete individual audit summaries (by beneficiary)
        E.   Copies of any medical policy related to focus of the review

    II.   Make sure you understand every denial or reduction of service.

III.   Make sure claim was actually paid to physician or other health care professional.

IV.   Review all applicable Medicare published articles:
     A.   Medicare updates, AMA CPT®
     B.   Look for conflicts

V.   Summarize each patient's office or hospital care:
     A.   Recap patients' medical history.
     B.   List diagnoses being treated, complications, and other changes that justify services performed.
     C.   Note all drugs being taken.
     D.   Determine and document medical necessity for each denied test or procedure, in chronological order.
     E.   Indicate any abnormal test results.

VI.   Photocopy results of any services denied for lack of documentation.

VII.   Take entire medical record to fair hearing or ALJ hearing.

VIII.   Supply medical articles to the hearing officer or ALJ that support the medical necessity for denied services. (This is strong evidence, particularly for an ALJ.) Another source of evidence for medical necessity of diagnostic tests is information from the *Physicians' Desk Reference*.

IX.   Be familiar with sections 1870 and 1879 of the Social Security Act:
     A.   Known as "Waiver of Liability"
     B.   Reviewer must make a finding whether physician knew or should have known services would not be considered medically necessary.
     C.   Was the physician notified in writing about the medical policy?
     D.   Are there conflicts in policy?
     E.   Was the claim paid under appeal?
     F.   Are there other claims paid, after review, with same diagnosis?
     G.   Is their notification through AMA CPT® book?
     H.   Were articles published by Medicare and disseminated to physicians covering billing guidelines and other relevant policies?
     I.   Locate any medical articles that support treatment and/or frequency.
     J.   Has Medicare carrier published frequencies on the denied service?

Medicare Integrity Program

Earlier we mentioned the Medicare Integrity Program as a relatively new effort to prevent fraud and abuse. The Health Insurance Portability and Accountability Act of 1996 enacted the Medicare Integrity Program (MIP), which provides CMS with new authorities to contract with entities beyond, but also including, the current carriers and intermediaries to improve performance in program safeguard functions. The functions of the so-called *Program Safeguard Contractors* include medical review, cost report audit for hospitals and other facilities, data analysis, education, and fraud detection and prevention. Among other strategies to improve performance, MIP will lead to new prepayment edits, postpayment analyses, and audit targets.

The excerpt below from the *Federal Register* (March 20, 1998;63:13590-13608) illustrate the program's goals.

The Medicare Integrity Program

The Health Insurance Portability and Accountability Act of 1996 (Public Law 104-191) was enacted on August 21, 1996. Section 202 of Public Law 104-191 adds a new section 1893 to the Act establishing the Medicare integrity program (MIP). This program is funded from the Medicare Hospital Insurance Trust Fund for activities related to both Part A and Part B of Medicare. **Specifically, section 1893 of the Act expands our contracting authority to allow us to contract with eligible entities to perform Medicare program integrity activities performed currently by intermediaries and carriers.** These activities include medical, fraud, and utilization review; cost report audits; Medicare secondary payer determinations; overpayment recovery; education of providers, suppliers, beneficiaries, and other persons regarding payment integrity and benefit quality assurance issues; and developing and updating a list of durable medical equipment items that, under section 1834(a)(15) of the Act, are subject to prior authorization. [boldface added]

Congress established section 1893 of the Act to strengthen our ability to deter fraud and abuse in the Medicare program in a number of ways. First, it provides a separate and stable long-term funding mechanism for MIP activities. Historically, Medicare contractor budgets had been subject to wide fluctuations in funding levels from year to year. The variations in funding did not have anything to do with the underlying requirements for program integrity activities. This instability made it difficult for us to invest in innovative strategies to control fraud and abuse. Our contractors also found it difficult to attract, train, and retain qualified professional staff,

including auditors and fraud investigators. A dependable funding source allows us the flexibility to invest in innovative strategies to combat fraud and abuse. **It will help us shift emphasis from post-payment recoveries on fraudulent claims to prepayment strategies designed to ensure more claims are paid correctly the first time.** [boldface added]

Second, to allow us to more aggressively carry out the MIP functions and to require us to use procedures and technologies that exceed those currently being used, section 1893 greatly expands our contracting authority. Previously, we had a limited pool of entities with whom to contract. This limited our ability to maximize efforts to effectively carry out the MIP functions. Section 1893 now permits us to attract a variety of offerors with potentially new and different skill sets and will allow those offerors to propose innovative approaches to implement MIP to deter fraud and abuse. By using competitive procedures, as established in the FAR, our ability to manage the MIP activities is greatly enhanced, and the Government can seek to obtain the best value for its contracted services.

Third, section 1893 requires us to address potential conflicts of interest among potential MIP contractors before entering into any contracting arrangements with them. By requiring offerors/contractors to report situations that may constitute conflicts of interest, we can minimize the number of situations where there is either an actual or an apparent conflict. This is a concern particularly when intermediaries and carriers processing Medicare claims are also private health insurance companies. . . .

Detection of Potential Fraud and Abuse

Potential fraud and abuse may be detected in the following ways.

- Pattern of billing more office visits, injections, specific surgeries, specific endo-scopies, etc, than other physicians of the same specialty in the same locality, particularly more services per beneficiary

- Pattern of billing higher levels of evaluation and management codes than peers (or other codes with levels, times, etc)

- Complaints from patients, their families, or other sources indicating services billed were not rendered (this could occur to a consultant who saw a patient in the hospi-tal, but the patient was not aware of the service rendered because of his or her poor condition)

- Complaints from a disgruntled employee, an ex-spouse, an irate patient, a competi-tor, etc

- The Office of Inspector General hotline (800 HHS-TIPS)

- Carrier receipt of an altered bill

- Receipt of a claim for services rendered after a patient's death

- Inappropriate billing of supplies

- Complaints from other physicians or competitors

- Carrier utilization screens (one nursing home visit per month, etc)

- Aberrant utilization patterns and focused medical review data analysis: the focused medical review software package provided by CMS to all carriers supposedly defines referral patterns and source of all referrals per physician and provides CPT® utiliza-tion package comparison of all physicians in descending order

- Anonymous tips from employees (former or current)

- *Qui tam* suits

- Fraud alerts from other carriers

- Violation of Medicare charge limits

- Responses to fraud alerts published by the Department of Justice, CMS/HCFA, and Office of Inspector General

- Claim record data and common working file edits

Increasingly, physicians and some others may be brought into an investigation or audit because of the organizations with which they are associated. Physician practice groups at teaching hospitals are a good example.

The point is, as physicians and others become part of larger organizations, they become a bigger target. Obviously, a large organization that has a lot going on is more likely to violate—unknowingly or knowingly—one or more of the many complex rules that apply to government and other health programs. Finally, severe penalties levied on a large organization can adversely impact anyone associated with the organization regardless of personal wrongdoing. This is another example of the importance of an effective compliance program.

Endnotes

1. The government uses the term *provider* when referring collectively to physicians, hospitals, home health agencies, psychologists, suppliers, and other health care professionals and entities.

2. Remember, while claims may "kick out" because you see nursing home patients more than once in a month or you provide more than four electrocardiograms, and the like, you can still get paid if your documentation justifies medical necessity for such care. For example, your patient who resides in a nursing home may have developed a serious condition necessitating five visits during the month. Use ICD-9 codes appropriately and make sure your medical record documentation clearly indicates the necessity for the visits.

3. The manuals and CD-ROMs can be purchased from the National Technical Information Service, US Department of Commerce, by calling 800 363-2068. Because there are a number of ordering options and prices, use of the Web site www.ntis.gov/products/families/cci/ will facilitate getting the right manual for your purposes. An order form is available at www.ntis.gov/pdf/NCCOrderForm82.pdf. Some Medicare carriers have published some of the correct coding information in their monthly newsletter.

4. You should make sure that your physician specialty is listed correctly with Medicare (and other payers); otherwise, you might be compared to physicians of a specialty with markedly different billing profiles.

5. Carriers do not always extrapolate overpayments. Consultants report being involved in a number of audits where they have been able to keep the settlement related only to the services actually reviewed in the audit sample.

6. Details about what Medicare carriers can do when making an overpayment request are available in the Medicare Carriers Manual. These are available on the internet at www.cms.hhs.gov/manuals/14_car/3btoc.asp. Sections 7100–7170 include many of the details applicable to demand letters and other aspects related to overpayment requests.

7. Usually this is a relatively small sample. Medicare carriers vary as to the size of their routine sample. Consultants have reported a sample as small as 10 dates of service per physician, up to more than 100; 15 to 30 seems to be a common sample size for these routine audits.

8. If initial audit results are adverse, one may want to verify that the audit consisted of a *random* sample large enough to be statistically valid. This is critically important if the carrier chooses to extrapolate findings from the small sample to recoup payments from similar services over several years.

9. The time period from the initial letter requesting records to receipt of results varies considerably. Consultants report time periods from a few months to considerably more than a year.

10. Consultants report that this letter is not always sent, although it is part of CMS/ HCFA's carrier guidelines.

8

Medical Necessity Denials

Most physicians encounter a "medical necessity" denial when a claim fails to pass a Medicare carrier's prepayment edits. Medical necessity denials may also occur during a postpayment audit if the auditor determines that medical services were not necessary or a less intense service was more appropriate than the level billed. Repeated denials of claims through prepayment edits have been used as a basis for auditing a practitioner's records.

Noncovered Services vs Medical Necessity Denials

First, it is important to understand the difference between a noncovered service and one that is deemed not medically necessary. Under Medicare rules, some services are always excluded from coverage; thus, reimbursement is never available from Medicare. However, some services that are normally covered may be deemed not reasonable and necessary for a patient's current condition. These services would likely be denied as not medically necessary (other terms used for these denials are "medically unnecessary" or "not reasonable and necessary").

The following is an illustration of a situation that could produce a medical necessity denial:

Evaluation and management (E/M) services are normally covered. In most cases, a claim for an E/M service will be covered and paid by a Medicare carrier. However, five 99214

E/M visits for treatment of a common cold could result in denial of payment (or recoupment after an audit) for visits that a carrier might consider medically unnecessary.[1]

Payment Edits

For some CPT® codes, carriers have a list of ICD-9 diagnosis codes for which they will make payment. These are called *diagnosis* or *payment edits*.[2] Payment will be denied if a claim is submitted with an ICD-9 code that is not on the list. Other prepayment edits compare factors such as frequency to time (eg, number of events within a time frame). As an illustration, one carrier's guidelines for chest x-rays, including a listing of covered diagnoses, are provided at the end of this chapter.

When a claim fails to pass one of these computerized prepayment edits, denial notices will often indicate that the service has been deemed medically unnecessary or "not reasonable and necessary." These denials can be appealed if the physician believes the service was necessary.

Some carriers do a good job of releasing these covered diagnosis code edits in newsletters and other announcements. Sometimes, carrier representatives will release the information in response to a telephone inquiry (even if they do not release the diagnosis in formal publications). While physicians should bill only with these "approved" ICD-9 codes when it reflects their patient's condition, knowledge of the denial screens will help them bill appropriately or understand the denial.

Unfortunately, some carriers do not release many edits, particularly those unrelated to diagnosis codes. These carriers fear that physicians will tend to provide services up to the edit parameters. Keeping track of denials by Medicare carriers within the physician's office is a way to gain knowledge about these edits, but this knowledge should only be used to improve the accuracy of claims.

There is a Web site—www.lmrp.net—where CMS provides copies of each carrier's Local Medical Review Policies. These policies are extremely important in helping medical practices avoid prepayment denials for medical necessity and postpayment recoupments where medical necessity is questioned as result of an audit. While other carrier's policies are not necessarily binding in your area, you may be alerted to billing situations that should be reviewed for appropriateness. There is also a site where proposed/draft LMRP's are posted, www.draftlmrp.net.

Recommendation: Someone in every medical practice should be specifically responsible for reviewing payer newsletters and the LMRP Web sits for draft, newly adopted, or revised medical review policies. If the draft seems unreasonable, you should offer comments and contact appropriate medical societies, if necessary, to ensure adequate input into policy development. Make sure that someone is responsible for reviewing draft or adopted policies with respect to your current coding and billing practices. Change those practices if necessary.

Failing a medical necessity edit is *not* absolute. Medical necessity can still be established through review of documentation at a later date. The carrier's edits may have missed the inclusion of certain diagnoses that clearly justify a service. Perhaps the edits are too simplistic to weigh the need for a test or procedure when a patient has multiple diagnoses, more common treatments have failed, or complications arise. Medical necessity denials are often reversed on appeal, although appeals can be an administrative hassle at times.

As an example, many carriers have in the past denied nursing home claims for more than one or two visits in a month unless there is an indication that something unusual happened. For example, a patient may become very ill, necessitating a number of visits. A patient may fall, necessitating more visits than the average. Sometimes, using a different ICD-9 code that explains complications or an exacerbation of a chronic illness will help justify additional visits. Other times, the physician may have to ask that the denial be reconsidered on the basis of a letter of explanation or submission of medical record documentation.

This is also an example of why reviewing your Medicare carrier's Local Medical Review Policies is so important (as well as reviewing policies developed by other carriers). As this edition of this book is being written, there is a draft LMRP posted at the CMS maintained Web site, www.draftlmrp.net, that includes the following comments about subsequent nursing home visits:

Utilization Guidelines

Coverage for subsequent nursing facility care without a specific indication will be generally accepted as follows:

- One physician visit each 30 days for the first 90 days after admission and every 60 days thereafter.

Coverage for subsequent nursing facility care for evaluation of specific medical conditions will be considered reasonable and necessary if they would require the skill of a physician to evaluate the patient or were of such severity or duration as would generally occasion an office visit.

More frequent follow-up would require documentation of:

- Patient instability or change in condition that the physician documents is significant enough to require a timely medical or mental status evaluation and/or

physical examination to establish the appropriate treatment intervention and/or change in care plan;

- Therapeutic issues that require a timely follow-up evaluation to assess effectiveness of therapy or treatment including recent surgical or invasive diagnostic procedures, pressure ulcer evaluation, psychotropic medication regimens, or (for the terminally ill) comfort measures.

The following clinical situations are examples of conditions where weekly or more frequent visits may be considered reasonable and necessary:

- One physician visit per week for the following clinical situations

  - Stage III or IV pressure sore;

- Unstable COPD during acute management;

- Unstable angina follow-up;

- Urosepsis (not UTI) treatment (probably 2 visits before moving to routine follow-up);

- Rehabilitation patient not responding to expected progression of therapy;

- Unstable dementia or psychiatric problem requiring further medication titration;

- Unstable diabetes—initial therapy;

- Resolving herpes zoster or dermatitis (probably 2 visits before moving to routine follow-up);

- IV medications without complication;

- Pain regimen titration (beyond OTC's);

- Follow-up of fairly stable acute medical condition until off Part A level coverage.

- Two to three physician visits per week for the following clinical situations:

  - Presenting problem not responding to present regimen (probably no more than 2 visits before moving to weekly follow-up, if stabilizes);

  - Initial post-hospitalization for cardiac event (probably no more than 2 visits before moving to routine follow-up);

  - IV medications requiring titration;

  - Resolving pneumonia—x 1 week then weekly follow-up;

  - Resolving infected surgical wound;

- Ischemic limb with amputation as possible consideration if not responding to current treatment;

- Anti-coagulation therapy in DVT (not prophylaxis) patient;

- Unstable seizure disorder medication regimen titration or evaluation of TIAs.

- One physician visit daily for the following clinical situations:

  - Stage III or IV pressure sore with new secondary infection (probably no more than 2 visits before moving to weekly follow-up);

  - Unstable clinical situations such as recent transfer from hospital of patient with:

    Changing vital signs associated with their acute problem

    Ventilator dependent—until stable

    IV medications which require daily adjusting (probably no more than 2 visits before moving to 2 or 3 times per week follow-up)

    Infected surgical wound—2-3 visits then three times per week

- Any condition that would require hospitalization if not evaluated daily;

- Hyperglycemic, hyperosmotic diabetic situations elected to be treated at facility;

- End of life events requiring daily pain titration—last stages of death and VERY SHORT TERM.

Please remember that the LMRP above is only a Draft posted at draftlmrp.net during a comment period. It has not been published as an adopted local policy, and if it is ultimately adopted, would apply to services in that carrier's locality.

For Medicare to consider an item or service medically necessary, it must have been established as safe and effective, and services must be:

1   Consistent with the symptoms or diagnosis of the illness or injury under treatment

2   Necessary and consistent with generally accepted professional medical standards (ie, not experimental or investigational) and furnished by competent personnel in an appropriate setting for the patient's condition

Importance of the Distinction Between Noncovered and Medically Unnecessary Services

Physicians can bill their patients for noncovered services in the same manner in which they would bill a non-Medicare patient. If the service is truly noncovered:

- The physician is not restricted to an approved amount or a charge limit.

- The physician does not have to submit a claim to Medicare (unless requested to do so by the patient).

- The physician does not have to have the patient sign an Advance Beneficiary Notice (ABN) waiver form (assuming carriers make a clear and proper distinction between noncovered and medically unnecessary services). On the other hand, the physician's ability to collect for services deemed medically unnecessary often depends on whether the patient was *notified in writing prior to service* that denial was likely.

Services Considered Included in Payment for Other Services

Another type of denial that has become common in recent years has to do with the concept of bundled services.[3] A *bundled service* is one that is considered to be included in the allowance for other services.

Medicare rules consider payments for most telephone calls to be included within the allowance for other services. Thus, a telephone call between a physician is not separately payable under Medicare because it is considered to be included in the payment for other services, such as hospital visits (made either before or after the call). Similarly, Medicare will no longer pay for ventilation management on the same day that an E/M service is billed (the physician can bill for either the ventilation management or the E/M service, but not both).

The Introduction to the *National Correct Coding Policy Manual for Part B Medicare Carriers* describes unbundling as follows:

There are two types of unbundling; the first is unintentional which results from a misunderstanding of coding, and the second is intentional, when this technique is used by providers to manipulate coding in order to maximize payment. Unbundling is essentially the billing of multiple procedure codes for a group of procedures that are covered by a single comprehensive code.

Correct coding means reporting a group of procedures with the appropriate comprehensive code. Examples of unbundling are described below:

- Fragmenting one service into component parts and coding each component part as if it were a separate service. For example the correct CPT-4 comprehensive code to use for upper gastrointestinal endoscopy with biopsy of stomach is CPT-4 code 43239. Separating the service into two component parts, using CPT-4 code 43235 for upper gastrointestinal endoscopy and CPT-4 code 43600 for biopsy of stomach is inappropriate.

- Reporting separate codes for related services when one comprehensive code includes all related services. An example of this type is coding the total abdominal hysterectomy with or without removal of tubes, with or without removal of ovary (CPT-4 code 58150) and salpingectomy (CPT-4 code 58700) and oophorectomy (CPT-4 code 58940) rather than using the comprehensive CPT-4 code 58150 for all three related services.

- Breaking out bilateral procedures when one code is appropriate. In this example, a bilateral mammography is coded correctly using CPT-4 code 76091 rather than submitting CPT-4 code 76090-RT for right mammography and CPT-4 code 76090-LT for left mammography incorrectly.

- Separating a surgical approach from a major surgical service. For example, a provider should not bill CPT-4 code 49000 for exploratory laparotomy and CPT-4 code 44150 for total abdominal colectomy for the same operation because the exploration of the surgical field is included in the CPT-4 code 44150.

Policy Manual Conditions & Format

The National Correct Coding Policy Manual has been developed with the following conditions applied: All policies and edits were formulated with the scenario of the same physician billing all of the CPT-4 codes involved.

The services are for the same beneficiary and provided on the same day. . . .

Each chapter consists of the Manual divided into two sections: Mutually Exclusive Procedures and Comprehensive and Component Procedures. Mutually Exclusive Procedures are those which cannot be performed during the same operative or patient session. The procedure code combinations in this category are divided into Column I and Column 2 procedures. The Column 2 procedure will not be reimbursed when it is rendered by the same provider on the same date of service since it cannot be performed during the same operative or patient session as the Column I procedure.

Comprehensive and Compound Procedure code combinations are divided into Column I and Column 2 procedures. The Component procedure (Column 2) will not be reimbursed when it is rendered by the same provider on the same date of service since it is a part of the Comprehensive procedure.

IMPORTANT: It is critical to search for each procedure code as the Comprehensive code in order to determine if in fact your procedure code combinations are found in the CCI edit list.

Many other guidelines besides those published in the *Manual* may prohibit billing one code with another. The *Manual* is revised periodically to update guidelines and correct any errors in previous editions. The *Manual* is a useful tool in dealing with Medicare and even other payers, but it is only one source of coding information.

Whenever Medicare denies payment for a service—and the reason for the denial is that the service is included within the allowance for another service—it is very difficult to achieve payment, and the patient should not be billed.[4] Again, the rationale is that the allowance for another CPT® code includes payment for the denied code.

> Notice that services denied as included in the payment for another service are not considered noncovered services. Therefore, it is generally inappropriate to bill patients for these services, because the care represented by the denied code is considered included within the allowance for another service (even on nonassigned claims).

Some other examples of services that will be denied by Medicare as included within the allowance of other services are 15850, Removal of sutures; 99000-99001, Specimen handling; 99050, Services after hours; and 99371-99373, Physician telephone calls.

Sometimes, CPT® codes are removed from bundled status. In 1994, physician care plan oversight (99375 and 99378) was considered to be included within the allowance for other services in all cases. However, in 1995, care plan oversight became covered and separately billable under Medicare for home health care services and hospice services (of course, there are special Medicare guidelines when these codes are used).

When a Claim Is Denied for Medical Necessity

One of the most confusing Medicare issues relates to services deemed medically unnecessary (ie, not reasonable and necessary). Part of the confusion has to do with a lack of communication among government officials, carriers, patients, physicians, and staff. More important, however, confusion is due to the way the denials are initiated and communicated to physicians and patients.

How It Works in Practice

How do carriers make a determination that a service is medically unnecessary? Generally, the initial denial notice is a result of the claim not passing a computer edit developed to weed out services with a high probability of being "not reasonable and necessary." These computer edits do not recognize all the circumstances of the encounter and are not always consistent with other guidelines. Often, such denials can be overturned by properly exerting the physician's appeal rights.

Many services denied as medically unnecessary are, in fact, legitimate medical procedures that have failed a carrier's computer screens. Other denials relate to care that should be more appropriately described as noncovered, ie, items and services always excluded from coverage under Part B of Medicare.

Billing for Services That May Be Deemed Medically Unnecessary

Nonparticipating physicians who do not accept assignment must refund to patients any amounts collected (including deductible and coinsurance amounts) for services or procedures that are determined by Medicare to be medically unnecessary. Similarly, participating physicians or nonparticipating providers who accept assignment and collect the copayment at the time of service for services deemed not medically necessary must refund the copayment.

This provision applies to both medical necessity denials and medical necessity reductions. For example, if Medicare determines that a less costly diagnostic procedure would have been sufficient to obtain the same results, the carrier may then require a refund to the patient equal to the amount the physician collected that exceeded the physician's limiting charge for the less extensive procedure (or a refund of the copayment if collected at the time of service). Thus, it is important for physicians to use their independent medical judgment to determine the necessity for the particular procedure or service to be performed in the context of the patient's needs.

Note that a refund must be made within 30 days of notification by the Medicare carrier. However, a refund is not required if either of the following two conditions is met:

1   The physician did not know and could not reasonably have been expected to know that payment may not be made for the services or procedures because they were not reasonable and necessary, or

2   Before the services or procedures were furnished, the patient was informed that Medicare payments might not be made for the specific services or procedures because they could be deemed medically unnecessary, and the patient agreed to pay the physician for the services or procedures.

In essence, physicians are not required to make a refund for medical necessity denials if their patients agree in advance to pay for the service (yes, it does seem impractical to have to tell patients that a service about to be performed could be medically unnecessary). Having a patient sign a waiver of liability form—the form is now commonly called an Advanced Beneficiary Notice (ABN)—is sufficient acknowledgment that the patient has agreed to pay for the service, even if it is denied as "not reasonable and necessary".[5]

To qualify as a proper ABN and avoid having to make a refund, the notification must meet these criteria:

- It was obtained before the service
- It identifies the actual services to be performed
- It includes reasons for believing a denial is possible

Most Medicare carriers allow physicians to attach the modifier "-GA"—or a similar modifier the carrier may accept—to the CPT® code for which a proper ABN was signed by the patient.

Advanced Beneficiary Notice (ABN)

As this edition of *Health Care Fraud and Abuse* is being written, we are in a transition period from the original ABN established under legislation passed in 1986 to a revised form that is supposed to be used exclusive after October 1, 2002. You should review your Medicare carrier's announcements to ensure full compliance with the new instructions. As of August 2002, one can still use the original Waiver of Liability form or the newly adopted ABN form.

As a little history, prior to the enactment of the Omnibus Budget Reconciliation Act of 1986 (OBRA '86), Medicare beneficiaries were liable (ie, had to pay the physician or other provider) for any services determined not to be "reasonable and necessary" under section 1863(a)(1) of the Social Security Act. OBRA '86 added the limitation of liability provision (or waiver of liability provision) to the Social Security Act. This provided beneficiaries with protection from liability when they, in good faith, received services from a Medicare provider for which Medicare payment is subsequently denied as "not reasonable and necessary."

A waiver of liability statement/form signed by the patient was required to "protect" beneficiaries, physicians, and other providers by advising that an anticipated service may not be covered under Medicare because it was not reasonable and necessary. Waivers were to be signed by the beneficiary and dated prior to having services performed.

This entire Waiver of Liability process, including the forms suggested by Medicare agencies, were quite confusing to patients and physicians. In the past two years, CMS has taken efforts to improve the situation, although the basic principles have not changed dramatically.

Medicare's Waiver of Liability

The original waiver of liability form that the government has recommended since the 1980s is displayed below:

Dear Patient:

Medicare will only pay for services that it determines to be "reasonable and necessary" under section 1862(a)(1) of Medicare law. If Medicare determines that a particular service, although it would otherwise be covered, is not "reasonable and necessary" under Medicare program standards, Medicare will deny payment for that service. I believe that, in your case, Medicare is likely to deny payment for:

CPT Code _____   **Procedure (Specify)** _____

_____

for the following reasons: _____

_____

_____

Beneficiary Agreement:

I have been notified by my physician that he or she believes that, in my case, Medicare is likely to deny payment for the services identified above for the reasons stated. If Medicare denies payment, I agree to be personally and fully responsible for payment.

_____   _____
Date   **Medicare Beneficiary**

Medicare requires that the reason(s) the service is likely to be denied must be indicated on the waiver notification form. Some of the acceptable reasons are listed below:

- Medicare usually does not pay for this many visits or treatments.

- Medicare usually does not pay for this service.

- Medicare usually pays for only one nursing home visit per month.

- Medicare usually does not pay for this injection.

- Medicare usually does not pay for this many injections.

- Medicare does not pay for this because it is a treatment that has yet to be proved effective.

- Medicare does not pay for this office visit unless it was needed because of an emergency.

- Medicare usually does not pay for like services by more than one doctor during the same period.

- Medicare usually does not pay for this many services within this period of time.

- Medicare usually does not pay for more than one visit a day.

- Medicare usually does not pay for such an extensive procedure.

- Medicare usually does not pay for like services by more than one doctor of the same specialty.

- Medicare usually does not pay for this equipment.

- Medicare usually does not pay for this lab test.

Medicare carrier announcements would usually state that the law does not require that the notice take the exact form displayed above; however, HCFA/Medicare has determined that this form meets statutory requirements.

When Medicare denies a claim as "not medically necessary," the physician has 30 days to either refund the beneficiary or request a review of the decision. (The request for review may be made any time within 6 months of the decision. However, the refund must be made to the patient if the request for review is not made within the first 30 days.)

New ABN Form

In June 2002, CMS published a revised Advance Beneficiary Notice (ABN), which may be used in connection with Medicare claims. The new ABNs are part of what CMS calls the Beneficiary Notices Initiative (BNI). You should watch for detailed announcements from your Medicare carrier.

Form CMS-R-131 is the new ABN that was approved by the Office of Management and Budget on June 18, 2002. There are actually two CMS-R-131 forms, the General Use form (ABN-G) and the Laboratory Tests form (ABN-L). Both CMS-R-131 ABN forms are standard forms that—unlike the prior notices—are not supposed to be modified by the physician's office. Both forms contain special boxes to handle the specific circumstances of the patient encounter requiring the notice. The CMS Web site, www.cms.hhs.gov/medicare/bni/, contains the forms, including Spanish translations, and instructions.

Following is a reproduction of the general use ABN form:

Patient's Name: _____   Medicare # (HICN): _____

ADVANCE BENEFICIARY NOTICE (ABN)

NOTE: You need to make a choice about receiving these health care items or services.

We expect that Medicare will not pay for the item(s) or service(s) that is described below. Medicare does not pay for all of your health care costs. Medicare only pays for covered items and services when Medicare rules are met. The fact that Medicare may not pay for a particular item or service does not mean that you should not receive it. There may be a good reason your doctor recommended it. Right now, in your case, **Medicare probably will not pay for –**

Items or Services:

Because:

The purpose of this form is to help you make an informed choice about whether or not you want to receive these items or services, knowing that you might have to pay for them yourself. Before you make a decision about your options, you should **read this entire notice carefully.**
• Ask us to explain, if you don't understand why Medicare probably won't pay.
• Ask us how much these items or services will cost you (**Estimated Cost: $**_____), in case you have to pay for them yourself or through other insurance.

PLEASE CHOOSE **ONE** OPTION. CHECK **ONE** BOX. **SIGN & DATE** YOUR CHOICE.

☐ **Option 1. YES.   I want to receive these items or services.**
I understand that Medicare will not decide whether to pay unless I receive these items or services. Please submit my claim to Medicare. I understand that you may bill me for items or services and that I may have to pay the bill while Medicare is making its decision. If Medicare does pay, you will refund to me any payments I made to you that are due to me. If Medicare denies payment, I agree to be personally and fully responsible for payment. That is, I will pay personally, either out of pocket or through any other insurance that I have. I understand I can appeal Medicare's decision.

☐ **Option 2. NO.   I have decided not to receive these items or services.**
I will not receive these items or services. I understand that you will not be able to submit a claim to Medicare and that I will not be able to appeal your opinion that Medicare won't pay.

_____   _____
       Date   **Signature of patient or person acting on patient's behalf**

NOTE: Your health information will be kept confidential. Any information that we collect about you on this form will be kept confidential in our offices. If a claim is submitted to Medicare, your health information on this form may be shared with Medicare. Your health information which Medicare sees will be kept confidential by Medicare.

OMB Approval No. 0938-0566   Form No. CMS-R-131-G   (June 2002)

Some key excerpts of CMS's ABN instruction to Medicare carriers are reproduced at the end of this chapter. Additional information related to ABNs is available at www.cms.gov.

The Appeals Process for Prepayment Denials

Many physicians overlook the appeals process. When a physician has a justifiable position, reviews and hearings are an avenue to claims payment. Claim denials are often reversed through reviews or hearings. The success rate substantially increases with proper documentation and when information is organized in a format that helps reviewers make the right decision.

Although review and hearing determinations are not officially binding on subsequent claim denials, a favorable result will at least improve a physician's position in future disputes. It is hoped that carriers will reevaluate their position to allow favorable decisions to become precedent.

Initial Review

An initial review is the first step in the appeals process. A physician may request an initial review by asking that the claim be reopened for review after receipt from the carrier of a denial, reduction in service, incorrect payment, etc. In this phase, the physician should copy the explanation of benefits or carrier's denial letter, highlight the portion of the claim in controversy, and clearly explain the issue.

A physician may request the review by letter or by using HCFA Form 1964. Recently, some carriers have developed special review request forms, which seem to work very well. Many carriers even allow telephone reviews in certain cases.

Essentially, a review is an *informal* reevaluation of the original claim. It is intended to be a complete reassessment by another reviewer; however, unless requests are carefully documented, initial reviews often result in a "rubber stamp" of the initial determination.

Generally, a 6-month period is allowed from the date of the initial denial or other determination in controversy to request a review (sometimes this period can be extended if good cause can be demonstrated). Although 6 months are allowed on denials for medical necessity, the physician is required to refund any overpayment within 30 days or refund any collections from the patient pending adjudication of the appeal (as discussed earlier in this section).[6]

Technically, the carrier must complete the review within 45 days of receipt of the request. Unfortunately, carriers generally interpret this as 45 working days (and carriers often fail to meet even this less restrictive deadline). The carrier's finding should include information on what factors were considered. The review determination will be final unless the physician decides to request a fair hearing, the next step in the process.

Medical Necessity Denials

When claims are denied or downcoded under medical necessity guidelines, a review of an initial determination may be requested by sending a letter to the carrier (or by completing HCFA Form 1964).

The physician's explanation should be geared toward substantiating medical necessity of the service. Substantiating information should be organized, highlighted, and summarized such that a reviewer can pick out salient points within *10 seconds*. That is the extent of most reviews before the claim is rubber-stamped—"another specially trained individual has reviewed your claim and the initial decision (denial) is correct."

We suggest that a short cover letter accompany operative reports, lab tests, medical records, etc. The first paragraph of an appeal request should succinctly demonstrate medical necessity. The second paragraph should explain exactly which services were performed; this explanation should meet the criteria in CPT® for the service in question.

Try to avoid short statements like, "In my opinion services were necessary" or "I do not understand why this claim was denied." Reviewers respect a physician's opinion, but only if it is presented logically, as discussed above.

This approach often works for appeals to payers other than Medicare as well.

Some initial reviewers will uphold the denial on the basis of the original determination. If a carrier begins falling into the pattern of upholding the original determination, physicians should exert their appeal rights further. Physicians often overturn denials at the hearing level when initial reviews prove unsuccessful. Consultants report hearing officers saying, "Doctor, I can't explain why they denied this claim and your subsequent appeal; it's clear the service was appropriate . . . you will be paid."

Medicare carriers generally follow their internal processing manuals when conducting initial reviews. These manuals may contain incorrect interpretations of Medicare regulations and guidelines. Hearing officers are not necessarily bound by internal processing manuals; however, they are bound by Medicare regulations and HCFA's *Medicare Carriers Manual*.

Fair Hearing

A physician who is dissatisfied with the initial review determination may request a fair hearing if the amount in dispute is greater than $100. Several similar claims may be accumulated to meet this threshold. HCFA Form 1965 or a letter is used to request a hearing.[7] The physician should be notified within 10 days that his or her request has been received. Hearings are supposed to be completed within 120 days.[8]

Two or more physicians may aggregate claims when determining whether they meet the threshold amount for requesting an appeal. While the rules are somewhat confusing, the aggregated claims do not necessarily have to involve the same issue or the same patient, nor do the physicians have to be in the same practice.

A hearing can be conducted in person or by telephone or based on the record (ie, written documentation). Consultants report success with each type.

Physicians should not be intimidated; hearings are relatively informal, although proceedings will be audiotaped (except in the case of on-the-record hearings).[9] Usually hearings are conducted in a small office with only the hearing officer and appellant(s) present.

Consultants indicate that hearings conducted in person are the most effective, especially when the issue has a major impact on the physician's practice.[10] For example, under old pathology coding guidelines, one carrier began denying many claims for pathology evaluations of multiple skin lesion specimens. The carrier's rationale was that the specimens were from the same anatomic site; therefore, only one charge should be paid.

In one hearing, a pathologist took several specimen bottles. The physician explained to the hearing officer (verbally and *visually*) that he received separately packaged specimens, each had to be examined individually, and the pathology report had to designate the results of each specimen so that the surgeon would know which lesions required removal.

The hearing officer—who had no medical training—was able to visualize the clinical aspects of the pathologist's examinations. The hearing officer agreed with the pathologist and ordered full payment on about $50,000 worth of old claims. The carrier also modified its processing manual to prevent denials in the future.

Physicians should appear reasonable and make sure they are on firm ground before requesting a hearing. They should find out if the adverse determination was based on internal processing manuals, regional HCFA policies, HCFA's *Medicare Carrier Manual*, regulations, or law (or even a reviewer's whim). The first is the easiest to overturn.

At hearings conducted in person, oral arguments may be presented. Physicians do not have to go (although it often helps), and they can be represented by an attorney, consultant, office manager, or others familiar with the process. The physician can take witnesses, including patients, although care should be used in deciding whether to take a patient. Photographs and testimonials may also be helpful. The physician can take all evidence in his or her possession and examine all pertinent evidence in the carrier's possession before the hearing. Any documentation submitted should be carefully organized for clarity. Highlighting, page numbers, and exhibit numbers may be used to improve the presentation.

Remember, the hearing officer is not always familiar with all aspects of the hearing. Most controversies are confusing, and the hearing officer is likely to have limited clinical experience and limited knowledge of some portions of Medicare law. Physicians may actually know more about the rules and regulations that apply to their practice or specialty. Most hearing officers are reasonable and can be persuaded, provided the physician's arguments are within regulations.

Denial patterns can often be corrected during the hearing process. Well-presented arguments addressing the overall reason for the denials being appealed will often lead to education of carrier employees. Carriers are monitored by HCFA for the number of overturned denials. This rating impacts the carrier's bonus for accuracy and efficiency. Most carriers are happy to address claims denial practices that result in a high rate of reversal at the hearing level.

Additional Appeals

If still dissatisfied with the hearing officer's determination, the physician may request another hearing before an administrative law judge (ALJ) if the amount in dispute is at least $500 (again, claims can be accumulated).[11] After receipt of the fair hearing officer's determination, the physician has 60 days to request a decision by an ALJ. This request is filed with the Social Security Administration. (The letter disclosing the hearing officer's determination should include instructions for advancing to the next phase of the appeals process.)

Again, the physician should not be intimidated by an ALJ. This level is somewhat more formal but is not a major court case. Again, ALJ appeals can be held in person or on the record. An attorney is not necessary, although issues such as admissibility of evidence and limitation of liability arise that may be best handled by an attorney. ALJ appeals can be held at local Social Security Administration offices.

An ALJ is bound by the facts previously presented, law, and Medicare regulations; however, ALJs are not necessarily bound by HCFA's *Carrier Manual* and other directives. Thus, there is even more room for interpretation than at the hearing and carrier review levels. Nevertheless, the physician's arguments have to be persuasive.

If still dissatisfied, physicians have further appeals rights through the Social Security Office's Appeals Council and the courts; however, qualifying becomes more difficult and costly.

A physician may request that an ALJ's decision be overturned by going to the Appeals Council. Generally, use of an attorney is recommended (although not required) at this point because the physician must show that the ALJ made an error of law or abused his or her discretion, findings were not supported by the facts, and the like. Obviously, an attorney will be needed to proceed to federal courts.

Amount in Controversy

Most of the various levels of appeal require that the dollars in controversy be above a certain threshold—$100, $500, etc. Several claims can be accumulated to meet these thresholds.

To determine amounts that apply toward the various appeal thresholds, take amounts disallowed by the carrier, subtract any remaining deductibles, and reduce the remainder by the 20% coinsurance if applicable. That is, the $100 and $500 thresholds are based on the check Medicare would have written had the original claim been paid correctly at the level charged less what was actually paid.

Final Advice on Reviews and Hearings

Reviews and hearings should not be requested every time a denial is received, but physicians should pursue appeal rights when on firm ground. Although appealed decisions are not binding in future situations, they often establish some precedent. Again, physicians should not be intimidated by the hearing process. Their accomplishments will ultimately help all physicians as well as their patients.

Requests for reviews and hearings should be well documented. Accurately frame the issues involved and clearly explain why the carrier's payment or denial is wrong. Make it difficult for reviewers to "rubber-stamp" initial denials.

Also, spend a little extra time documenting requests for initial reviews. Do not waste this level of the administrative appeals process, because the next step—a fair hearing—is a little more involved (but worth the effort when you are right).

Sample Coverage Policy: Chest X-ray

The following is an example of one Medicare carrier's coverage policy for chest x-rays, including covered ICD-9 diagnosis codes that are used as prepayment edits. The actual list of covered ICD-9 codes is much longer than presented here. Physicians should check their carrier's current coverage policy.

Subject: Chest x-ray
Policy Number: 1234
Description: Chest x-rays are noninvasive diagnostic studies to aid in the diagnosis of lung disease, cardiac conditions, bony abnormalities and chest wall conditions.
Policy Type: Local Medical Review Policy
HCPCS Section Benefit Category: Radiology

HCPCS Codes:

| 71010 | Radiologic examination, chest; single view, frontal |
| 71020 | Radiologic examination, chest; two views, frontal and lateral |

HCFA'S National Policy: Title XVIII of the Social Security Act, section 1862(a)(7). This section excludes routine physical examinations. Title XVIII of the Social Security Act, section 1862(a)(1)(A). This section allows coverage and payment for only those services that are considered to be medically reasonable and necessary.

Indications & Limitations of Coverage and/or Medical Necessity:

1. Medicare provides coverage for chest x-rays that are medically necessary based on signs, symptoms, illness or injuries or diseases.

2. Specific symptoms or findings such as cough, hemoptysis, dyspnea, recent conversion of a T.B. skin test from negative to positive, or fever of undetermined origin constitute medical necessity for performing chest x-rays.

3. Medical conditions with manifestations involving chest structures such as metastatic carcinoma or congestive heart failure are indications for performing a chest x-ray.

4. Chest x-rays are covered when performed to follow-up an invasive procedure such as thoracentesis or central venous line placement.

5. Preoperative chest x-rays are covered if the patient is scheduled for major surgery and has risk factors which make the x-rays necessary. The risk factors must be clearly stated in the patient's medical record.

ICD-9 Codes that Support Medical Necessity:

[Note: For illustrative purposes only; many ICD-9 codes have not been reproduced here.]

010.00-018.96	Tuberculosis
031.0-031.9	Diseases due to other mycobacteria
038.0-038.9	Septicemia
039.1	Pulmonary actinomycosis
042	Human immunodeficiency virus disease (use additional codes for all manifestations of HIV—excludes asymptomatic HIV infection status, exposure to HIV and non-specific serologic evidence of HIV)
093.0-093.9	Cardiovascular syphili
112.4	Candidiasis of lung
112.5	Disseminated candidiasis
140.0-149.9	Malignant neoplasm of lip, oral cavity or pharynx
170.0-176.9	Malignant neoplasm of bone, connective tissue, skin and breast
780.2	Syncope and collapse
780.31-780.39	Convulsions (08/25/98)
780.4	Dizziness and giddiness
780.6	Pyrexia of unknown origin
781.2	Abnormality of gait
781.3	Lack of coordination
781.4	Transient paralysis of limb
783.2	Abnormal loss of weight
922.1	Contusion of chest wall (08/25/98)
V10.00-V10.9	Personal history of malignant neoplasm (10/01/99)
V12.01	Personal history of tuberculosis
V12.6	Personal history of diseases of respiratory system
V58.69	Long-term (current) use of other (high risk)medications (1/1/96)
V67.51	Follow-up exam following treatment with high risk medication

V72.81   Pre-operative cardiovascular examination (This ICD-9 code may be used when a medically necessary pre-operative chest x-ray was performed. The medical record must document the risk factors that necessitated the chest x-ray.)

V72.82   Pre-operative respiratory examination (This ICD-9 code may be used when a medically necessary pre-operative chest x-ray was performed. The medical record must document the risk factors that necessitated the chest x-ray.)

Reasons for Denial: Any conditions not meeting the criteria in this policy.

Noncovered ICD-9 Code(s): All ICD-9 codes not listed in the "ICD-9 Codes that Support Medical Necessity" section of this policy.

Sources of Information: Carrier newsletters, other carrier medical directors, advisory committee members and written comments from practicing physicians.

Coding Guidelines: Documentation describing the medical necessity for performing the chest x-ray must be present in the patient's medical record. The chest x-ray should be linked to the appropriate ICD-9 diagnosis code in each instance. If chest x-rays are performed for screening purposes as part of routine examinations, append the CPT® code with modifier 5E to receive proper denial. [*Note: Do not use this modifier unless required by your carrier.*] The physician may then bill his/her customary charge to the patient.

Documentation Requirements: Documentation for performing all chest x-rays is expected to indicate clear and concise medical necessity in the patient's medical record. These medical records are subject to audit review.

Other Comments: All [Physician Current Procedural Terminology] (CPT®) five digit numeric codes and descriptions are copyright ©1995 American Medical Association. All rights reserved.

CAC Notes: This policy does not reflect the sole opinion of the carrier Medical Director. This policy was developed considering comments from the medical community via the Carrier Advisory Committees.

Revision Date: 10/19/95

Revision Number: A

The information that follows is a detailed discussion of the new ABN form and CMS's instructions to Medicare carriers; however, it is not the complete document.

These instructions will be communicated to physicians some time in August to November 2002 (assuming no further delays). Readers should carefully review carrier announcements to ensure compliance with ABN instructions. It appears that CMS and carriers will be making greater efforts to educate beneficiaries on this topic.

Program Memorandum Department of Health & Human Services (DHHS) Intermediaries/Carriers

Centers for Medicare & Medicaid Services (CMS)
Transmittal AB-02-114 Date: JULY 31, 2002

. . . **The purpose of the ABN is to inform a Medicare beneficiary, before he or she receives specified items or services that otherwise might be paid for, that Medicare probably will not pay for them on that particular occasion.** The ABN, also, allows the beneficiary to make an informed consumer decision whether or not to receive the items or services for which he or she may have to pay out of pocket or through other insurance. In addition, the ABN allows the beneficiary to better partici-pate in his/her own health care treatment decisions by making informed consumer decisions. If the physician or supplier expects payment for the items or services to be denied by Medicare, the physician or supplier must advise the beneficiary before items or services are fur-nished that in their opinion the beneficiary will be person-ally and fully responsible for payment.

To be "personally and fully responsible for payment" means that the beneficiary will be liable to make pay-ment "out-of-pocket," through other insurance coverage (e.g., employer group health plan coverage), or through Medicaid or other Federal or non-Federal payment source. The physician or supplier must issue notices each time, and as soon as, they make the assessment that Medicare payment probably or certainly will not be made. If a physician or supplier fails to provide a proper ABN in situations where one is required, you may find the physician or supplier to be liable under the provisions of LOL or RR, where such provisions apply, unless the physician or supplier can show that they did not know and could not reasonably have been expected to know that Medicare would deny payment.

To be acceptable, an ABN must be on the approved Form CMS-R-131, must clearly identify the particular item or service, must state that the physician or supplier believes Medicare is likely (or certain) to deny payment for the particular item or service, and must give the physician's or supplier's reason(s) for their belief that Medicare is likely (or certain) to deny payment for the item or service.

1. Reason for Predicting Denial.—Statements of rea-sons for predicting Medicare denial of payment at a level of detail similar to those in the *Medicare Carriers Manual*, Part 3 §7012, Item 15.0.ff., "Medical Necessity" are acceptable for ABN purposes.

Simply stating "medically unnecessary" or the equivalent is not an acceptable reason, insofar as it does not at all explain why the physician or supplier believes the items or services will be denied as not reasonable and necessary. To be acceptable, the ABN must give the beneficiary a reasonable idea of why the physician or supplier is predicting the likelihood of Medicare denial so that the beneficiary can make an informed consumer decision whether or not to receive the service and pay for it personally.

The use on the ABN-G, in the customizable "Because:" box, of lists of reasons for denial which the particular

physician or supplier has found are frequently applicable, with check-off boxes or some similar method of indicat-ing the selection of the reason(s), is an acceptable prac-tice. For example, the three reasons included on the ABN-L form may be used, with slight modification, on the ABN-G form: "Medicare does not pay for this item or service for your condition"; "Medicare does not pay for this item or service more often than *frequency limit*"; and "Medicare does not pay for services which it consid-ers to be experimental or for research use."

Listing several reasons which apply in different situations without indicating which reason is applicable in the bene-ficiary's particular situation generally is not an acceptable practice, and such an ABN may be defective and may not protect the physician or supplier from liability. However, if more than one reason for denial could apply (e.g., exceed-ing a frequency limit and "same day" duplication; cases where the reason for denial could depend upon the result of a test; etc.), do not invalidate an ABN on the basis of citing more than one reason for denial. . . .

2. Routine Notices Prohibition—Generic and Blanket Notices.—In general, the "routine" use of ABNs is not effective. By "routine" use, we mean giving ABNs to beneficiaries where there is no specific, identifiable rea-son to believe Medicare will not pay. Physicians and sup-pliers should not give ABNs to beneficiaries unless the physician or supplier has some genuine doubt that Medicare will make payment as evidenced by their stated reasons. Giving routine notices for all claims or services is not an acceptable practice. If you identify a pattern of rou-tine notices in situations where such notices clearly are not effective, write to the physician or supplier and remind them of these standards. In general, routinely given ABNs are defective notices and will not protect the physician or supplier from liability. However, in certain cir-cumstances, ABNs may be routinely given to beneficiar-ies because all or virtually all beneficiaries may be at risk of having their claims denied in those circumstances.

Section I.1.A.2.d.ff specify those circumstances in which ABNs may be routinely given.

   a. Generic ABNs: "Generic ABNs" are routine ABNs to beneficiaries which do no more than state that Medicare denial of payment is possible, or that the physician never knows whether Medicare will deny payment. Such "generic ABNs" are not con-sidered to be acceptable evidence of advance ben-eficiary notice. The ABN must specify the service and a genuine reason that denial by Medicare is expected.

ABN standards likewise are not satisfied by a generic document that is little more than a signed statement by the beneficiary to the effect that, should Medicare deny payment for anything, the beneficiary agrees to pay for the service. "Generic ABNs" are defective notices and will not protect the physician or supplier from liability.

b. Blanket ABNs: A physician or supplier should not give an ABN to a beneficiary unless the physician or supplier has some genuine doubt regarding the likelihood of Medicare payment as evidenced by its stated reasons. Giving ABNs for all claims or items or services (i.e., "blanket ABNs") is not an acceptable practice. Notice must be given to a beneficiary on the basis of a genuine judgment about the likelihood of Medicare payment for that individual's claim.

c. Signed Blank ABNs: A physician or supplier is prohibited from obtaining beneficiary signatures on blank ABNs and then completing the ABNs later. An ABN, to be effective, must be completed before delivery to the beneficiary. Hold any ABN that was blank when it was signed to be defective notice that will not protect the physician or supplier from liability.

d. Routine ABN Prohibition Exceptions: ABNs may be routinely given to beneficiaries and considered to be effective notices which will protect physicians and suppliers only in the following exceptional circumstances: i. Services Which Are Always Denied for Medical Necessity—In any case where a national coverage decision provides that a particular service is never covered, under any circumstances, as not reasonable and necessary under §1862(a)(1) of the Act (e.g., at present, all acupuncture services are denied as not reasonable and necessary), an ABN that states in the "Because:" box that: "Medicare never pays for this *item/service*" may be routinely given to beneficiaries, and no claim need be submitted to Medicare. If the beneficiary demands that a claim be submitted to Medicare, submit the claim as a demand bill in accordance with Section 1.3.G. ii.

A. Experimental Items and Services.—When any item or service which Medicare considers to be experimental (e.g., "Research Use Only" and "Investigational Use Only" laboratory tests) is to be furnished, since all such services are denied as not reasonable and necessary

under §1862(a)(1) of the Act because they are not proven safe and effective, the beneficiary may be given an ABN-G that states in the "Because:" box that: "Medicare does not pay for services which it considers to be experimental or for research use" or an ABN-L with a test listed in the third column," Medicare does not pay for experimental or research use tests." Alternative, more specific, language with respect to Medicare coverage for clinical trials may be substituted as necessary in the ABN-G "Because:" box or as the caption for the right column of the customizable portion of the ABN-L at the user's discretion. iii. Certain Frequency Limited Items and Services - When any item or service is to be furnished for which Medicare has established a statutory or regulatory frequency limitation on coverage, or a frequency limitation on coverage on the basis of a national coverage decision or on the basis of your local medical review policy (LMRP), because all or virtually all beneficiaries may be at risk of having their claims denied in those circumstances, the physician or supplier may routinely give ABNs to beneficiaries. In any such routine ABN-G, the physician or supplier must state the frequency limitation in the ABN-G "Because:" box (e.g., "Medicare does not pay for this item or service more often than *frequency limit*"). iv. Medical Equipment and Supplies Denied Because the Supplier Had No Supplier Number or the Supplier Made an Unsolicited Telephone Contact - Given that Medicare denials of payment under §1834(j)(1) of the Act on the basis of a supplier's lack of a supplier number, and under §1834(a)(17)(B) of the Act, the prohibition on unsolicited telephone contacts, apply to all varieties of medical equipment and supplies and to all Medicare beneficiaries equally, the usual prohibition on provision of routine notices to all beneficiaries does not apply in these cases. See Section 1.2.D.1 & 2.

B. Determining Whether or Not the Beneficiary is Liable.—In deciding whether the beneficiary or his/her authorized representative knew, or could reasonably have been expected to know, that payment would not be made for items or services s/he received, the beneficiary's allegation that s/he did not know, in the absence of evidence to the contrary, will be acceptable evidence for LOL purposes. However, there may be evidence that will rebut such an allegation. For example, within the previous twelve months a beneficiary received a denial notice stating that a service was excluded from coverage, that previous denial notice, if it pertains to a similar or reasonably comparable service, would constitute evidence that the beneficiary did have knowledge of exclusion.

While evidence of beneficiary knowledge generally must be based on written notice, §1879(a)(2) of the Act specifies only that knowledge must not exist in order to apply the LOL protection. If it is clear and obvious that a beneficiary in fact did know, prior to receiving a service or item, that Medicare payment for that service or item would be denied, the administrative presumption favorable to the beneficiary is rebutted. For example, if a beneficiary admits he or she had prior knowledge that payment would be denied, no further evidence is required; the absence of a written notice is moot.

The failure of any physician or supplier to furnish an ABN to a beneficiary is not sufficient to afford the beneficiary the protection of the LOL provision if you have proof that the beneficiary, nonetheless, had the requisite knowledge that payment would be denied. In any case in which you have such evidence of prior knowledge on the beneficiary's part, old the beneficiary liable under the LOL provision. The most likely reason to find that the beneficiary knew or could reasonably have been expected to know that Medicare would not pay is where, before the item or service was furnished, the physician or supplier notified the beneficiary by properly delivering the approved Form CMS-R-131, of the likelihood that Medicare would not pay for the specific service. In a case where a beneficiary received an ABN and, upon initial determination, the claim was paid as covered, that original ABN cannot be used as evidence of knowledge to hold the beneficiary liable in a later case relating to a similar or reasonably comparable service in which the same reason for denial applies, since the original ABN was belied by the favorable payment decision. In a case where RR applies, in order for the beneficiary to be held liable, it is necessary that after being informed, the beneficiary agreed to pay the physician or supplier for the service personally or through other insurance, as evidenced by a signed agreement to pay. (See §7300.5 of the MCM for instructions on determining liability for assigned claims for physician and supplier services for which payment is denied as "not reasonable and necessary.")

Do not accept generic ABNs or blanket ABNs as effective notice to beneficiaries for either LOL or RR purposes.

C. Delivery of ABN.—Delivery of an ABN occurs when the beneficiary or authorized representative (i.e., the person acting on the beneficiary's behalf) both has received the notice and can comprehend its contents. All notices must include an explanation written in lay language of the physician's or supplier's reason for believing the items or services will be denied payment. Do not accept an incomprehensible notice or any notice which the individual beneficiary or his/her authorized representative is incapable of understanding due to the particular circumstances (even if others may understand).
1. The physician or supplier should hand-deliver the ABN

to the beneficiary or authorized representative. Delivery is the physician's or supplier's responsibility. (Consider delivery of an ABN by a physician's or supplier's staff or employees to be delivery by the physician or supplier.) If the beneficiary alleges non-receipt of notice and the physician cannot show that notice was received by the beneficiary, do not find that the beneficiary knew or could reasonably have been expected to know that Medicare would not pay; i.e., hold the physician or supplier liable and the beneficiary not liable. The ABN must be prepared with an original and at least one copy.

The physician or supplier must retain the original and give the copy to the beneficiary or authorized representative. (In a case where the physician or supplier that gives an ABN is not the entity which ultimately bills Medicare for the item or service, e.g., when a physician draws a test specimen and sends it to a laboratory for testing, the physician or supplier should give a copy of the signed ABN to the entity which ultimately bills Medicare.) The copy is given to the beneficiary immediately after the beneficiary signs it. Legible duplicates (carbons, etc.), fax copies, electronically scanned copies, or photocopies will suffice. This is a fraud and abuse prevention measure. If a beneficiary is not given a copy of the ABN and if the beneficiary later alleges that the ABN presented to the carrier by the physician or supplier is different in any material respect from the ABN he/she signed, give credence to the beneficiary's allegations.

2. Do not consider a telephone notice to a beneficiary, or authorized representative, to be sufficient evidence of proper notice for limiting any potential liability, unless the content of the telephone contact can be verified and is not disputed by the beneficiary. If a telephone notice was followed up immediately with a mailed notice or a personal visit at which written notice was delivered in person and the beneficiary signed the written notice accepting responsibility for payment, accept the time of the telephone notice as the time of ABN delivery.

3. Do not consider delivery of a notice to be properly done unless the beneficiary, or authorized representative, was able to comprehend the notice (i.e., they were capable of receiving notice). A comatose person, a confused person (e.g., someone who is experiencing confusion due to senility, dementia, Alzheimer's disease), a legally incompetent person, a person under great duress (for example, in a medical emergency) is not able to understand and act on his/her rights, therefore necessitating the presence of an authorized representative for purposes of notice. A person who does not read the language in which the notice is written, a person who is

not able to read at all or who is functionally illiterate to read any notice, a blind person or otherwise visually impaired person who cannot see the words on the printed page, or a deaf person who cannot hear an oral notice being given by phone, or could not ask questions about the printed word without aid of a translator, is a person for whom receipt of the usual written notice in English may not constitute having received notice at all (this is not an exclusive list). This may be remedied when an authorized representative has no such barrier to receiving notice. However, in the absence of an authorized representative, the physician or supplier must take other steps to overcome the difficulty of notification. These may include providing notice in the language of the beneficiary (or authorized representative), in Braille, in extra large print, or by getting an interpreter to translate the notice, in accordance with the needs of the beneficiary or authorized representative to act in an informed manner. If the beneficiary was not capable of receiving the notice, hold that the beneficiary did not receive proper notice, hold that the beneficiary is not liable, and hold the physician or supplier liable.

4. **Hold that a beneficiary did not receive proper notice in any case where you find that the physician or supplier refused to answer inquiries from a beneficiary, or authorized representative, who requested further information and/or assistance in understanding and responding to the notice, including the basis for his/her/its assessment that items or services may not be covered.** In the case of a beneficiary complaint about not receiving sufficient information about the cost of a service or item for which an ABN was given, follow the guidance in Section I.3.E.1.b.vi in determining whether the physician or supplier was sufficiently responsive.

5. a. **A patient must be notified far enough in advance of receiving a medical service so that the patient can make a rational, informed consumer decision without undue pressure.** The purpose of this timely delivery rule is to avoid putting the beneficiary into a position in which she/he is already committed to receiving the item or service before receiving notice of the likelihood of denial of payment by Medicare.

   b. **As a general rule, ABN delivery should take place before a procedure is initiated and before physical preparation of the patient (e.g., disrobing, placement in or attachment of diagnostic or treatment equipment) begins.** This criterion does not constitute a blanket prohi-

bition on giving an ABN to a beneficiary after she/he has entered an examination room, a draw station, a DMEPOS sales room, etc., and is ready to receive services or items. We recognize, for example, that situations may arise during an encounter when a physician (or supplier) sees a need for a previously unforeseen service, expects that Medicare will not pay for it, and wishes to give an ABN.

This is permissible, provided that the beneficiary is capable of receiving notice in accordance with paragraph 3 above, and has a meaningful opportunity to act on it (e.g., the beneficiary is not under general anesthesia). Where it is foreseeable that the need for service for which Medicare likely would not pay may arise during the course of an encounter, and the beneficiary is either certain or likely not to be capable of receiving notice during the initial service (e.g., the beneficiary will be under anesthesia), it is permissible to give an ABN before any service is initiated; such an ABN would not violate the general prohibition of routine ABNs in Section I.1.A.2. Also, in a case where a physician draws a test specimen and sends it to a laboratory for testing, and did not give the beneficiary an ABN, the laboratory may contact the beneficiary and give him/her an ABN without violating this timely delivery rule, so long as testing of the specimen has not begun.

   c. **If a beneficiary alleges she/he was coerced into accepting medical items or services by receiving the ABN at the last moment, investigate the facts.** If the physician or supplier clearly and obviously violated this timely delivery rule, hold that the notice was not properly delivered in advance of furnishing the item or service and that the beneficiary therefore is not liable.

6. In the case of an ABN on which the physician's or supplier's identifying information in the header of the ABN form identifies the physician or supplier that obtained the ABN, rather than the physician or supplier that is billing for the services (e.g., when one laboratory refers a specimen to another laboratory which then bills Medicare for the test; when a physician executes an ABN with his or her own identifying information in the header in conjunction with ordering a laboratory test for which the testing laboratory will submit the claim to Medicare), consider the ABN form to be valid so long as it was otherwise properly executed.

D. Effect of Furnishing ABNs and Collection from Beneficiary.—

1. When ABNs are properly used by physicians and suppliers, the ABNs also protect them from liability under the several statutory provisions which limit beneficiaries' liability. A beneficiary who has been given a proper written ABN, before an item or service was furnished, giving notice of the likelihood (or certainty) that Medicare would not pay for the specific item or service and of the reason therefore and who, after being so informed, has agreed to pay the physician or supplier for the item or service, will be held liable. That is, that beneficiary will be found to have known in advance that Medicare would not pay, and the physician or supplier will be free to bill and collect the related charges from the beneficiary.

A beneficiary who has been given such a proper ABN and who, after being so informed, refused to sign the ABN at all but demanded and received the item or service, may be held liable under LOL, but not under RR (see Section I.1.B, above).

2. Failure to meet the ABN standards and procedures will expose a physician or supplier to the risk of potential financial liability for denied items or services in cases where, in the absence of a proper ABN, the beneficiary would be held not to have known, nor to reasonably have been expected to have known, that his/her claims for the denied items and services he/she received were likely to be denied by Medicare. A physician or supplier held liable for such denied charges will be precluded from collecting from the beneficiary and may be required to make refunds to the beneficiary, or face possible sanctions for failure to do so.

If you suspect that a physician or supplier is not furnishing ABNs with the intent to induce or coerce referrals for other items and/or services paid for by Medicare whereby anti-kickback statutes could be implicated, or if you suspect that a physician or supplier is doing so for any fraudulent, abusive, or otherwise illegal purposes, refer the case to the CMS regional office. In the case of a physician or supplier that does not obtain an ABN, when giving an ABN would have been appropriate, because the physician or supplier had no opportunity to do so (e.g., when a laboratory receives a specimen for testing, does not see the patient, and the specimen's testing is time-sensitive, such that the patient cannot be contacted about an ABN before the test is performed), do not consider the physician's or supplier's failure to obtain an ABN under such circumstances as indicative of fraud or abuse on that sole basis.

3. **A physician or supplier who supplies a defective ABN (one which does not meet the standards in Section I.ff) will not be protected from liability.** A beneficiary who received a defective ABN should not be liable and the physician or supplier who/which gave the defective ABN should be held liable. Certain ABN standards may vary on the basis of the particular type of denial (e.g., as not reasonable and necessary, as violating the prohibition on unsolicited telephone contacts) and on the basis of whether the claim is assigned or unassigned. Section I.2 provides particular standards which apply to specific types of denials.

4. When an ABN was properly executed and given timely to a beneficiary (who, if RR applies, agreed to pay in the event of denial by Medicare) and, in fact, Medicare denies payment on the related claim (whether assigned or unassigned), the physician or supplier may bill and collect from the beneficiary for that service (see MCM §3045.2, Physician's Right to Collect from Enrollee on Assigned Claim). Medicare does not limit the amount which the physician or supplier, participating or nonparticipating, may collect from the beneficiary in such a situation. Medicare charge limits do not apply to either assigned or unassigned claims when collection from the beneficiary is permitted on the basis of an ABN. A beneficiary's agreement to "be personally and fully responsible for payment" means that the beneficiary agrees to pay out-of-pocket or through any other insurance that the beneficiary may have, e.g., through employer group health plan coverage, Medicaid or other Federal or non-Federal payment source.

5. When an ABN was given to a beneficiary for a service for which Medicare pays in more than one part to different entities, e.g., for a radiological test with a technical component and a professional component, if the specification of the service on the ABN reasonably includes both components, that ABN, from either party, will serve as evidence of knowledge for LOL and RR. It is not necessary that both parties to the service give separate ABNs. If the beneficiary asks for a cost estimate, the estimate should include both parts of the service.

6. **ABNs may not be used to shift liability to a beneficiary in the case of services or items for which full payment is bundled into other payments; that is, where the beneficiary would otherwise not be liable for payment for the service or item because bundled payment is made by Medicare.** Using an ABN to collect from a beneficiary where full payment is made on a bundled basis would constitute double billing. An ABN may be used to shift liability to a beneficiary in the case of services or items for which partial payment is bundled

into other payments; that is, where part of the cost is not included in the bundled payment made by Medicare.

7. Health Insurance Portability & Accountability Act of 1996 (HIPAA) Sanctions and the Use of ABNs.—Section 231(e)(4) of HIPAA adds to the Social Security Act a new §1128A(a)(1)(E) which provides for civil monetary penalties when claims are submitted "for a pattern of medical or other items or services that a person knows or should know are not medically necessary." This HIPAA sanction provision and the ABN provisions are not related and should not be confused with one another, but also are not mutually exclusive. Concerns have been raised by the physician and supplier communities that the use of ABNs could be construed by CMS or another agency pursuing enforcement activities as documenting such a pattern of medically unnecessary care. You may assure physicians and suppliers inquiring about this matter that the use of ABNs will not run them afoul of the HIPAA sanctions. The HIPAA sanctions are meant to deal with fraudulent claims for patently unnecessary medical care. . . .

E. Approved Notice Language.—The OMB-approved ABNs for use with Part B items and services (viz., OMB Approval No. 0938-0566, Form No. CMS-R-131) satisfy the requirements under both LOL and RR for the physician's or supplier's advance beneficiary notice and the beneficiary's agreement to pay. The use of any other ABNs or modified ABNs may be ineffective in protecting physicians and suppliers from liability.

Section I.2 Special Rules.—

A. Exception for Repetitive Notices.—**A single ABN covering an extended course of treatment is acceptable provided the ABN identifies all items and services for which the physician or supplier believes Medicare will not pay.** If, as the extended course of treatment progresses, additional items or services are to be furnished for which the physician or supplier believes Medicare will not pay, the physician or supplier must separately notify the patient in writing (i.e., give the beneficiary another ABN) that Medicare is not likely to pay for the additional items or services and obtain the beneficiary's signature on the ABN. Items or services (e.g., laboratory tests) provided on a regularly scheduled basis under a "standing order" may be considered, for these beneficiary notice purposes only, as an extended course of treatment; and a single ABN may suffice (e.g., for all the tests furnished the beneficiary which are contemplated by that order), as described above, with a new ABN being required only when additional items or services, which are not specified by the initial course of

treatment ABN and for which noncoverage is expected, are to be furnished to the beneficiary. When an ABN is to be given for a "standing order" the physician or supplier must specify in the "Items or Services:" box of the ABN-G, or in the appropriate column of the customizable box beginning "Medicare probably will not pay..." on the ABN-L, the pertinent facts (e.g., frequency and duration) of the standing order (see Section I.3.E.1.b.v.).

One year is the limit for use of a single ABN for an extended course of treatment; if the course of treatment extends beyond one year, a new ABN is required for the remainder of the course of treatment. An ABN, once signed by the beneficiary, may not be modified or revised. When a beneficiary must be notified of new information, a new ABN must be given.

B. **Guidelines for Situations Where the Beneficiary is in a Medical Emergency or Is Otherwise Under Great Duress.—**
An ABN-G or ABN-L should not be obtained from a beneficiary in a medical emergency or otherwise under great duress (i.e., when circumstances are compelling and coercive) since that individual cannot be expected to make a reasoned informed consumer decision. In genuine emergencies, the beneficiary/victim and his or her family/friends (authorized representative) are under great duress by the emergency circumstances, to sign anything in order to obtain help. On the other hand, there is a risk that beneficiaries might actually forego needed emergency services if faced with a financial burden which they believe they cannot bear. A requirement for delivery of a notice is that the beneficiary, or authorized representative, must be able to comprehend the notice, i.e., they must be capable of receiving notice (see Section I.1.C.3). A person under great duress is not able to understand and act on his or her rights. If the beneficiary is not capable of receiving the notice, then the beneficiary has not received proper notice and cannot be held liable where the LOL or RR provisions apply, and the physician or supplier may be held liable.

1. Emergency Medical Treatment and Active Labor Act (EMTALA) Situations.—An ABN should not be given to a beneficiary in any case in which EMTALA (§1876 of the Act) applies, until the hospital has met its obligations under EMTALA, which includes completion of a medical screening examination (MSE) to determine the presence or absence of an emergency medical condition, or until an emergency medical condition has been stabilized. CMS published this policy in the November 10, 1999 OIG/HCFA Special Advisory Bulletin on the Patient Anti-Dumping Statute:

"A hospital would violate the patient anti-dumping statute if it delayed a medical screening examination or necessary stabilizing treatment in order to prepare an ABN and obtain a beneficiary signature. The best practice would be for a hospital not to give financial responsibility forms or notices to an individual, or otherwise attempt to obtain the individual's agreement to pay for services before the individual is stabilized. This is because the circumstances surrounding the need for such services, and the individual's limited information about his or her medical condition, may not permit an individual to make a rational, informed consumer decision."

This policy applies in any case in which EMTALA applies, not only to EMTALA cases seen in emergency rooms (ERs). Giving ABNs to beneficiaries under great duress is not permitted, regardless of the particular treatment setting or location. Even when a beneficiary does not appear to have a life threatening condition, rather, he or she is seeking primary care services at an ER, an ABN should not be given to the beneficiary in any case in which EMTALA applies until the hospital has met its obligations under EMTALA. An ABN that is otherwise appropriate may be given to a Medicare beneficiary who is seen in the ER after completion of an MSE, but an ABN should not be given unless there is a genuine reason to expect that Medicare will deny payment for the services because giving routine "blanket" ABNs to beneficiaries is not permitted (see §I.1.A.2.b.). There always must be a reason for expecting that Medicare will deny payment for the services furnished to the individual beneficiary on a specific occasion, and that reason must appear on the ABN. EMTALA does not prohibit asking payment questions entirely, rather, only doing so before screening/stabilization. After screening/stabilization, EMTALA no longer applies and ABNs may be given, when otherwise appropriate, to beneficiaries who come to emergency care settings after they have received a medical screening examination and are stabilized.

2. Other Situations.—A physician or supplier may not shift liability to a beneficiary under great duress by giving an ABN to the beneficiary. ABNs given to any individual who is under great duress cannot be considered to be proper notice. It is inconsistent with the purpose of advance beneficiary notice, which is to facilitate an informed consumer decision by a beneficiary whether or not to receive an item or service and pay for it out-of-pocket, to attempt to obtain beneficiaries' signatures on ABNs during medical emergencies and other compelling, coercive circumstances where a rational, informed consumer decision cannot reasonably be made. For that reason, physicians and suppliers may not use ABNs to shift

financial liability to beneficiaries in emergency care situations. Ambulance companies may not give ABN-Gs to beneficiaries or their authorized representatives in any emergency transport because such beneficiaries are under great duress. Skilled nursing facilities may not give ABN-Gs in the case of "middle-of-the-night" emergencies or in any other emergency circumstances, since the beneficiary clearly cannot make an informed consumer decision (see Section I.2.G).

Consider any ABN-G or ABN-L given in any kind of coercive circumstances, including medical emergencies, to be defective. In all such coercive situations, find that the beneficiary did not know and could not reasonably have been expected to know that Medicare would not make payment. Determine the physician's or supplier's liability by the appropriate knowledge standards which are used in cases where ABNs are not given and beneficiary agreements to pay are not obtained (see §§7300.5.B, 7330.D.1 of the MCM, and Section II.5). This policy regarding duress applies in any case in which a beneficiary is under great duress and cannot make an informed consumer decision. **This is the basis for the "last moment delivery" policy that a beneficiary must be notified well enough in advance of receiving a medical service so that the beneficiary can make a rational, informed consumer decision.** In any case of such "last moment delivery" of an ABN, the delivery may not be considered timely and the beneficiary may not be held liable (see Section I.1.C.5 regarding "last moment delivery" of the ABN).

C. ABNs for Claims Affected by the Physicians' Services Refund Requirement.—Under §1842(1) of the Act, the prohibition against billing for unassigned physician services which are denied on the basis of §1862(a)(1) of the Act as not reasonable and necessary, the physicians' services Refund Requirement provision, a refund is required under certain circumstances, unless a proper ABN-G was given the beneficiary and the beneficiary agreed to pay. (See §7330 of the MCM for instructions on determining situations where a refund under §1842(1) of the Act is required.)

D. ABNs for Claims Affected by the Medical Equipment and Supplies Refund Requirement.—
[Several sections are not reproduced here. The complete document is available at http://www.cms.gov/medlearn/refabn.asp]

G. ABN Standards for Services in Skilled Nursing Facilities (SNF).—Skilled nursing facilities may not give ABNs to beneficiaries in the case of "middle-of-the-night" emergencies, since the beneficiary is under duress and clearly cannot make an informed consumer decision. . . .

H. ABN Standards for Items and Services for Which ABNs Are Not Required.—Physicians and suppliers need use ABNs only when Medicare is expected (or certain) to deny payment on the basis of one of the following statutory exclusions: §1862(a)(1) & (9); §1834(a)(17)(B); §1834(j)(1); and §1834(a)(15) of the Act. ABNs are not required in the case of statutorily excluded items and services not listed above.

Examples of exclusions for which ABNs are not required include, but are not limited to:

- Personal comfort items;

- Routine physicals and most tests for screening;

- Most shots (vaccinations);

- Routine eye care, eyeglasses and examinations;

- Hearing aids and hearing examinations;

- Cosmetic surgery;

- Most outpatient prescription drugs;

- Orthopedic shoes and foot supports (orthotics);

- Dental care and dentures (in most cases);

- Routine foot care and flat foot care;

- Services under a physician's private contract;

- Services paid for by a governmental entity that is not Medicare;

- Health care received outside of the USA;

- Services by immediate relatives;

- Services required as a result of war;

- Services for which the patient has no legal obligation to pay;

- Home health services furnished under a plan of care, if the agency does not submit the claim;

- Items and services excluded under the Assisted Suicide Funding Restriction Act of 1997;

- Items or services furnished in a competitive acquisition area by any entity that does not have a contract with the Department of Health and Human Services (except in a case of urgent need);

- Physicians' services performed by a physician assistant, midwife, psychologist, or nurse anesthetist, when furnished to an inpatient, unless they are furnished under arrangements by the hospital;

- Items and services furnished to an individual who is a resident of a skilled nursing facility or of a part of a facility that includes a skilled nursing facility, unless they are furnished under arrangements by the skilled nursing facility;

- Services of an assistant at surgery without prior approval from the peer review organization; and

- Outpatient occupational and physical therapy services furnished incident to a physician's services. (See §1862(a) of the Act for a more complete listing.)

ABNs also are not required when Medicare is expected to deny payment for an item or service which may be a Medicare benefit but for which the coverage requirements (not listed above) are not met, e.g., when a service is covered only in a qualifying setting and the service in question was not provided in such a qualifying setting. In situations in which ABNs are not required, the lack of an ABN, by itself, will not prevent a physician or supplier from collecting from a beneficiary. In situations in which ABNs are not required, physicians and suppliers are neither required to nor prohibited from voluntarily giving some sort of notice to beneficiaries anyway, as a prudent customer service, however, since standard ABN forms include language asking for a claim to be submitted to Medicare, physicians and suppliers who wish to give notice in these situations should not use the CMS-R-131 ABN forms.

Section I.3 The Proper Use of the ABN (CMS-R-131).—

A. When An ABN Should Be Given.—

1. Whether an ABN should be given in a particular instance depends on the physician's or supplier's expectation of Medicare payment or denial.

   a. If the physician or supplier expects Medicare to pay, an ABN should not be given.

   b. If the physician or supplier "never knows whether or not Medicare will pay," an ABN should not be given.

   c. If the physician or supplier expects Medicare to deny payment, the next question is: "On what basis is denial expected?"

      i. If the item or service is not a Medicare benefit (e.g., routine physical and tests in the absence of signs and symptoms, routine foot care, dental care), neither the ABN-G nor the ABN-L should be given.

      ii. If Medicare is expected to deny payment for an item or service which is a Medicare benefit because it does not meet a technical benefit requirement (e.g., an ambulance service denied due to an unapproved destination, diabetic care shoes not prescribed by a podiatrist or other qualified physician), neither the ABN-G nor the ABN-L should be given.

iii. If Medicare is expected to deny payment (entirely or in part) for the item or service because it is not reasonable and necessary under Medicare program standards (viz., "medical necessity denials" under §1862(a)(1) of the Act), the ABN-G or the ABN-L, as appropriate, should be given (this is applicable to all assigned Part B items and services, and to unassigned physicians' services and medical equipment and supplies). Certain screening tests (mammography, pap smear, pelvic exam, glaucoma, prostate cancer, colorectal cancer) have frequency limits under §1862(a)(1) of the Act, therefore, LOL applies and ABNs should be given when Medicare denial of payment for frequency is expected for any of these tests.

iv. If Medicare is expected to deny payment for medical equipment and supplies because it is not covered: (i) under §1834(a)(17)(B) of the Act, violation of the prohibition on unsolicited telephone contacts; (ii) under §1834(j)(1) of the Act, supplier number requirements not met; or (iii) under §1834(a)(15) of the Act, failure to obtain advance determination of coverage, the ABN-G should be given (this is applicable to both assigned and unassigned medical equipment and supplies).

2. **Do not find a physician or supplier to have violated the prohibition on routine ABNs solely on the basis of the number of ABNs which the physician or supplier gives to beneficiaries, when those ABNs are justified by the physician or supplier having a genuine reason to give an ABN.** Some physicians or suppliers (e.g., a physician furnishing acupuncture services) may give ABNs to most or all of their Medicare patients without violating the routine ABNs prohibition.

B. **To Whom An ABN May Be Given.**—An ABN may be given to a Medicare beneficiary or to the beneficiary's authorized representative, that is, to a person who is acting on the beneficiary's behalf when the beneficiary is temporarily or permanently unable to act for himself or herself. (See the definition of an authorized representative for ABN purposes in Section I.1.F.)

C. **How An ABN May Be Given.**—Delivery of an ABN occurs when the beneficiary or authorized representative (i.e., the person acting on the beneficiary's behalf) both has received the notice and can comprehend its contents. An incomprehensible notice, or a notice which the individual beneficiary or his/her authorized representative is incapable of understanding due to the particular circumstances (even if others may understand), cannot be used to fulfill notice requirements. (See the applicable standards for delivery of an ABN in Section I.1.C.)

D. **Choosing The Form To Use.**—Physicians and suppliers must use the OMB-approved ABNs (ABN-G and ABN-L) for use with Part B items and services. The ABN-G may be used for all situations, including laboratory tests, by all physicians and suppliers. The ABN-L may be used for laboratory tests, by any person or entity furnishing laboratory tests.

E. **Filling Out The Forms.—**

1. Form Instructions for ABN-G and ABN-L—

a. Format of Insertions on ABN.—The physician or supplier must ensure that the readability of the ABN facilitates beneficiary understanding. No insertion into the blanks and boxes of the ABN, if typed or printed, should use italics nor any font that is difficult to read. An Arial or Arial Narrow font, or a similarly readable font, in the font size range of 10 point to 12 point, is recommended. Black or dark blue ink on a white background is strongly recommended. A visually high-contrast combination of dark ink on a pale background is required. Low-contrast combinations and block shading are prohibited. If insertions are handwritten, they must be legible. In all cases, both the originals and copies of ABNs must be legible and high-contrast. When Spanish language ABNs are used, the physician or supplier should make insertions on the form in Spanish to the best of their ability. If this is impossible, the physician or supplier needs to take other steps as necessary to ensure that the beneficiary understands the notice.

b. **Filling in the Form.—**

i. The ABN's header should have the identifying information of the billing entity. If the billing entity is a group practice, then the group practice may have its identifying information in the header. It may be prudent for each member of a group practice to also include their name in the header, but it is not required. A laboratory should put its own identifying information in the header where a client physician is delivering the ABN form to a beneficiary on behalf of the laboratory. ABNs included on laboratory requisition forms should have the identifying information of the laboratory in the header, not the client physician's information, even when stocks of the ABNs are provided to client physicians for their use in ordering tests. The physician or supplier puts his/her/its name, address, and telephone number at the top of the notice header; and may elect to include his/her/its logo (if any). Within these general rules, a notice header may be customized by the physician or supplier.

ii. "Patient name" Line—The physician or supplier enters the name of the patient, not substituting the name of an authorized representative.

iii. "Medicare Health Insurance Claim Number (HICN) Line"—The physician or supplier enters the patient's Medicare HICN. Do not invalidate an ABN solely for the lack of a Medicare HICN unless the beneficiary recipient of an ABN alleges that the ABN was signed by someone else of the same name and you cannot resolve the matter with certainty.

iv. ABN-G Customizable Boxes—In the section of the ABN-G beginning "We expect that Medicare will not pay for the item(s) or service(s) …", in the first box "Items or Services:", the physician or supplier specifies the health care items or services for which he/she/it expects Medicare will not pay. **The items or services at issue must be described in sufficient detail so that the patient can understand what items or services may not be furnished. HCPCS codes by themselves are not acceptable as descriptions.** The use on the ABN of a list of the items and/or services which the particular physician or supplier frequently furnishes, with check-off boxes or some similar method of identifying the particular items or services for which denial is predicted, is an acceptable practice. Listing several items and/or services without indicating which is/are applicable in the beneficiary's particular situation is not an acceptable practice and such an ABN is defective and will not protect the physician or supplier from liability. In the second box "Because:", the physician or supplier gives the reason why they expects Medicare to

deny payment. The reason(s) must be sufficiently specific to allow the patient to understand the basis for the expectation that Medicare will deny payment. The physician or supplier may customize these two boxes for their own use.

v. ABN-L(Lab) Customizable Boxes—In the section of the ABN-L beginning "Medicare probably will not pay…", the physician or supplier specifies the laboratory tests for which he/she/it expects Medicare will not pay in the customizable boxes. The laboratory tests at issue must be described in sufficient detail so that the patient can understand what laboratory tests may not be furnished. The use of standard laboratory test descriptions is permitted. HCPCS codes by themselves are not acceptable as descriptions. ABN-L has been designed with three columns with the specific reasons for expected denial captioning these columns. The physician or supplier enters or preprints laboratory tests in these three columns; the use of check off boxes is permitted. This format allows the physician or supplier to customize the ABN-L with a preprinted list of tests linked to the captioned reasons for denial. The boxes containing three columns for laboratory tests and reasons for expecting denial on the ABN-L may be customized by the physician or supplier, except that the captions (reasons) for the left and center columns may not be revised while the right column (experimental and research use exclusion) may be revised or deleted at the discretion of the user. Use of the right column to specify the frequency and/or duration of a standing order is permissible (see §I.2.A). Use of a fourth category, "Other:" is permissible.

vi. **"Estimated Cost" Line**—The physician or supplier may provide the patient with an estimated cost of the items and/or services. The patient may ask about the cost and jot down an amount in this space. The physician or supplier should respond to such inquiries to the best of their ability. The lack of an amount on this line, or an amount which is different from the final actual cost, does not invalidate the ABN; an ABN should not be considered to be defective on that basis. In the case of an ABN which includes multiple items and/or services, it is permissible for the physician or supplier to give estimated amounts for the individual items and/or services rather than an aggregate estimate of costs. Amounts may be provided either with the description of items and services or on the "Estimated Cost" line.

vii. Options 1 & 2 Boxes—**The patient must personally select an option.** Do not accept as evidence of beneficiary notice any ABN on which the physician or supplier has pre-selected an option; pre-selecting options is prohibited.

viii. In the "Date" blank, the patient, or his or her authorized representative, should enter the date on which he or she signed the ABN. If the date is filled in by the physician or supplier and the beneficiary or his or her authorized representative does not dispute the date, you should accept that date. Do not reject ABNs simply because the date is typed or printed. In the "Signature of patient ..." blank, the patient, or person acting on his or her behalf, must sign his or her name.

2. **Signature Requirements** for ABN-G and ABN-L.—

a. The beneficiary himself or herself may sign an ABN. In the case of a beneficiary who is incapable or incompetent, his or her "authorized representative," as defined for ABN purposes in Section I.1.F may sign an ABN. The policy enunciation in Section I.1.F of who may be an "authorized representative" supersedes the previous policy that "generally applicable rules of the Medicare program with respect to who may sign for a beneficiary apply to signing notices, including ABNs." The regulations on signature requirements for claims purposes at 42 CFR 424.36(b) do not apply to ABNs except that, with respect solely to ABNs for unassigned claims for physicians' services, someone eligible to sign for the beneficiary under CFR §424.36(b), who is an "authorized representative" as defined for ABN purposes in Sections I.1.F and I.1.F.3 notwithstanding, may sign an ABN.

b. If the beneficiary's (or authorized representative's) signature is absent from an ABN, in case of a dispute as to the beneficiary's (or authorized representative's) receipt of the ABN, give credence to the beneficiary's (or authorized

representative's) allegations regarding the ABN, except as specified in Section I.3.F.2.

c. The physician or supplier must obtain the signed and dated ABN from the beneficiary, either in person or, where this is not possible, via return mail from the beneficiary or authorized representative acting on the beneficiary's behalf as soon as possible after the ABN has been signed and dated. The beneficiary retains the patient's copy of the signed and dated ABN and returns the original. The physician or supplier retains the original ABN. These copies will be relevant in case of any future appeal. Do not require physicians and suppliers to routinely submit copies of all ABNs to you.

F. Resolving Beneficiary Problems.—

1. A beneficiary who has been given either ABN-G or ABN-L (or the person acting on the beneficiary's behalf) may decide to receive the item or service. In this case, the beneficiary should select option 1 to indicate that he/she is willing to be personally and fully responsible for payment. When a beneficiary decides to decline an item or service, he/she should select Option 2. There is no third option. The beneficiary cannot properly refuse to sign the ABN at all and still demand the item or service. If a beneficiary refuses to sign a properly executed ABN, the physician or supplier should consider not furnishing the item or service, unless the consequences (health and safety of the patient, or civil liability in case of harm) are such that this is not an option. If the beneficiary refuses to sign the ABN, the physician or supplier should annotate the ABN, and have the annotation witnessed, indicating the circumstances and persons involved.

2. In the case of claims to which Limitation on Liability protections under §1879(a), (b), and (c) of the Act apply, if the physician or supplier does furnish the item or service, the beneficiary's signature is meant to attest to receipt of the ABN; it has "agreement to pay" language so that it is absolutely clear to the beneficiary what the implications for him or her are. Once the beneficiary has read a properly executed ABN, he or she is "on notice"; that is, the beneficiary "knew, or could reasonably have been expected to know, that payment could not be made." The beneficiary has two legitimate choices: a) To obtain the service and be prepared to pay out of pocket, that is, personally or by any other insurance coverage, or b) Not to obtain the service. If the beneficiary demands the service and refuses to pay, the physician or supplier should have a second person witness the provision of the ABN and the beneficiary's refusal to sign. They

should both sign an annotation on the ABN attesting to having witnessed said provision and refusal. Where there is only one person on site (e.g., in a "draw station"), the second witness may be contacted by telephone to witness the beneficiary's refusal to sign the ABN by telephone and may sign the ABN annotation at a later time. The unused patient signature line on the ABN form may be used for such an annotation; writing in the margins of the form is also permissible. The physician or supplier should file as having given the ABN, with a GA modifier. The beneficiary will be held liable per §1879(c) of the Act in case of a denial.

3. In the case of claims to which Refund Requirement protections under §§1834(a)(18), 1834(j)(4), 1842(l), or §1879(h) of the Act apply, if the physician or supplier does furnish the item or service, the beneficiary's signature is meant to attest both to receipt of the ABN and to the beneficiary's agreement to pay. The beneficiary both must receive a properly executed ABN so that he or she is "on notice" (that is, the beneficiary "knew, or could reasonably have been expected to know, that payment could not be made") and must agree to pay. The beneficiary has the same two legitimate choices: a) To obtain the service and be prepared to pay out of pocket, that is, personally or by any other insurance coverage, or b) Not to obtain the service. If the beneficiary demands the service and refuses to pay (in other words, selects Option 1 but will not sign or else marks out the agreement to pay language), the physician or supplier must take into account the fact that it will not be able to collect from the beneficiary in deciding whether or not to furnish the items or services. Although there would be little point in having a second person witness the provision of the ABN and the beneficiary's refusal to agree to pay (because the requirement that the beneficiary agree to pay still would not be fulfilled), the physician or supplier may annotate the ABN, as described in paragraph 2, above. The physician or supplier, if the items or services are furnished despite the beneficiary's refusal to pay, should file the claim using the GZ modifier, that is, as not having obtained a signed ABN, since it was not completed properly by the beneficiary.

Do not hold the beneficiary liable per §§1834(a)(18), 1834(j)(4), 1842(l), or §1879(h) of the Act in case of a denial. Do not hold the physician or supplier liable.

4. In either case (F.2 and F.3, above), the beneficiary who does receive an item or service, of course, always has the right to a Medicare determination and the claim must be filed with Medicare in accordance with §1848(g)(4) of the Act.

G. Demand Bills—A demand bill is a complete, processable claim which must be submitted promptly to Medicare by the physician or supplier at the timely request of the beneficiary, the beneficiary's representative, or, in the case of a beneficiary dually entitled to Medicare and Medicaid, a state as the beneficiary's subrogee. A demand bill is requested usually, but not necessarily, pursuant to notification of the beneficiary (or representative or subrogee) of the fact that the physician or supplier expects Medicare to deny payment of the claim. When the beneficiary (or representative or subrogee) selects an option on an ABN that includes a request that a claim be submitted to Medicare, no further demand is necessary; a demand bill must be submitted. When a beneficiary chooses Option 1 on an ABN-G or an ABN-L and receives the item or service, claims submission is mandatory. The physician or supplier must submit a claim to you, billing as covered, for an initial determination. On such a claim, a **GA modifier** must appear on the CMS-1500 in item 24D. The GA modifier indicates that an ABN was furnished by the physician or supplier and is on file in their office and it also documents the physician's or supplier's expectation that Medicare will not pay the claim. (**The GA modifier is mandatory; it must be used anytime an ABN was obtained.** The use of the GZ modifier is optional. A GZ modifier may be included on the CMS-1500 in item 24D if the physician or supplier wishes to indicate that denial for medical necessity is expected but an ABN was not obtained. Reject as unprocessable any claim line item including both the GA and GZ modifiers, as they are mutually exclusive.) Do not change your process for making an initial determination on the basis that a claim was submitted with a GA or GZ modifier. The provision of an ABN and/or the inclusion of a GA or GZ modifier by the physician or supplier only represent the physician's or supplier's assessment that Medicare will deny payment. You must make your initial determination on the usual bases. You may not auto-deny any claim solely on the basis of a GA or GZ modifier. After you have denied payment on a claim, take into account the presence of the GA or GZ modifier in determining the liability of the beneficiary and the physician or supplier. If you receive a claim that does not include a GA modifier, but a properly executed ABN is submitted with the claim, you should add the GA modifier to the claim yourself.

[For the complete Program Memorandum, please see http://www.cms.gov/medlearn/refabn.asp]

Endnotes

1. Even five 99211s could be deemed medically unnecessary.

2. Sometimes the term *screen* is used instead of *edit*.

3. Probably the most memorable example of a bundled service has now been changed because of the uproar it caused among physicians. In 1992, payment for interpretation of electrocardiograms was considered included within the allowance for E/M codes. Thus, in 1992 and 1993, no separate payment was made for electrocardiogram interpretations provided "during, as a result of, or in conjunction with any visit or consultation" (including critical care and all sites of visits). HCFA's rationale was that the payment for E/M codes included an increment to cover such services as electrocardiogram interpretations. Effective January 1, 1994, however, Medicare once again began paying physicians for electrocardiogram interpretation and E/M codes billed on the same day.

4. A few services have been removed from the "bundled" list because of appeals filed by individual physicians or efforts by medical societies and other groups.

5. Today, the waiver is called an advance beneficiary notice (ABN), but readers may find older Medicare carrier newsletters and other publications that use the term *waiver of liability*.

6. In this section, we are discussing a denial of an *initial* claim submission. The time frames are different in the case of postpayment audits. If you are dealing with a postpayment audit, carefully read your carrier's instructions as to how you should handle your specific circumstances. Their "demand" letter should include a description of your appeal rights.

7. Some carriers have developed special forms for requesting hearings.

8. Technically, you can go directly to the hearing level if the carrier does not process your initial claim within 60 days. Some physicians use this fact to speed up claim processing when backlogs occur (although it is not likely a hearing will be granted).

9. In an effort to streamline the hearing process, some carriers require most "first" hearings to be conducted in writing. If you are dissatisfied with the results, you are afforded an opportunity to appear in person or conduct the hearing by telephone (before another hearing officer). Check the fine print on denial notifications for applicability of these requirements in your area.

10. We have experienced excellent results with telephone as well as in-person hearings. Consequently, telephone reviews are a good compromise when inordinate time, travel, etc, are required. In many areas, in-person hearings are available at a site within 60 miles of your office (often at a local Social Security office).

11. Usually you have to go through the hearing level to get to an administrative law judge. Generally, you will find that each successive level of the appeals process results in less bias in the decision by reviewers.

How to Minimize Risk of an Audit

Avoiding an audit is really not difficult, especially in light of how few audits actually occur in relation to the number of physicians and others filing claims. Anecdotal evidence from fraud and abuse consultants seems to indicate that there has been a lull in audits starting in 2000. There are several theories cited—statistics that indicate Medicare payment errors have been reduced by about half since 1996; significant changes in requirements for carrier random sampling; efforts devoted to the privacy and security provisions under HIPAA; the tragic events of September 11, 2001; and shifting of some enforcement priorities; etc.

But there is no verifiable proof that the rate of audits, particularly carrier-initiated audits, have declined permanently. Therefore, this is not the time to relax or postpone meaningful compliance efforts. Physicians still need to take action to keep audit risk low. The possibility always exists that a physician might be selected for a random audit or that someone will allege that a physician is involved in fraudulent and abusive activities. Proactive steps should be taken to minimize the risk.

The next few chapters address doing things the right way to avoid audits, ensure proper medical record documentation so that the physician survives an audit if one occurs, and establish a compliance program suited to the size of the operation so as to minimize the long-term risk.

The recommendations are mostly common sense. The real art is making sure to do these things and that efforts are effective. By following these steps, physicians may actually see an increase in income because there is diminished pressure to downcode claims because of uncertainty about what is right.

The first chapter asked the question, Are you really sure that your billing processes are appropriate? An example was cited in which a well-meaning billing clerk routinely upcoded evaluation and management (E/M) codes above what the physician marked on encounter forms because she "found that this would get the practice reimbursement closer to what they charged."

By performing a simple self-audit, this physician could have spotted the problem early enough to prevent any serious consequences.[1] If physicians do not want to perform these self-audits, consulting firms can do it for them or help them set up an effective audit protocol. Consultant referrals are available through a free service operated by AMA Solutions (800 366-6968).

Ways to Minimize Audit Exposure

1   Communicate effectively with your patients about the treatment you are rendering or the tests you are ordering. The well-informed patient is less likely to question the necessity or appropriateness of care and is less likely to contact a toll-free hotline because of a misunderstanding.

     If patients will receive a separate bill from a clinical lab, tell them. If you are a consultant who stops by and sees a heavily sedated patient in the hospital, leave your card, explain to the family who you are (explain that the attending physician requested your consultation), if necessary write the patient a letter, and get your billing statements processed in a reasonable period of time. Work with the hospital or referring physicians to make sure patients understand they will receive a separate bill for your professional services if you are a pathologist, radiologist, anesthesiologist, or the like. Put an explanation on statements.

2   Keep detailed and legible records that substantiate everything. Document all complaints, symptoms, and an extensive assessment of the problems and course of treatment for each of these. Learn and follow the documentation guidelines for E/M codes and any other special documentation requirements promulgated by Medicare carriers or other payers.

3   Train your staff well and conduct random audits on your billing and coding procedures to ensure accuracy in the process and provide for early detection of any problems. Remember, physicians are responsible for the actions of their personnel. The fact that errors are made will not protect you from liability—certainly with respect to recoupment—in the event of an audit. If you are limited in time for such activity, obtain the services of an outside consultant to ensure unbiased results.

Many practice management consultants recommend that physicians—rather than billing staff—select CPT® codes because physicians are most aware of what services were provided. This can be accomplished by designing a superbill or other encounter form that lists common codes. If necessary, billing staff can look over the codes to make sure the physician's choice seems appropriate and meets special payer guidelines.

Regarding ICD-9 codes, it is generally easier for the physician to pick from a billing sheet indicating common diagnoses for the specialty. If physicians do not use a billing form with ICD-9 codes, they should write, in a designated place in the record, diagnoses that can be easily translated to ICD-9 codes. (See the next two chapters on CPT® and ICD-9 coding for some ideas on how to make billing work better in your office.)

Of course, ICD-9 codes need to be related to CPT® codes if multiple CPT® codes are provided. Write an "A" or "1" by the first CPT® code and an "A" or "1" by the diagnosis codes that justify that service. Write a "B" or "2" by the next, etc.

One of the most revealing audit techniques is to start with payer Explanation of Benefits (EOBs) and identify original claims that were denied or for which additional information was requested. Then research to determine what happened to the claims. If it was paid, what information was sent to the payer that prompted them to pay? Was that information correct and included in the documentation or was it "manufactured" to get the claim paid?

If the claim was not ultimately paid, what happened? Was the original claim filed incorrectly? Did staff do a creditable job of dealing with the denial or are improvements necessary?

One can easily see that looking at how denials are handled will provide a lot of information about the effectiveness of your billing activities from a fraud and abuse standpoint and from a collection standpoint. This type of analysis may: help you identify situations where one can avoid denials in the first place; indicate situations where physicians can document critical information to facilitate claims filing and follow-up; indicate billing circumstances that require study to improve results; etc. Expert billing consultants use this type of analysis to identify fraud and abuse risks and potential lost income from ineffective follow-up.

4   Your billing and coding personnel should be required to maintain a high level of competency through seminar attendance on a regular basis and through review of all billing information supplied by the carrier. As a general rule, do not expect to hire inexperienced personnel with hopes of training them (unless it is truly an entry-level position). Coding and billing are too complicated to expect anyone to become proficient in a short period of time.

Take advantage of coding certification programs for key staff. This will improve proficiency, awareness, and instill a sense of professionalism that will certainly pay for itself each and every year.

5   Implement a fraud and abuse compliance program. A well-thought-out and well-executed plan can minimize the risk that your practice will be the subject of an audit. (Chapters 12 through 14 cover the essential elements of a compliance program.)

6   All AMA CPT® codes used should reflect the service provided and not the anticipated reimbursement. In the next chapter, we discuss some of these coding situations and the importance of documentation to support the code selected. E/M codes are an obvious example. As another illustration, a number of services are designated by one code for *simple* services and another code for *complex* services. Complex services may have allowances 5 to 15 times those of simple services. Sometimes the CPT® code's definition makes it difficult to distinguish between the two, but your documentation ought to make it clear which was performed.

7   Do not necessarily assume that Medicare's payment of a particular procedure or item guarantees the service to be covered or appropriate in your patient's situation. Strictly speaking, payment indicates only that there are no prepayment edits or screens to prevent inappropriate payments.

Obviously, payment indicates a better chance of coverage than a denial; however, there have been recoupments where a carrier has shown that it clearly notified physicians a given service was not covered but some claims were paid in error anyway. On the other hand, there have also been cases in which the carrier officials and/or government regulators decided not to pursue recoupment because physicians had no way of knowing that the payment was incorrect (often a medical society became involved on behalf of a number of physicians).

The real point here is that if you think you have been paid incorrectly, do not use the fact that you have been getting paid as an excuse to keep billing the carrier.

8   Be wary of advice from vendors or manufacturer representatives on Medicare billing protocol or coverage issues. In most instances, these individuals have a vested interest in providing an answer that justifies the purchase of their product. Any coverage issues should be verified, in writing, with the carrier's medical policy department.

9   Stay informed of changes and updates in reimbursement policy. All educational material sent to you from a carrier should be reviewed thoroughly and on a timely basis. Any issues that relate to your practice should be noted and necessary changes made immediately.

You and your billing staff should review *every* carrier newsletter to see if there is any announcement impacting the services you perform. If you miss an expected carrier newsletter, call your carrier and request another. If you are new to coding in a given physician specialty, go back and review several years' worth of carrier newsletters. Several carriers maintain Web sites in which old newsletters and other coverage policies are available. If you start reviewing 3 years ago, make sure you read every issue in between in case guidelines changed. It is also worth reading other carriers' newsletters to improve your understanding of Medicare and other payers' guidelines.

It is also worth getting a copy of the annual issue of the *Federal Register* that updates the relative values for the next calendar year (it is usually published in late November or early December). This issue includes discussions of any major policy revisions related to coding. Also, review any specialty society publications that discuss coding and other issues (such as self-referrals) that could be related to fraud and abuse.

Finally, take advantage of the Internet resources that are available today such as: www.lmrp.net; your carrier's Web site; the various federal government and Medicaid program sites; etc.

10   Never bill for services that were not rendered or documented.

11   All diagnoses used on claims should be documented in medical records. Carriers often issue coverage policies that provide specific ICD-9 codes that are considered covered for designated CPT® codes. Do not use these "covered" codes just to get your claims paid unless they truly reflect a patient's condition and documentation in the medical record. Do not let staff get denials paid by putting one of the covered diagnoses on the claim without checking to make sure it is appropriate.

12   Consider obtaining a copy of your Medicare utilization profile at least once per year to see how your practice looks on paper. Make sure E/M codes are selected appropriately.

13   Contact the Medicare Part B provider registration department and determine if the carrier has your specialty designated with the appropriate two-digit specialty code. In addition, ensure that all location suffixes are appropriate for satellite offices.

14   Review all Medicare and Medicaid rejections and denials as they are received. A timely appeal will often result in payment. If your claims are being rejected for medical necessity reasons, you need to determine whether changes in your billing or coding are warranted (again, don't just put the codes on claims that will get you paid unless they are appropriate).[2] All rejections should be reviewed before an appeal is filed to make sure the potential for success is real.

15   As much as possible, you should be careful with whom you associate.[3] You could be putting yourself in jeopardy by being a physician in a large group where some physicians are billing inappropriately or in which the group is engaging in illegal self-referrals or kickback arrangements.

Consultants recommend that large groups appoint a committee charged with the responsibility of reviewing billings and other activities for potential fraud and abuse implications. This committee is an important part of the compliance program recommended for group practices.

16   If you use a billing service, monitor them just as you would your own staff to ensure that they are billing services as you intend. There is nothing uglier than a fraud and abuse investigation that pits physicians against a billing service.

Again, it is recommended that physicians should normally control the codes and other information that goes on claim forms. In any event, monitor the billing service and perform some checks or audits to make sure you are protected.

Once again, do not be tempted to rationalize things that you think may be fraudulent or abusive by saying, "Well, my billing service said it was all right." It is not that simple.

17   A physician, or a staffer well trained in billing and/or medical records, should review all documentation before it is sent to a payer to ensure that it properly reflects the encounter.

18   Review Chapters 4 and 5 regarding illegal kickbacks and self-referrals. If you are involved in any arrangement that causes concern, talk with your attorney. Watch for the final regulations with respect to Stark II self-referral legislation. Pay particular attention to the provisions regarding income distribution arrangements tied directly to ordering diagnostic tests within a group.

19   Now, more than ever, if you are concerned about something related to fraud and abuse, talk to someone who can provide a reliable answer. Although many carriers are helpful when physicians ask questions, it is also a good idea to seek opinions from others. It is not a good idea in today's climate to call your carrier and say, "For years I have been billing like this . . . is that all right?"

Self-auditing Records

Every practice should perform a chart audit as part of a compliance program. CPT® and ICD-9 codes that were placed on insurance claim forms should be compared to the documentation in medical records. Documentation should clearly support the services billed. Physicians should participate in these audits.

Physicians should be very critical and carefully compare the codes billed to the CPT® description. It is surprising how often minor errors occur. Obviously, this increases audit exposure and may be costing the practice money. For example, if records indicate that a lesion of 0.5 cm was removed, the code billed must not be for a larger lesion (0.6 cm or larger) and the code for the method of removal must be appropriate (ie, shaving, destruction, or excision). If a level 4 office visit was billed, records must meet CPT® and payer guidelines by properly addressing history taking, the extent of the examination, and the complexity of medical decision making.

Documentation is important from a number of perspectives, including patient care, professional liability exposure, reimbursement enhancement, audit exposure, and research. Physicians should be concerned not just about government programs or reimbursement. Many managed care plans include documentation audits as part of their overall quality management program.

Some plans audit records of potential participants. Others routinely audit records to ensure that physicians are meeting quality standards. Thus, poor medical record documentation could result in failure to meet a health plan's quality standards.

Look at more than Evaluation and Management codes. Too many billing consultants concentrate on E/M codes. There are many other audit targets and risk areas.

Go back and look at some of the risks illustrated in Chapter 2 and audit billings for those risks that apply to your practice. Think of other potential risks or problems experienced in the past that should be reviewed in an audit. Don't think of audits as merely identifying errors or improper billing practices. Look at all aspects of billing activities to identify those aspects that are handled well and those that need improvement. Re-audit significant billing activities—just because something was working correctly during the last period audited does not mean it will be working correctly during the next audit period.

Finally, review the information in Chapter 13 related to auditing as covered in the OIG's *Compliance Guidance*.

Frequency Distributions and Billing Profiles

One of the most common ways that Medicare carriers and others determine audit targets is through what is called "profiling." Medicare has amassed a large database that includes frequency distributions of CPT® code usage by physician specialty. It is relatively easy for their computer systems to compare a specific physician's code usage to the average for the specialty (either in the payer locality or with national data).

Those physicians who exhibit a pattern markedly different from the average are called *outliers*. Outliers have significantly higher chances of an audit. Data are available through Medicare Part B Extract Summary System reports (referred to as BESS data) by physician specialty. A medical practice can also monitor code frequency distributions over time to determine if there are any significant changes that need to be investigated.

Frequency distributions should be computed for the practice as a whole—without regard to payer—and by major payer grouping, particularly distributions for Medicare beneficiaries, Medicaid, CHAMPUS, etc. Thus, Medicare data for a practice would be compared to BESS data because frequency distributions may be different for elderly vs younger patients.

Tables 9-1 and 9-2 and Figures 9-1 and 9-2 display frequency distributions for a medical practice for services to Medicare patients. This example indicates that the group may be undercoding because there is very little usage of higher levels of service compared to peers. Of course, actual medical records would have to be examined to determine if documentation supports usage of higher-level codes.

Also, the example is for the group as a whole. Frequency data for individual physicians should also be compared to identify individuals who may be outliers.

Table 9-1 New Patient Evaluation and Management Codes

	CPT Code	Actual Billed	Percent	National Percent	Simulated Billings
New Patients	99201	0	0.00%	6.27%	8
	99202	106	79.70%	24.89%	33
	99203	27	20.30%	33.58%	45
	99204	0	0.00%	22.33%	30
	99205	0	0.00%	12.93%	17

Amounts and percentages are for illustration only.

Figure 9-1 New Patient Utilization

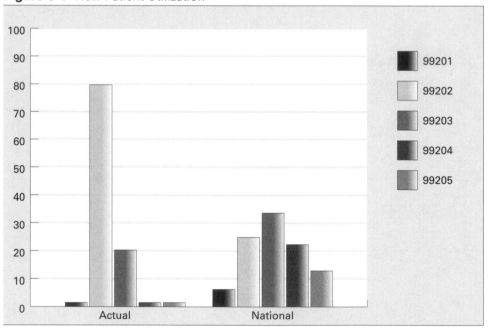

Table 9-2	Established Patient Evaluation and Management Codes				
	CPT Code	Actual Billed	Percent	National Percent	Simulated Billings
Established Patients	99211	0	0.00%	5.12%	33
	99212	539	84.75%	17.03%	108
	99213	73	11.48%	51.37%	329
	99214	24	3.77%	21.66%	138
	99215	0	0.00%	4.46%	28

Amounts and percentages are for illustration only.

Figure 9-2 Established Patient Utilization

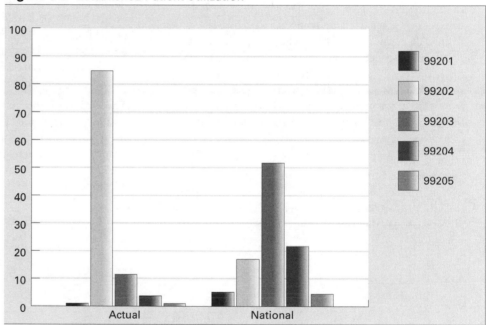

Endnotes

1. In fact, most good medical practice computer systems will produce a utilization report that displays the number of encounters in the time period (ie, month, quarter, etc) and the CPT® and ICD-9 codes billed. By simply looking at this report for 2 minutes, the physician should have realized that billing staff was sending out claims with a higher number of 99214 codes than he or she normally checked off on encounter forms.

   Additionally, the report helps physicians identify what their billing pattern looks like. They might spot other things, such as many claims going out with poorly defined diagnosis codes. This might prompt them to be a little more specific in their diagnosis coding to accurately portray the severity of the patient's condition. A self-audit might also improve a practice's internal control (ie, help the physician spot anything suspicious that might indicate inappropriate application of funds [a nice way of saying *embezzlement*]).

   Obviously, another approach to this self-audit would be to take encounter forms and compare them to paid explanations of benefits. This would have identified the billing irregularity cited, as well as helped the physician gauge the overall effectiveness of the billing operation.

2. As an example, with most Medicare carriers, appending a -25 modifier to an E/M code when a minor procedure—such as a sigmoidoscopy—is performed will allow payment for the visit code and procedure. The -25 modifier means that documentation indicates a significant, separately identifiable E/M service was performed on the day of the sigmoidoscopy. However, documentation often indicates that the sigmoidoscopy was scheduled at a previous visit and all the physician did on the day of the procedure was to perform it and briefly discuss the outcome with the patient. That probably does not justify payment of the E/M code under Medicare rules, but many carriers will pay it if the -25 modifier is used. An audit will likely reveal it was billed inappropriately, however.

3. The Office of Inspector General maintains a Web site that includes a cumulative sanction report that reflects the status of physicians and others who have been excluded from participation in the Medicare and Medicaid programs: www.oig.hhs.gov/fraud/exclusions/listofexcluded.html.

Chapter 10

CPT® Coding

During the past 30 years, a system of coding has evolved for reporting physician and other health care services. At the heart of this reporting system is a coding structure developed by the American Medical Association (AMA) called Physician's Current Procedural Terminology (CPT®).

The foreword to the CPT® 2002 book provides this description of the coding system:

> Current Procedural Terminology, Fourth Edition (CPT®) is a listing of descriptive terms and identifying codes for reporting medical services and procedures performed by physicians. The purpose of the terminology is to provide uniform language that will accurately describe medical, surgical, and diagnostic services, and will thereby provide an effective means of reliable nationwide communication among physicians, patients, and third parties. CPT® 2002 is the most recent revision of a work that first appeared in 1966.
>
> CPT® descriptive terms and identifying codes currently serve a wide variety of important functions in the field of medical nomenclature. CPT is the most widely accepted nomenclature for the reporting of physician procedures and services under government and private health insurance programs. CPT® is also useful for administrative management purposes such as claims processing and for the development of guidelines for medical care review. The uniform language is likewise applicable to medical education and research providing a useful basis for local, regional, and national utilization comparisons.

In the next chapter, we discuss another component of the coding system, ICD-9, which is a mechanism for reporting signs, symptoms, and medical conditions that essentially explain the reason(s) a particular medical service was performed and reported by means of a CPT® code or codes.

CPT® codes explain *what* service you performed.

ICD-9 codes explain *why* you performed that service.

Much of the government's efforts to identify fraud or abuse begin with analysis of data involving CPT® and/or ICD-9 codes. Improper coding, whether intentional or not, will increase one's chances of becoming the target of an audit or overpayment request. A basic understanding of the coding system and periodic monitoring of billing activities will help ensure proper reimbursement.

Before looking more closely at CPT®, we should mention another coding system that has been developed by the government to report durable medical equipment, prosthetics, medications, medical supplies, and the like. Technically, these codes are level II of what is generally referred to as HCPCS (Health Care Financing Administration [HCFA] Common Procedure Coding System). CPT® is essentially level I of the HCPCS system under the government's scheme. Level II HCPCS codes are assigned by the government; it is becoming increasingly common for private payers to accept some of these codes, particularly for injectable medications.

Most level II HCPCS codes describe supplies and injectable medications. However, a few codes are used to report procedures or services performed by physicians. For example, M0064 is used by a psychiatrist to report a visit to a Medicare beneficiary for a brief office visit for the sole purpose of monitoring or changing drug prescriptions used in the treatment of mental, psychoneurotic, and personality disorders.

In recent years, it has become common for the AMA to add codes to CPT® for physician services assigned a level II HCPCS code on an interim basis by the government.

Here are a few more examples of level II HCPCS codes:

J0290　　Injection ampicillin sodium 500 mg

J1642　　Injection heparin sodium (Heparin Lock Flush) per 10 units

V2115　　Lenticular (myodisc) per lens, single vision

R0070　　Transportation of portable x-ray equipment and personnel to home or nursing home, per trip to facility or location, one patient seen

G0008　　Administration of influenza virus vaccine

Again, CPT® is the heart of the system used to report physician services. The next few pages provide a brief discussion of CPT® in the context of fraud and abuse.

We cannot discuss this complex topic in depth in this book, but it is essential that physicians and their administrative staff understand CPT® and ICD-9 to avoid audit exposure. Chapters 10 and 11 only cover some of the basics, focusing primarily on the importance of documentation and selecting the correct codes to ensure accuracy and minimize audit exposure. In the event of an audit, physicians will need to demonstrate that the CPT® codes billed were actually performed and reflect medically necessary services. Physicians should keep up with the coding guidelines that impact the services they provide.

An important aspect of fraud and abuse—and the management of a practice—is ensuring that claim forms submitted to insurance companies, Medicare, managed care organizations, and other health plans are coded correctly. CPT® coding will impact ultimate reimbursement and audit exposure. ICD-9 codes should justify services provided and will impact payer profiling. For example, if a practice performs more electrocardiograms than the "average" physician, its claims and/or documentation should indicate that it had more patients with symptoms or conditions requiring such diagnostic tests.

Medical record documentation should provide all the information to support services reported with these codes and indicate the quality of care delivered. While there are excellent physicians who provide very little written documentation, payers are more likely to review records than in the past. These reviews are designed to ensure proper billing and to assess the quality of care provided.

CPT® Coding Background

Again, this chapter is not meant to be an exhaustive discussion of CPT® coding. While CPT® codes are accepted by almost all third-party payers, interpretation of individual codes and applicable reimbursement policies often varies among payers.

You should purchase a new copy of the AMA's CPT® code book annually.

On receipt of each year's edition, turn to Appendix B before doing anything else. Appendix B summarizes all changes to codes as listed in the previous year's book. Code changes impacting your practice could require modification to billing slips, other forms, computer programs, fees, etc, to ensure that you and/or your patients are paid quickly and appropriately.

The AMA publishes CPT® codes. Codes, descriptions, and various coding guidelines are determined by a 16-member editorial panel. There is also an AMA CPT® Advisory Committee with representatives from many medical specialty societies and the Health Care Professionals Advisory Committee, with representation from various health care professions.

In the context of this book, the CPT® coding system provides the mechanism for communicating (ie, billing) the medical services performed to third-party payers for reimbursement and statistical purposes. There is an inherent level of complexity in any system designed to report the thousands of medical services performed in today's modern medical practice. Unfortunately, the process of achieving reimbursement becomes very complex when third-party payers apply varying rules and interpretations when adjudicating a health insurance claim.

The complexity in the reimbursement process is especially apparent under government programs such as Medicare, where many rules have been changed in recent years and carrier interpretation and enforcement of some guidelines vary from state to state (notwithstanding standardization efforts). In recent years, Medicare has dramatically changed billing rules relating to the global surgical package, services considered to be bundled within other services, and documentation requirements for evaluation and management (E/M) services. To add to the confusion, an increasing number of third-party payers are adopting Medicare's rules to some extent.

Under resource-based and other reimbursement schemes, physicians must use the code that best describes the service performed. Otherwise, they will forgo income or increase audit exposure. As a simple example, physicians will not achieve fair reimbursement if they use a code for fracture reduction *without* manipulation when manipulation was actually performed. The CPT® descriptors must be read carefully to avoid making an error that could mean the difference between adequate and inadequate reimbursement, and increased audit exposure.

It is critical to stay abreast of changes in CPT® and payer billing guidelines related to coding. Each year there are hundreds of changes to CPT®—new codes added, existing codes deleted, and code descriptions changed. Similarly, payers will periodically change how they view certain codes and other billing guidelines. Maintaining current knowledge is imperative for the long-term survival and safety of a practice.

A prime example of payer policy changes occurred in 1992 and 1993, when Medicare stopped paying separately for interpretation of electrocardiograms in most circumstances (even though separate reporting was clearly appropriate under CPT® guidelines). Fortunately, the rules changed in 1994 to allow separate billing. Similarly, carriers considered angiography to be included within the allowance for cardiac catheterization prior to 1992; now carriers pay separately for angiography. In 1992, oncologists could not bill for chemotherapy by push *and* infusion method on the same day. In 1993, the rules changed to allow billing of both methods.

Private payers' billing policies may even be less well defined than Medicare's rules. As reimbursement levels become more restrictive and physicians participate with more plans, they will need to watch for distinctions among codes and guidelines that improve reimbursement without increasing audit liability.

The way billing is done can increase the chances of an audit. Using the same E/M code repeatedly, without regard to the actual level of care provided, will not only impact reimbursement but could significantly increase audit exposure. The same can be said regarding the use of consultation codes, selection of "fragmented" surgical codes, ignoring policies regarding global surgical fees, and the like.

It is not our intent to make it sound as though there is a Medicare auditor ready to pounce on every physician, because there is not. However, those who continually misuse the system stand a greater chance of an audit with potential recoupments, sanctions, and financial penalties. Not monitoring the billing aspects of the practice increases the odds of inappropriate billing mistakes, which could lead to an audit.

At times, Medicare carriers can take a tough stance. The following advisory statements were published in the April 1993 *Medicare Bulletin* for Tennessee, and basic points still apply today:

> Inappropriate billing practices—whether intentional or accidental—can have severe consequences. The limits of punishment for inappropriate Medicare billing are substantial. Physicians and their staff should remember the absolute imperative for totally accurate billing systems, whether working with Medicare and Medicaid programs, third-party payers, or other reimbursement systems. **Physicians are ultimately responsible for the acts of their employees, including billing and accounting staffs.** [boldface added]

As part of a settlement agreement between a physician and the US Attorney's office in a case involving inappropriate billing to Medicare, a Wisconsin physician had to publish the following statement to "educate" his colleagues about the seriousness of the issue:

> I paid Medicare for my mistake. My mistake was not ensuring the accuracy of the Medicare Claims that I was submitting. I left the task of preparing the claim forms to my clerical staff and signed the forms they prepared. Even though I did not intend to take advantage of the Medicare program, I was held accountable for the improper claims I signed. I have refunded the amount that I was overpaid, and paid an additional $65,000 in penalties. Don't make the same mistake I did. —*Wisconsin Medical Journal*

CPT® and ICD-9 Coding Under Managed Care

CPT® and ICD-9 coding is not particularly different under managed care. If the plan reimburses physicians on a fee-for-service basis, physicians will have to select appropriate codes to submit on claim forms. Most plans accept the standard CMS/HCFA 1500 claim form.

Obviously, CPT® does not play the same role under capitated systems. In fact, some plans simply require physicians in capitated systems to complete a simple encounter form for each patient visit. If it is an office visit, the physician merely checks an encounter block for office visit.[1] If it is a hospital visit, the physician checks a hospital encounter block. There are usually blocks for electrocardiograms, x-rays, etc.

However, in most capitated plans there are services that may be billable outside the capitation payment. In addition, some plans have stop-loss provisions that may make it necessary to code services accurately to take full advantage of such protection. It is also in the physician's and the plan's interest to use CPT® accurately to record what is performed and monitor quality of care and costs.

There is inconsistency among managed care plans in terms of payer rules for billing physician services. Plans differ as to the codes they accept. For example, some plans will pay additionally when the special service codes are reported for after-hours services or services on holidays. Others will not, and patients usually cannot be billed for these codes.

Some plans subscribe to many of Medicare's basic billing policies. Other plans do not have formal rules (particularly for the more difficult coding situations), and they seem to make rules up as needed. Plans vary as to how they reimburse for multiple surgical procedures on the same day, what is included in the global surgical fee, whether they routinely downcode higher levels of E/M services, the extent to which they cover preventive care, what they pay for supplies and injectable drugs, whether they pay separately for specimen collections, under what circumstances they will cover assistants at surgery, claim submission deadlines, and the like.

Managed care organizations will often review medical record documentation before paying large claims, claims for services that may be noncovered, claims with many surgical procedures performed on the same day, and other claims that may raise questions regarding medical necessity. Therefore, particular attention should be paid to documentation in medical records.

Some plans produce very good manuals that delineate common billing rules. Some have representatives who will try to answer physicians' questions. Unfortunately, some plans fare poorly in these respects.

Physicians should review the plan's billing manual very carefully. If coding situations common to their practice are not addressed sufficiently, they should call and talk to the plan's director of provider relations. It may be a good idea to meet with personnel who set the plan's coding policies.

In meeting with the payer, physicians should be careful what they say, exhibit a pleasant attitude, and indicate that they want to code correctly. They should avoid the appearance that they may really be looking for a "coding edge."

While physicians may have appeal rights, some managed care plans will simply terminate a participation agreement with physicians they suspect of coding improperly. If a physician is lax in selecting appropriate diagnosis codes, a plan might label him or her as a "high-cost" physician because the diagnoses do not adequately explain the patient's condition and treatment required.

Physicians are well advised to employ staff with extensive experience in Medicare, coding, dealing with insurance companies (particularly managed care plans), and other billing- and reimbursement-related activities. Things are changing too rapidly and there is too much money involved to entrust this responsibility to someone who is not prepared.

Physicians must stay abreast of new code changes and how payers interpret and apply policies to current codes. Otherwise, they will forgo income or increase audit exposure by billing for a service a payer says was not really performed. Worse, they may agree it was performed but still deny full coverage because it is deemed medically unnecessary.

Again, there are plans that pay little attention to coding on claims as long as things are reasonable. Other plans can be quite picky. Good documentation will help the physician support and justify most of his or her claims.

Use of Medicare Rules When Billing Other Payers

As mentioned earlier, payers vary as to their billing guidelines and coverage policies. Sometimes offices bill private insurers under Medicare's guidelines. Many private payers will cover supplies and other services that Medicare considers included within the payment for E/M codes or surgical procedures. There are private payers that allow physicians to bill for a specimen collection (36415) *and* a handling code (99000) when using a reference lab to perform tests. Some private insurers do not require or recognize CPT® modifiers (-24, -25, -57, -58, -59, -78, -79), which are an integral part of Medicare's global surgical policy.

On the other hand, Medicare will at times pay for CPT® codes that some private payers will not. Some private payers have more restrictive rules—at least in terms of the services that can be billed separately—under their global surgery policies.

Increasingly, Medicare's billing policies are becoming standards for private insurers. Thus, knowledge of Medicare's rules may make it easier to determine other payers' policies and payment guidelines in similar circumstances. As discussed earlier, *The National Correct Coding Policy Manual for Part B Medicare Carriers* is a valuable tool for determining when one service is reimbursable when billed with another performed on the same day; however, the manual's edits do not necessarily apply to non-Medicare payers.

E&M Documentation Guidelines

In June of 2000 the Centers for Medicare and Medicaid Services (CMS), then the Health Care Financing Administration, issued draft Evaluation and Management Documentation Guidelines. These guidelines were revised in December 2000. They focused on correct documentation of E&M encounters with Medicare beneficiaries and offered an alternative approach through clinical examples. CMS contracted with Aspen Systems Corporation to develop clinical example which were intended to illustrate acceptable E&M Documentation practices, provide guidance for clinical practitioners and to promote consistent medical review of E&M claims by Medicare Carriers. The clinical examples were to illustrate the guidelines for various levels of physical examination and medical decision-making. Aspen developed clinical examples for 16 medical specialties from de-identified medical records obtained from Medicare Carriers throughout the country. In May 2001 Aspen introduced the examples and their methods to organized medicine to begin an in depth review by physicians and Carrier Medical Directors

At the time of the introduction, specialty societies had many questions regarding how the clinical examples would be used in practice, the availability of Carrier feedback to the specialties, coordination between Carriers and specialty societies, and next steps. Also, the possibility that the clinical examples were based on medical records that were "downcoded" was raised as a serious concern. Since medical records were not available for some specialties, pediatrics, the issue was raised of the ability to develop sufficient clinical examples for all E&M services for all specialties. The participating specialty societies and Carriers were given a short timeframe (60 days) to review a large volume of clinical examples.

On June 26, the AMA hosted a specialty society meeting designed to collect broad specialty society reaction to the CMS/Aspen clinical examples. This meeting resulted in a specialty sign-on letter to Thomas Scully, Administrator of CMS. The letter attempted to capitalize on the Bush Administration's efforts to reduce the regulatory burden on physicians and called on CMS to re-examine the need for documentation guidelines and their commitment to the development of clinical examples. The letter made the point that it would be more appropriate for organized medicine to develop their own examples that accurately reflect appropriate levels of patient care, rather than use those suggested by the CMS contractor.

On July 19 the Department of Health and Human Services responded to medicine's concerns indicating that they were willing to address the E&M documentation burden. CMS stopped all work on the Aspen project and the 2000 Documentation

Guidelines (Carriers will continue to use either the 1995 or the 1997 Documentation Guidelines). The announcement was a direct response to advocacy efforts by the AMA and the specialty societies and represents a significant concession to the physician community. In follow-up statements CMS indicated that they believed that E&M coding should also be reviewed and it was their belief that physicians may be having problems with the E&M descriptors and CPT® coding guidelines.

The AMA, through the CPT® Editorial Panel, is responsible for maintaining CPT® codes and thus, the preferred approach is to address ambiguities with the code descriptors and coding guidelines through the established CPT® Panel process. The Panel opted to form an E&M Workgroup to address CMS's concerns. Initial discussions were held with CMS on the proposed scope and composition of the Workgroup. The Federal Advisory Committee Act (FACA) has prevented CMS from organizing its own task force and the Workgroup provides a viable approach to resolve CMS's coding concerns, CMS is supportive of the Workgroup and will participate in its deliberations. In November at the CPT® Annual Advisory Committee and Editorial Panel Meeting, the issue of a Panel E&M Workgroup was discussed. Advisors from the specialty societies were given the Workgroups prospective charge and scope of work that was developed through detailed discussions with CMS. Following the Advisors discussion, the Panel voted unanimously to form a Workgroup that would report back to the Panel in November 2002 through the normal Advisory Committee process.

CPT® Editorial Panel, E&M Workgroup

The Panel's E&M Workgroup includes representatives from several specialties, the Practicing Physician Advisory Council, a Carrier Medical Director, the Blue Cross Blue Shield Association, representatives from the CMS Center for Medicare Management and the Office of Program Integrity, and the AMA Board Ad Hoc Task Force on E&M Documentation Guidelines. The charge of the Workgroup is to enhance the functionality and utility of CPT® Evaluation and Management (E&M) codes by recommending changes in code descriptors, codes selection criteria and/or code levels in order to improve understanding among physicians. E&M codes must reflect current clinical practice and continue to describe physician work, while reducing the need for documentation guidelines and ensuring that any remaining documentation guidelines are oriented toward facilitating patient care. The mission of the Workgroup was to develop a coding system that physicians can use to report their services while practicing medicine according to the needs of the patient.

Since the beginning of the year, the E&M Workgroup has met six times, conducted an open meeting with public testimony, studied public and private sector E&M utilization data, and surveyed over 300 practicing physicians on their use and understanding of E&M codes (see the following internet site for more information www.ama-assn.org/cpt). At the August 2002 CPT® Editorial Panel the E&M

Workgroup chair, Douglas Wood, MD, presented the Workgroup's recommendations for a new framework for E&M codes, proposed code level instructions and code descriptor language, and follow-up development efforts on clinical examples. The CPT® Editorial Panel accepted the recommendations of the E&M Workgroup for the purpose of collecting input from the CPT®/HCPAC Advisory Committee. Advisor opinion forms have been sent to all 112 members of the CPT®/HCPAC Advisory Committee to allow comment and modifications to the proposed new framework and language for E&M instructions and codes. In addition, the Panel believes that the nature of E&M codes is such that potential changes to the codes requires input beyond the national medical specialty societies involved in the CPT®/HCPAC Advisory Committee. As a result, an opinion form containing the proposed new framework and language for E&M instructions and codes has been sent to all state medical association executives to allow input.

The CPT® Editorial Panel will meet in November to consider the input of all national medical specialty societies and state medical associations on the new framework and language. Based on this input and their own judgement the panel will develop and vote on a new framework and language for E&M instructions and codes. A follow-up process is currently being conducted to develop and review clinical examples to aid in the appropriate use of the new E&M codes. All new clinical examples must be reviewed for cross specialty work comparability and code level accuracy.

Surgery Section of CPT®

The surgery section of CPT® (code range, 10000-69979) is the longest, with codes and notes covering more than 300 pages. Achieving coding accuracy requires a thorough knowledge of CPT® codes and guidelines, monitoring of special payer billing requirements, and good communication between physicians and billing staff. Unfortunately, many third-party payers offer little assistance when difficult coding situations arise.

Several factors determine which code is most descriptive of the surgical procedure performed. As an example, the selection of the right code for some procedures depends on the surgical approach. Thus, 58800 is appropriate for drainage of an ovarian cyst, vaginal approach; 58805 is appropriate for an abdominal approach. In other cases, the right code depends on whether the procedure is complicated, deep, more involved than routine procedures, performed on someone younger than 2 years, and the like.

Modifying Words and Phrases

Look for words like "with" or "without" in CPT® 's description to accurately report the procedures performed. These words can make a substantial difference in selecting the correct code, reimbursement, and potential audit liability. Similar words and phrases are as follows:

Closed vs open	Each (ie, each digit)
Simple vs complicated	One or more sessions
Benign vs malignant	Separate procedure
Unilateral vs bilateral	List/charge in addition to
Deep vs superficial	Charge or list separately
Excision vs destruction	

These modifying words and phrases can substantially change the meaning of a code and ultimate reimbursement. For example, codes for closed reduction *with* manipulation often pay 20% to 30% more than codes for closed reduction *without* manipulation. A false claim could occur if a service with greater reimbursement than the procedure actually performed is billed.

Similarly, using a code for a *deep* or *complex* procedure, when the code for a superficial or simple procedure accurately reflects the service performed, could result in an overpayment of 200% or more. This type of error could easily result in significant Medicare recoupment and interest penalties if Medicare extrapolates coding errors over all of the claims a physician has filed with this code.

Physicians should help staff (and themselves) by providing specific and complete documentation in medical records.

Other Examples of Code Definitions

- 32604   "Thoracoscopy, diagnostic (separate procedure); pericardial sac with biopsy" is a more extensive procedure than

  32603   "Thoracoscopy, diagnostic (separate procedure); pericardial sac without biopsy."

- A procedure that entails *revision* of a graft is more complicated than one that does not.
    35875   Thrombectomy of arterial or venous graft (other than hemodialysis graft or fistula)
    35876   with revision of arterial/venous graft

- A *complex* surgery will have greater reimbursement than a surgery that is considered *simple*.
    61680   Surgery of intracranial arteriovenous malformation; supratentorial, simple
    61682   supratentorial, complex

An even more common example is wound repairs—simple, intermediate, and complex.

- *Attaching* muscles to an implant involves enough additional effort to warrant more reimbursement than a procedure in which muscles are not attached.

    65103   Enucleation of eye; with implant, muscles not attached to implant

    65105   with implant, muscles attached to implant

- The *location* of a laceration might have an impact on the amount of effort required to repair it. Medicare's allowance for 41251 (repair, posterior 1/3 of tongue) is greater than 41250 (anterior 2/3 of tongue). Reimbursement for wound repairs varies by complexity of repair and location—trunk, face, extremities, etc. Similarly, skin grafts, lesion excisions, and biopsies vary greatly depending on the location.

- Occasionally, CPT® provides a special code for billing postoperative complications.

    32100   Thoracotomy, major; with exploration and biopsy

    32120   for postoperative complications

- The type of *approach* taken during a procedure can often add to its complexity and thus impact reimbursement.

    43420   Closure of esophagostomy or fistula; cervical approach

    43425   transthoracic or transabdominal approach

- The spellings of some medical procedures are quite similar. Choosing the incorrect code can adversely affect reimbursement or audit exposure.

    92230   Fluorescein angioscopy with interpretation and report

    92235   Fluorescein angiography (includes multiframe imaging) with interpretation and report

Notes to CPT® Codes

In many cases, special notes appear near specific codes in the CPT® book. These notes can be critical to improving reimbursement and reducing audit exposure.

Here are some examples:

- The notes associated with some CPT® codes help improve coding accuracy.

    11100   Biopsy of skin . . . ; single lesion

    11101   each separate/additional lesion

    CPT® Note: (For biopsy of conjunctiva, use 68100; eyelid, use 67810)

- Some notes in CPT® actually indicate that a specific code should be billed in addition to a primary procedure.

    35601   Bypass graft, with other than vein; carotid

    35681   Bypass graft, composite, prosthetic and vein

    CPT® Note: List separately in addition to code for primary procedure.

Examples of the Variety of Codes

In CPT®, there may be a variety of codes from which to choose. As an example, below are listed some codes related to skin lesions and suturing. Reimbursement varies widely for these services. Note that there are other codes related to skin surgeries that are not listed here (eg, codes for Mohs surgery, tissue rearrangement, skin grafts, and the like).

A. Paring or cutting, corn or callus   11055-11057

    The correct code depends on the number of lesions.

B. Shaving epidermal or dermal lesions   11300-11313

C. Excision of benign lesions   11400-11471

D. Excision of malignant lesions   11600-11646

For B through D above, the correct code and reimbursement depend on site of lesion—leg, neck, face, etc—and size in *centimeters* (lesion size, not excision size).

- Destruction, benign or premalignant lesions   17000-17250
- Destruction, malignant lesions   17260-17286

Includes electrocautery, cryosurgery, laser, and chemical treatment. Correct code and reimbursement depend on site of lesions, number of lesions, and whether benign or malignant.

- Skin biopsy   11100-11101
- Removal of skin tags   11200-11201
- Wound repairs/suturing (size, location, complexity)[2]

Adhesive strips	E/M Codes
Simple	12001-12021
Intermediate	12031-12057
Complex	13100-13160

Sample Technique for Handling Coding

The following technique is used in some practices to handle difficult coding situations and responses for denied claims and requests for additional information. This technique helps ensure correct reimbursement, minimize audit exposure, reduce administrative hassles, and promote efficiency:

- **Routine billing:** Billing staff submits claims for routine or common procedures on a daily basis. These billings are based on a system where the physician carefully describes the services performed and applicable diagnoses in a special place in medical records to facilitate code selection by staff. Better yet, physicians mark special check-off forms with preprinted CPT® and ICD-9 codes. Typically, these routine or common procedures account for 85% to 90% of claims.

- **Difficult billing:** The other 10% to 15% of claims represent situations where staff may have questions regarding the appropriate CPT® code for primary and secondary procedures, whether a -22 modifier for unusual services is warranted, the appropriate ICD-9 code, whether additional information is necessary, and the like. For these claims, staff write down their questions and put the medical record aside in a special file.

- **Review of difficult claims:** Every Friday afternoon, the coding staff, the office manager, and a physician(s) meet for about 30 minutes to review the claims in question. If supporting documentation is needed, the physician helps staff select the salient points. If a more specific diagnosis is needed, the physician helps. Where the correct CPT® code is in question (especially with complex surgical procedures), the physician helps. Similarly, the physician reviews denials or requests for additional information received during the week. An adequate response is developed.

These meetings promote efficiency by relieving staff of the need to track down physicians every time they have a question. Physicians are not bombarded during the day while they are concerned with patient care.

Some large practices designate only one physician to attend these meetings. In this case, it is beneficial if the responsibility can be rotated so that all physicians see the problems and complexity of billing in today's environment. All physicians must keep current on coding and reimbursement issues so that the meetings stay efficient and staff are not having to educate physicians.

These short meetings will help ensure accurate reimbursement, improve office efficiency, and significantly reduce claim filing errors. Additionally, the meetings will grow shorter because staff and physicians learn more about the types of billing problems that can be eliminated. Staff now have fewer claims to question, and physicians have learned how to document records to shorten the "Friday meeting."

Other practices have developed other innovative ways of improving coding efficiency and results in their office. The above example is only one illustration of how effective practices make things work. It is always helpful when physicians document medical records and billing slips to communicate to staff what procedure was actually performed.

Fragmentation/Unbundling

Medicare and some private insurers have become increasingly concerned with what they call *fragmentation* or *unbundling*. They use the term *fragmented bills* to refer collectively to claims in which physicians bill separately for services that are encompassed in a single procedure code or in a global fee. In light of this, an increasing number of billings of several surgical procedure codes are denied as they are deemed "related" by reviewers. At this time, Medicare is the most restrictive in this area, but billing consultants are reporting that an increasing number of commercial insurers are denying payment for similar reasons.

The *National Correct Coding Policy Manual for Part B Medicare Carriers* discusses unbundling as follows:

> There are two types of unbundling; the first is unintentional which results from a misunderstanding of coding, and the second is intentional, when this technique is used by providers to manipulate coding in order to maximize payment. Unbundling is essentially the billing of multiple procedure codes for a group of procedures that are covered by a single comprehensive code.

> Correct coding means reporting a group of procedures with the appropriate comprehensive code. Examples of unbundling are described below:

> Fragmenting one service into component parts and coding each component part as if it were a separate service. For example the correct CPT-4 comprehensive code to use for upper gastrointestinal endoscopy with biopsy of stomach is CPT-4 code 43239. Separating the service into two component parts, using CPT-4 code 43235 for upper gastrointestinal endoscopy and CPT-4 code 43600 for biopsy of stomach is inappropriate.

> Reporting separate codes for related services when one comprehensive code includes all related services. An example of this type is coding the total abdominal hysterectomy with or without removal of tubes, with or without removal of ovary (CPT-4 code 58150) and salpingectomy (CPT-4 code 58700) and oophorectomy (CPT-4 code 58940) rather than using the comprehensive CPT-4 code 58150 for all three related services.

> Breaking out bilateral procedures when one code is appropriate. In this example, a bilateral mammography is coded correctly using CPT-4 code 76091 rather than submitting CPT-4 code 76090-RT for right mammography and CPT-4 code 76090-LT for left mammography incorrectly.

> . . . Separating a surgical approach from a major surgical service. For example, a provider should not bill CPT-4 code 49000 for exploratory laparotomy and CPT-4 code 44150 for total abdominal colectomy for the same operation because the exploration of the surgical field is included in the CPT-4 code 44150.

Some payers expect to see one surgical procedure code billed for upper or lower gastrointestinal endoscopy. Generally, the procedure code allowed is the one for the deepest level of penetration. In some cases, medical necessity can be proved for billing other codes if it is shown that more than casual observation was performed.

Florida's Medicare carrier provided some other examples of situations they would consider inappropriate billing:

- Florida's interpretation of procedure code 52601 for transurethral electrosurgical resection of prostate includes control of postoperative bleeding. Therefore, code 52606 for transurethral fulguration for postoperative bleeding should not be billed on the same day. The carrier goes further to say that 52606 should not be billed within the postoperative period. They also say that 52606 is included in the allowance for 52612-52650 when billed on the same day.

- Florida's carrier says that some ophthalmologists are incorrectly billing 36000 for injection of fluorescein in addition to the codes for fluorescein angioscopy (92230, 92235, 92287). Reimbursement for the injection procedure is included in the procedure codes for fluorescein angioscopy (according to their interpretation).

Fragmentation or unbundling is not common, and it is questionable whether physicians are reaping any real benefit if they, in fact, unbundle services (because incorrect coding combinations are usually denied by prepayment edit programs).

However, physicians should understand this concept to avoid inappropriate fragmentation and to ensure that other codes are billed when justified.

In an environment of managed care, it is imperative that surgeons understand each plan's billing guidelines, not just Medicare's. A physician cannot afford to be branded—because of coding errors, misunderstandings, or lack of communication on the payer's part—as an abuser, unbundler, overutilizer, or one who charges too much. Once this happens, regardless of the reason, it is difficult to get a plan to allow the physician to participate. Also, the physician should understand a plan's rules (assuming they have definitive guidelines) before evaluating payment rates.

Medicare Correct Coding Initiative

Below are comments from the July 2002 version of the *National Correct Coding Policy Manual for Part B Medicare Carriers* related to unbundling and other coding guidelines. As mentioned earlier, a few of the Medicare Correct Coding Initiative policies appear to be in conflict with previous Medicare guidelines. Physicians should watch for carrier announcements before assuming there has been a change in billing guidelines.

Introduction

The Physicians' Current Procedural Terminology (CPT) developed by the American Medical Association and HCPCS Level II codes developed by the Centers for Medicare and Medicaid Services (CMS) are listings of descriptive terms and identifying codes for reporting medical services and procedures performed by physicians. The codes in the *CPT Manual* are copyrighted by the AMA, and updated annually by the CPT Editorial Panel based on input from the AMA Advisory Committee which serves as a channel for requests from various providers and specialty societies. The purpose of both coding systems and annual updates is to communicate specific services rendered by physicians and other providers, usually for the purpose of claim submission to third party (insurance) carriers. A multitude of codes is necessary because of the wide spectrum of services provided by various medical care providers. Because many medical services can be rendered by different methods and combinations of various procedures, multiple codes describing similar services are frequently necessary to accurately reflect what service a physician performs. While often only one procedure is performed at a patient encounter, multiple procedures are performed at the same session at other times. In the latter case, the pre-procedure and post- procedure work does not have to be repeated and, therefore, a comprehensive code, describing the multiple services commonly performed together, can be defined.

Third party payers have adopted the CPT coding system for use by providers to communicate payable services. It therefore becomes more important to identify the various potential combinations of services to accurately adjudicate claims.

There are two sets of Correct Coding Initiative tables, comprehensive/component (correct coding) edits and mutually exclusive edits. All edits consist of code pairs that are arranged in column 1 and column 2 of the tables.

All edits are included in the comprehensive/component table except those meeting the criteria for mutually exclusive edits (Chapter I, Section R). Edits based on the Designation of Sex" criteria (Chapter I, Section S) are also included in the mutually exclusive tables. The column 2 code in both tables is not payable with the column 1 code unless the edit permits use of a modifier associated with CCI (Chapter I, Section H). The following policies encompass general issues/coding principles that are to be applied in all subsequent chapters. Specific examples are stated to clarify the policy but do not represent the only code or service that is included in the policy.

B. Coding Based on Standard of Medical/Surgical Practice

In order for this system to be effective, it is essential that the coding description accurately describe what actually transpired at the patient encounter. Because many physician activities are so integral to a procedure, it is impractical and unnecessary to list every event common to all procedures of a similar nature as part of the narrative description for a code. Many of these common activities reflect simply normal principles of medical/surgical care. These "generic" activities are assumed to be included as acceptable medical/surgical practice and, while they could be performed separately, they should not be considered as such when a code descriptor is defined. Accordingly, all services integral to accomplishing a procedure will be considered included in that procedure and, therefore will be considered a component & part of the comprehensive code.

Many of these generic activities are common to virtually all procedures. On other occasions, some are integral to only a certain group of procedures but are still essential to accomplish these particular procedures. Accordingly, it would be inappropriate to separately code these services based on standard medical and surgical principles. Some examples of generic services integral to standard of medical/surgical services would include:

- Cleansing, shaving and prepping of skin

- Draping of patient; positioning of patient

- Insertion of intravenous access for medication

- Sedative administration by the physician performing the procedure (see Chapter II, Anesthesia section, for the separate policy)

- Local, topical or regional anesthetic administered by physician

- Surgical approach, including identification of anatomical landmarks, incision, evaluation of the surgical field, simple debridement of traumatized tissue, lysis of simple adhesions, isolation of neurovascular, muscular (including stimulation for identification), bony or other structures limiting access to surgical field

- Surgical cultures

- Wound irrigation

- Insertion and removal of drains, suction devices, dressings, pumps into same site

- Surgical closure

- Application, management, and removal of postoperative dressings including analgesic devices (peri-incisional TENS unit, institution of Patient Controlled Analgesia)

- Preoperative, intraoperative and postoperative documentation, including photographs, drawings, dictation, transcription as necessary to document the services provided

- Surgical supplies, unless excepted by existing CMS policy

In the case of individual services, there are numerous specific services that may typically be involved in order to accomplish a comprehensive procedure. Generally, performance of these services represents the standard of practice for a more comprehensive procedure and the services are therefore to be included in that service. Because many of these services are unique to individual CPT coding sections, the rationale for correct coding will be described in that particular section. The principle of the policy to include these services into the comprehensive procedure remains the same as the principle applied to the generic service list noted above. Specifically, these principles include:

1. The service represents the standard of care in accomplishing the overall procedure.

2. The service is necessary to successfully accomplish the comprehensive procedure; failure to perform the service may compromise the success of the procedure.

3. The service does not represent a separately identifiable procedure unrelated to the comprehensive procedure planned.

Specific examples consist of:

Medical:

1. Procurement of a rhythm strip in conjunction with an electrocardiogram. The rhythm strip would not be separately reported if it was procured by the same physician performing the interpretation, since it is an integral component of the interpretation.

2. Procurement of upper extremity (brachial) Doppler study in addition to lower extremity Doppler study in order to obtain an "ankle-brachial index" (ABI). The upper extremity Doppler would not be separately reported.

3. Procurement of an electrocardiogram as part of a cardiac stress test. The electrocardiogram would not be separately reported if procured as a routine serial EKG typically performed before, during, and after a cardiac stress test.

Surgical:

1. Removal of a cerumen impaction prior to myringotomy. The cerumen impaction is precluding access to the tympanic membrane and its removal is necessary for the successful completion of the myringotomy.

2. Performance of a bronchoscopy prior to a thoracic surgery (e.g. thoracotomy and lobectomy). Assuming that a diagnostic bronchoscopy has already been performed for diagnosis and biopsy and the surgeon is simply evaluating for anatomic assessment for sleeve or more complex resection, the bronchoscopy would not be separately reported. Essentially, this "scout" endoscopy represents a part of the assessment of the surgical field to establish anatomical landmarks, extent of disease, etc. If an endoscopic procedure is done as part of an open procedure, it is not separately reported. However, if an endoscopy is performed for purposes of an initial diagnosis on the same day as the open procedure, the endoscopy is separately reported. In the case where the procedure is performed for diagnostic purposes immediately prior to a more definitive

procedure, the -58 modifier may be utilized to indicate that these procedures are staged or planned services.

Additionally, if endoscopic procedures are performed on distinct, separate areas at the same session, these procedures would be reported separately. For example, a thoracoscopy and mediastinoscopy, being separate endoscopic procedures, would be separately reported. On the other hand, a cursory evaluation of the upper airway as part of bronchoscopic procedure would not be separately reported as a laryngoscopy, sinus endoscopy, etc.

3. Lysis of adhesions and exploratory laparotomy reported with colon resection or other abdominal surgery. These procedures represent gaining access to the organ system of interest and are not separately reported.

C. Medical/Surgical Package

As a result of the variety of surgical, diagnostic and therapeutic non-surgical procedures commonly performed in medical practice, the extent of the *CPT manual* has grown. The need for precise definitions for the various combinations of services is further warranted because of the dependence of providers on CPT coding for reporting to third party payers. When a Resource-Based Relative Value System (RBRVS) is used in conjunction with CPT coding, the necessity for accurate coding is amplified.

In general, most services have pre-procedure and post-procedure work associated with them; when performed at a single patient encounter, the pre-procedure and post-procedure work does not change proportionately when multiple services are performed. Additionally, the nature of the pre-procedure and post-procedure work is reasonably consistent across the spectrum of procedures.

In keeping with the policy that the work typically associated with a standard surgical or medical service is included in the *CPT manual* code description of the service, some general guidelines can be developed. With few exceptions these guidelines transcend a majority of CPT descriptions, irrespective of whether the service is limited or comprehensive.

1. A majority of invasive procedures require the availability of vascular and/or airway access; accordingly, the work associated with obtaining this access is included in the pre-procedure services and returning a patient to the appropriate post-procedure state is

included in the procedural services. Intravenous access, airway access (e.g. HCPCS/CPT codes 36000, 36400, 36410) are frequently necessary; therefore, CPT codes describing these services are not separately reported when performed in conjunction with a more comprehensive procedure. Airway access is associated with general anesthesia, and no CPT code is available for elective intubation. The CPT code 31500 is not to be reported for elective intubation in anticipation of performing a procedure as this represents a code for providing the service of emergency intubation.

Furthermore, CPT codes describing services to gain visualization of the airway (nasal endoscopy, laryngoscopy, bronchoscopy) were created for the purpose of coding a diagnostic or therapeutic service and are not to be reported as a part of intubation services.

When vascular access is obtained, the access generally requires maintenance of an infusion or use of an anticoagulant (heparin lock) injection (e.g. CPT codes 90780 - 90784). These services are necessary for the maintenance of the access and are not to be separately reported. Additionally, use of an anticoagulant for access maintenance cannot be separately reported (e.g. CPT code 37201).

In some situations, more invasive access services (central venous access, pulmonary artery access) are performed with a specific type of procedure. Because this is not typically the case, the codes referable to these services may be separately reported.

Placement of central access devices (central lines, pulmonary artery catheters, etc.) involve passage of catheters through central vessels and, in the case of PA catheters, through the right ventricle; additionally, these services often require the use of fluoroscopic support. Separate reporting of CPT codes for right heart catheterization, first order venous catheter placement or other services which represent a separate procedure, is not appropriate when the CPT code that describes the access service is reported. General fluoroscopic services necessary to accomplish routine central vascular access or endoscopy cannot be separately reported unless a specific CPT code has been defined for this service.

2. When anesthesia is provided by the physician performing the primary service, the anesthesia services are included in the primary procedure (CMS Global Surgery Policy). If it is medically necessary for a separate provider (anesthesiologist/ anesthetist) to

provide the anesthesia services (e.g. monitored anesthesia care), a separate service may be reported.

3. Most procedures require cardiopulmonary monitoring, either by the physician performing the procedure or an anesthesiologist/certified registered nurse anesthetist. Because these services are integral and routine, they are not to be separately reported. This may include cardiac monitoring, intermittent EKG procurement, oximetry or ventilation management (e.g. CPT codes 93000, 93005, 93040, 93041, 94656, 94760, 94761, 94770). These services, when integral to the monitoring service, are not to be separately reported.

4. When, in the course of a procedure, a non-diagnostic biopsy is obtained and subsequently excision, removal, destruction or other elimination of the biopsied lesion is accomplished, a separate service cannot be reported for the biopsy procurement as this represents part of the removal. When a single lesion is biopsied multiple times, only one biopsy removal service should be reported. When multiple distinct lesions are non-endoscopically biopsied, a biopsy removal service may be reported for each lesion separately with a modifier, indicating a different service was performed or a different site was biopsied (see Section H of Chapter I for definition of the -59 modifier). The medical record (e.g. operative report) should indicate the distinct nature of this service. However, for endoscopic biopsies of lesions, multiple biopsies of multiple lesions are reported with one unit of service regardless of how many biopsies are taken. If separate biopsy removal services are performed on separate lesions, and it is felt to be medically necessary to submit pathologic specimens separately, the medical record should identify the precise location of each biopsy site. If the decision to perform a more comprehensive procedure is based on the biopsy result, the biopsy is diagnostic, and the biopsy service may be separately reported.

5. In the performance of a surgical procedure, it is routine to explore the surgical field to determine the anatomic nature of the field and evaluate for anomalies. Accordingly, codes describing exploratory procedures (e.g. CPT code 49000) cannot be separately reported. If a finding requires extension of the surgical field and it is followed by another procedure unrelated to the primary procedure, this service may be separately reported using the appropriate CPT code and modifiers.

6. When a definitive surgical procedure requires access through abnormal tissue (e.g. diseased skin,

abscess, hematoma, seroma, etc.), separate services for this access (e.g. debridement, incision and drainage) are not reported. For example, if a patient presents with a pilonidal cyst and it is determined that it is medically necessary to excise this cyst, it would be appropriate to submit a bill for CPT code 11770 (excision of pilonidal cyst); it would not, however, be appropriate to also report for CPT code 10080 (incision and drainage of pilonidal cyst), as it was necessary to perform the latter to accomplish the primary procedure.

7. When an excision and removal is performed ("-ectomy" code), the approach generally involves incision and opening of the organ ("-otomy" code). The incision and opening of the organ or lesion cannot be separately reported when the primary service is the removal of the organ or lesion.

8. There are frequently multiple approaches to various procedures, and are often clusters of CPT codes describing the various approaches (e.g. vaginal hysterectomy as opposed to abdominal hysterectomy). These approaches are generally mutually exclusive of one another and, therefore, not to be reported together for a given encounter. Only the definitive, or most comprehensive, service performed can be reported. Endoscopic procedures are often performed as a prelude to, or as a part of, open surgical procedures. When an endoscopy represents a distinct diagnostic service prior to an open surgical service and the decision to perform surgery is made on the basis of the endoscopy, a separate service for the endoscopy may be reported. The -58 modifier may be used to indicate that the diagnostic endoscopy and the open surgical service are staged or planned procedures.

9. When an endoscopic service is performed to establish the location of a lesion, confirm the presence of a lesion, establish anatomic landmarks, or define the extent of a lesion, the endoscopic service is not separately reported as it is a medically necessary part of the overall surgical service. Additionally, when an endoscopic service is attempted and fails and another surgical service is necessary, only the successful service is reported. For example, if a laparoscopic cholecystectomy is attempted and fails and an open cholecystectomy is performed, only the open cholecystectomy can be reported; if appropriate, a -22 modifier may be added to indicate unusual procedural services.

10. A number of CPT codes describe services necessary to address the treatment of complications of the

primary procedure (e.g. bleeding or hemorrhage). When the services described by CPT codes as complications of a primary procedure require a return to the operating room, they may be reported separately; generally, due to global surgery policy, they should be reported with the -78 modifier indicating that the service necessary to treat the complication required a return to the operating room during the postoperative period. When a complication described by codes defining complications arises during an operative session, however, a separate service for treating the complication is not to be reported. An operative session ends upon release from the operating or procedure suite (as defined in MCM '4821).

D. Evaluation and Management Services

All CPT and HCPCS Level II codes have a global surgery indicator. The separate payment for Evaluation and Management (E & M) services provided on the same day of service as procedures with a global surgery indicator of "000," "010," or "090" are covered by global surgery rules.

Procedures with a global surgery indicator of "XXX" are not covered by these rules. Many of these "XXX" procedures are performed by physicians and have inherent pre-procedure, intra-procedure, and post-procedure work usually performed each time the procedure is completed. This work should never be reported as a separate E & M code. Other "XXX" procedures are not usually performed by a physician and have no physician work relative value units associated with them. A physician should never report a separate E & M code with these procedures for the supervision of others performing the procedure or for the interpretation of the procedure. With most "XXX" procedures, the physician may, however, perform a significant and separately identifiable E & M service on the same day of service which may be reported by appending the -25 modifier to the E & M code. This E & M service may be related to the same diagnosis necessitating performance of the "XXXn procedure but cannot include any work inherent in the "XXXn procedure, supervision of others performing the "XXXn procedure, or time for interpreting the result of the "XXXn procedure.

E. Standard Preparation/Monitoring Service

Anesthesia services require certain other services to prepare a patient prior to the administration of anesthesia and to monitor a patient during the course of anesthesia. The advances in technology allow for intraoperative monitoring of a variety of physiological parameters. Additionally, when monitored anesthesia care is provided, the attention devoted to patient monitoring is of a similar level of intensity so that general anesthesia may be established if need be. The specific services necessary to prepare and monitor a patient vary among procedures, based on the extent of the surgical procedure, the type of anesthesia (general, MAC, regional, local, etc.), and the surgical risk. Although a determination as to medical necessity and appropriateness must be made by the physician performing the anesthesia, when these services are performed, they are included in the anesthesia service. Because it is recognized that many of these services may occur on the same date of surgery but are not performed in the course of and as part of the anesthesia provision for the day, in some cases these codes will be separately paid by appending the -59 modifier, indicating that the service rendered was independent of the anesthesia service.

F. Anesthesia Service Included in the Surgical Procedure

Under the National Global Surgical Policy, Medicare does not allow separate payment for the anesthesia services performed by the physician who also furnishes the medical or surgical service. In this case, payment for the anesthesia service is made through the payment for the medical or surgical service. For example, separate payment is not allowed for the surgeon's performance of a local or surgical anesthesia if the surgeon also performs the surgical procedure. CPT codes describing anesthesia services or services that are bundled into anesthesia should not be reported in addition to the basic procedure requiring the anesthesia services if performed by the same physician.

G. Coding Services Supplemental to a Principal Procedure (Add-on Codes)

The CPT coding system identifies certain codes which are to be submitted in addition to other codes. Generally, these are identified with the statement "list separately in addition to code for primary procedure" in parentheses and other times the supplemental code is to be used only with certain primary codes which are parenthetically identified. The basis for these CPT codes is to enable providers to separately identify a service that is performed in certain situations as an additional service or a commonly performed supplemental service complementary to the primary procedure. Incidental services that are necessary to accomplish the primary procedure (e.g. lysis of adhesions in the course of an open cholecystectomy) are not separately reported. Certain complications with an inherent potential to occur in an invasive procedure are, likewise, not separately reported unless resulting in the necessity for a significant separate procedure to be performed. For example, control of bleeding during a procedure is considered part of the procedure and is not separately reported.

Supplemental codes frequently specify codes or ranges of codes with which they are to be used. It would be inappropriate to use these with codes other than those specified. On occasion, a procedure described by a CPT code is modified or enhanced, either due to the unique nature of the clinical situation or due to advances in technology since the code was first published. When CPT codes are not labeled as supplemental codes in the manner described above, they are not to be reported unless the actual procedure is, in fact, performed. Using non-supplemental codes that approximate part of a more comprehensive procedure but do not describe a separately identifiable service is not appropriate.

Example: If, in the course of interpreting an echocardiogram, an ejection fraction is estimated, it would be inappropriate to code a cardiac blood pool imaging with ejection fraction determination (CPT code 78472) in addition to an echocardiography code (CPT code 93307.) Although the cardiac blood pool imaging does determine an ejection fraction, it does so by nuclear gaiting techniques which are not used in an echocardiogram. In other cases codes are interpreted as being supplemental to a primary code without an explicit statement in the *CPT manual* that the code is supplemental. Unless the code is explicitly identified in such a fashion, it would be improper as a coding convention to submit a primary procedure code as a supplemental code.

H. Modifiers

In order to expand the information provided by CPT codes, a number of modifiers have been created by the AMA, the CMS, and the local Medicare carriers. These modifiers, in the form of two characters, either numbers, letters, or a combination of each, are intended to transfer specific information regarding a certain procedure or service. Modifiers are attached to the end of a HCPCS/CPT code and give the physician a mechanism to indicate that a service or procedure has been modified

by some circumstance but is still described by the code definition.

Like CPT codes, the use of modifiers (either AMA, CMS or locally-defined modifiers) requires explicit understanding of the purpose of each modifier. It is also important to identify when the purpose of a modifier has been expanded or restricted by a third party payer. It is essential to understand the specific meaning of the modifier by the payer to which a claim is being submitted before using it.

There are modifiers created by either the AMA or the CMS which have been designated specifically for use with the correct coding and mutually exclusive code pairs. These modifiers are -El through -E4, -FA, -Fl through -F9, -LC, -LD, -LT, -RC, -RT, -TA, -Tl through -T9, -25, -58, -59, -78, -79, and -91. When one of these modifiers is used, it identifies the circumstances for which both services rendered to the same beneficiary, on the same date of service, by the same provider should be allowed separately because one service was performed at a different site, in a different session, or as a distinct service. The -59 modifier will be explained in greater detail in this section. In addition, pertinent information about three other modifiers, the -22, the -25, and the -58 is provided.

1. **-22 Modifier:** The -22 modifier is identified in the *CPT manual* as Aunusual procedural services.@ By definition, this modifier would be used in <u>unusual</u> circumstances; routine use of the modifier is inappropriate as this practice would suggest cases routinely have unusual circumstances. When an unusual or extensive service is provided, it is more appropriate to utilize the -22 modifier than to report a separate code that does not accurately describe the service provided.

2. **-25 Modifier:** The -25 modifier is identified in the *CPT Manual* as a "significant, separately identifiable evaluation and management service by the same physician on the same day of the procedure or other service". This modifier may be appended to an evaluation and management (E & M) code reported with another procedure on the same day of service. CCI includes edits bundling E & M codes into various procedures not covered by global surgery rules. If in addition to the procedure the physician performs a significant and separately identifiable E & M service beyond the usual pre-procedure, intra-procedure, and-post-procedure physician work, the E & M may be reported with the -25 modifier appended. The E & M and procedure(s) may be related to the same or different diagnoses.

3. **-58 Modifier:** The -58 modifier is described as a Astaged or related procedure or service by the same physician during the postoperative period. It indicates that a procedure was followed by another procedure or service during the post-operative period.@ This may be because it was planned prospectively, because it was more extensive than the original procedure or because it represents therapy after a diagnostic procedural service. When an endoscopic procedure is performed for diagnostic purposes at the time of a more comprehensive therapeutic procedure, and the endoscopic procedure does not represent ?scout@ endoscopy, the -58 modifier may be appropriately used to signify that the endoscopic procedure and the more comprehensive therapeutic procedure are staged or planned procedures. From the National Correct Coding Initiative perspective, this action would result in the allowance and reporting of both services as separate and distinct.

4. **-59 Modifier:** The -59 modifier has been established for use when several procedures are performed on different anatomical sites, or at different sessions (on the same day). The specific language according to the *CPT manual* is:

    59 Modifier: 'Distinct procedural service: Under certain circumstances, the physician may need to indicate that a procedure or service was distinct or independent from other services performed on the same day. Modifier -59 is used to identify procedures/services that are not normally reported together, but are appropriate under the circumstances. This may represent a different session or patient encounter, different procedure or surgery, different site or organ system, separate incision/excision, separate lesion, or separate injury (or area of injury in extensive injuries) not ordinarily encountered or performed on the same day by the same physician."

When certain services are reported together on a patient by the same physician on the same date of service, there may be a perception of "unbundling," when, in fact, the services were performed under circumstances which did not involve this practice at all. Because carriers cannot identify this based simply on CPT coding on either electronic or paper claims, the -59 modifier was established to permit services of such a nature to bypass correct coding edits if the modifier is present. The -59 modifier indicates that the procedure represents a distinct service from others reported on the same date of

service. This may represent a different session, different surgery, different site, different lesion, different injury or area of injury (in extensive injuries). Frequently, another, already established, modifier has been defined that describes this situation more specifically. In the event that a more descriptive modifier is available, it should be used in preference to the -59 modifier.

Example: If a patient requires placement of a flow directed pulmonary artery catheter for hemodynamic monitoring via the subclavian vein, it would be appropriate to submit the CPT code 93503 (Insertion and placement of flow directed catheter, e.g. Swan-Ganz for monitoring purposes) for the service. If, later in the day, the catheter must be removed and a central venous catheter is inserted through the femoral vein, the appropriate code for this service would be CPT code 36010 (Introduction of catheter, superior or inferior vena cava). Because the pulmonary artery (PA) catheter requires passage through the vena cava, it may appear that the service for the PA catheter was being "unbundled" if both services were reported on the same day. Accordingly, the central venous catheter code should be reported with the -59 modifier (CPT code 36010-59) indicating that this catheter was placed in a different site as a different service on the same day.

Other examples of the appropriate use of the -59 modifier are contained in the individual chapter policies.

The -59 modifier is often misused. The two codes in a code pair edit often by definition represent different procedures. The provider cannot use the -59 modifier for such an edit based on the two codes being different procedures. However, if the two procedures are performed at separate sites or at separate patient encounters on the same date of service, the - 59 modifier may be appended.

Example: The comprehensive/component code edit with comprehensive code 85102 (bone marrow biopsy) and component code 85095 (bone marrow, aspiration only) are two separate procedures when performed at separate anatomic sites or separate patient encounters. In these circumstances, it would be acceptable to use the -59 modifier. However, if both 85102 and 85095 are performed at the same site at the same patient encounter which is the usual practice, the -59 modifier should NOT be used. Although 85102 and 85095 are different procedures, they are bundled when performed at the same site and same patient encounter.

I. HCPCS/CPT Procedure Code Definition

The format of the *CPT manual* includes descriptions of procedures which are, in order to conserve space, not listed in their entirety for all procedures. The partial description is indented under the main entry, and constitutes what is always followed by a semicolon in the main entry. The main entry then encompasses the portion of the description preceding the semicolon. The main entry applies to and is a part of all indented entries which follow with their codes. An example is:

> 70120 Radiologic examination, mastoids; less than three views per side
>
> 70130 complete, minimum of three views per side

The common portion of the description is "radiologic examination, mastoids" and this description is considered a part of both codes. The distinguishing part of each of these codes is that which follows the semicolon. In the course of other procedure descriptions, the code definition specifies other procedures that are included in this comprehensive code. CPT procedure code 29855 is an example of this. By stating in the code description that the code includes arthroscopy, it follows that the surgical knee arthroscopy(CPT code 29871) cannot be reported with CPT code 29855 or vice versa. In addition, a code description may define a correct coding relationship where one code is a part of another based on the language used in the descriptor. Some examples of this type of correct coding by code definition are:

1. "Partial" and 'complete" CPT codes are reported. The partial procedure is included in the complete procedure.

2. "Partial" and "total" CPT codes are reported. The partial procedure is included in the total procedure.

3. "Unilateral" and "bilateral" CPT codes are reported. The unilateral procedure is included in the bilateral procedure.

4. "Single" and "multiple" CPT codes are reported. The single procedure is included in the multiple procedure.

J. HCPCS/CPT Coding Manual Instruction/Guideline

Each of the six major sections of the *CPT manual* and several of the major subsections include guidelines that are unique to that section. These directions are not all inclusive or limited to definitions of terms, modifiers, unlisted procedures or services, special or written reports, details about reporting separate, multiple or starred procedures and qualifying circumstances. These instructions appear in various places and are found at the beginning of each major section, at the beginning of subsections, and before or after a series of codes or individual codes. They define items or provide explanations that are necessary to appropriately interpret and report the procedures or services and to define terms that apply to a particular section. Notations are made in parentheses when CPT codes are deleted or cross-referenced to another similar code so that the provider has better guidance in the appropriate assignment of a CPT code for the service.

K. Separate Procedure

The narrative for many CPT codes includes a parenthetical statement that the procedure represents a "separate procedure." The inclusion of this statement indicates that the procedure, while it can be performed separately, is generally included in a more comprehensive procedure and the service is not to be reported when a related, more comprehensive, service is performed. The "separate procedure" designation is used with codes in the surgery (CPT codes 10000-69999), radiology (CPT codes 70000-79999) and medicine (CPT codes 90000-99199) sections. When a related procedure is performed, a code with the designation of "separate procedure" is not to be reported with the primary procedure.

Example: If the code identified as a "separate procedure" is reported with a related procedure code, such as when a sesamoidectomy, thumb or finger (CPT code 26185) is reported with an excision or curettage of a bone cyst or benign tumor of the proximal, middle, or distal phalanx of the finger with autograft (CPT code 26215), then the sesamoidectomy (separate procedure) should not be reported. By definition the "separate procedure" is commonly performed as integral and part of a larger service and usually represents a procedure that the physician performs through the same incision or orifice, at the same site, or using the same approach.

In the case where a ?separate procedure is performed on the same day but at a different session, or different site, this code may be reported with a more comprehensive service but the -59 modifier should be included indicating that this service was, in fact, a separate service.

In other sections of the *CPT manual*, the word "separate" is used in a phrase identified as "separate or multiple procedures" with a different meaning.

L. Family of Codes

In a family of codes, there are two or more component codes that are not reported separately because they are included in a more comprehensive code as members of the code family. Comprehensive codes include certain services that are separately identifiable by other component codes. The component codes as members of the comprehensive code family represent parts of the procedure that should not be listed separately when the complete procedure is done. However, the component codes are considered individually if performed independently of the complete procedure and if not all the services listed in the comprehensive codes were rendered to make up the total service. If all multiple services described by a comprehensive code are performed, the comprehensive code should be reported. It is not appropriate to report the separate component codes individually nor is it appropriate to report the component code(s) with the comprehensive code.

M. More Extensive Procedure

When procedures are performed together that are basically the same, or performed on the same site but are qualified by an increased level of complexity, the less extensive procedure is included in the more extensive procedure. In the following situations, the procedure viewed as the most complex would be reported:

1. "Simple" and "complex" CPT codes reported; the simple procedure is included in the complex procedure on the same site.

2. "Limited" and "complete" CPT codes reported; the limited procedure is included in the complete procedure on the same site.

3. "Simple" and "complicated" CPT codes reported; the simple procedure is included in the complicated procedure on the same site.

4. "Superficial" and "deep" CPT codes reported; the superficial procedure is included in the deep procedure on the same site.

5. "Intermediate" and "comprehensive" CPT codes reported; the intermediate procedure is included in the comprehensive procedure on the same site.

6. "Incomplete" and "complete" CPT codes reported; the incomplete procedure is included in the complete procedure on the same site.

7. "External" and "internal" CPT codes reported; the external procedure is included in the internal procedure on the same site.

N. Sequential Procedure

An initial approach to a procedure may be followed at the same encounter by a second, usually more invasive approach. There may be separate CPT codes describing each service. The second procedure is usually performed because the initial approach was unsuccessful in accomplishing the medically necessary service; these procedures are considered "sequential procedures". Only the CPT code for one of the services, generally the more invasive service, should be reported. An example of this situation is a failed laparoscopic cholecystectomy, followed by an open cholecystectomy at the same session. Only the code for the successful procedure, in this case the open cholecystectomy, should be reported.

O. With versus Without Procedure

In the *CPT manual*, there are various procedures that have been separated into two codes with the definitional difference being "with" versus "without" (e.g. with and without contrast). Both procedure codes cannot be reported. When done together the "without" procedure is included in the "with" procedure. An example would be a closed treatment of a fracture with manipulation and without manipulation. The CPT code without manipulation is included in the code with manipulation. Another example is a procedure described as under or requiring "anesthesia" and "without anesthesia." The "without anesthesia procedure code is included in the "under" or "requiring anesthesia" procedure code.

P. Laboratory Panel

When all components of a specific organ or disease oriented laboratory panel (e.g. CPT codes 80074,80061) or of a metabolic or electrolyte panel (e.g.. CPT codes 80048, 80051 and 80053) are reported separately, they must be included in the comprehensive panel code that includes the multiple component tests. The individual tests that make up a panel are not to be separately reported.

Example: CPT code 80090(TORCH antibody panel) includes the following tests:

CPT code 86644: Antibody—cytomegalovirus

CPT code 86694: Antibody—herpes simplex

CPT code 86762: Antibody—rubella

CPT code 86777: Antibody—toxoplasma

When all 4 tests are performed and medically necessary, the panel test (CPT code 80090) must be reported in place of the individual tests.

Q. Misuse of Column 2 Code with Column 1 Code

In general, CPT codes have been written as precisely as possible to not only describe a specific service or procedure but to also avoid describing similar services or procedures which are already defined by other CPT codes. When a CPT code is reported, the physician or non-physician provider must have performed all of the services noted in the descriptor unless the descriptor states otherwise. (Frequently, a CPT descriptor will identify certain services that may or may not be included, usually stating ?with or without a service.) A provider should not report a CPT code out of the context for which it was intended. Providers who are familiar with procedures or services described in areas or sections of CPT will understand the specific language of the descriptor as well as the intent for which the code was developed. On the other hand, a provider who, for example, is unfamiliar with an area of CPT may fail to understand the intent of certain codes. Either intentionally or unintentionally, a provider may report a service or procedure using a CPT code that may be construed to describe the service/procedure but, in no way, was intended to be used in this fashion.

CPT codes describing services or procedures that would not typically be performed with other services or procedures but may be construed to represent other services have been identified and paired with the latter (comprehensive) CPT codes. Additionally, pairs of codes have been identified which would not be reported together because another code more accurately describes the services performed.

Example: CPT code 20550 (?Injection, tendon sheath, ligament, trigger points, or ganglion cyst) is intended to

describe a therapeutic musculoskeletal injection. It would represent a misuse of the code to report this code with other procedures (e.g. 20520 for simple removal of foreign body in muscle or tendon sheath) when the only service provided was injection of local anesthesia in order to accomplish the latter procedure.

R. Mutually Exclusive Procedure

There are numerous procedure codes that are not to be reported together because they are mutually exclusive of each other. Mutually exclusive codes are those codes that cannot reasonably be done in the same session. An example of a mutually exclusive situation is when the repair of the organ can be performed by two different methods. One repair method must be chosen to repair the organ and must be reported. A second example is the reporting of an "initial" service and a "subsequent" service. It is contradictory for a service to be classified as an initial and a subsequent service at the same time.

CPT codes that are mutually exclusive of one another based either on the CPT definition or the medical impossibility/improbability that the procedures could be performed at the same session can be identified as code pairs.

These codes are not necessarily linked to one another with one code narrative describing a more comprehensive procedure compared to the component code, but can be identified as code pairs that should not be reported together.

In order to identify these code pairs, an independent table of mutually exclusive codes has been developed as part of the CCI. This table differs from the traditional table of comprehensive and component codes. While the codes are listed as column 1 and column 2 codes, this fact does not mean that the column 2 code is included in the column 1 code because the column 2 code is a component or part of the column 1 comprehensive code. Rather the two codes cannot be reported at the same time. In the processing of the code pair when reported together, in general the procedure with the lower work relative value unit will be allowed. Accordingly, the code for this procedure has been placed in column 1. In cases where the work relative value unit is 0 for one or both of the procedures or the procedure(s) is (are) not paid according to the physicians' fee schedule, the code with the lowest Medicare allowance in general has been inserted in column 1.

S. Designation of Sex

Many procedure codes have a sex designation within their narrative. These codes are not reported with codes having an opposite sex designation because this would reflect a conflict in sex classification either by the definition of the code descriptions themselves (as they appear in the *CPT manual*) or by the fact that the performance of these procedures on the same patient would be anatomically impossible.

The sections that this policy pertains to are the male and female genital procedures. Other codes indicate in their definition that a particular sex is required for the use of that particular code. An example of this situation would be CPT code 53210 for total urethrectomy including cystostomy in a female as opposed to CPT code 53215 for the male. Both of these procedures are not to be reported together. Some other examples of these code pairs are: 53210-53250, 52275-52270, and 57260-53620. These specific edits have been included in the Mutually Exclusive Table because both procedures of a code pair edit cannot be performed on a patient. (See Section R in this chapter for more explanation of mutually exclusive codes.)

T. Excluded Service

Because some procedures are identified as excluded from coverage under the Medicare program as "excluded services," there is no need to address the issue of correct coding with these codes. In the development of National Correct Coding Policy and Correct Coding Edits, these excluded services have been ignored.

U. Unlisted Service or Procedure

The codes listed after each section and/or subsection which end in -99 (or a single -9 in a few cases) are used to report a service that is not described in any code listed elsewhere in the *CPT manual*. Because of advances in technology or physician expertise with new procedures, a code may not be assigned to a procedure when the procedure is first introduced as accepted treatment. The unlisted service or procedure codes are then necessary to code the service. Every effort should be made to find the appropriate code to describe the service and frequent use of these unlisted codes instead of the proper codes is not appropriate. Correct code assignment would occur after the documentation has been reviewed and bundling of code pairs would then take place based on the changed code or correctly submitted code. The unlisted service or procedure codes have not been included in the Correct Coding Policy or Edits because of the multiple procedures that can be assigned to these codes.

V. Modified, Deleted, and Added Code Pairs/Edits

Correct coding (comprehensive/component) and mutually exclusive code pairs/edits have been developed based on the coding conventions defined in the American Medical Association's *CPT manual* instructions and CPT code descriptions, national and local Medicare policies and edits, the coding guidelines developed by national societies, the analysis of standard medical and surgical practice, and the review of provider billing patterns and current coding practice. Prior to initial implementation, the proposed code pairs/edits underwent scrutiny by Medicare Part B carriers and physicians including Carrier Medical Directors, representatives of the American Medical Association's CPT Advisory Committee, and other national medical societies. As a part of the ongoing refinement of the National Correct Coding Initiative, a process has been established to address annual changes in CPT and HCPCS Level II codes such as additions, deletions, and modifications of existing codes. Additionally, ongoing changes occur based on changes in technology, and standard medical practice, and from continuous input from the AMA, and various specialty societies. During the refinement process, correspondence is received from the AMA, national medical societies, CMS Central and Regional Offices, Contractor Medical Directors, Medicare Part B carriers, individual providers, physicians' consultants and other interested parties. The comments and recommendations are evaluated and considered for possible modification or deletion of existing code pairs/edits or additions of new code pairs/edits. Subsequently based on the contributions from these sources, CMS Central Office decides which code pairs/edits are modified, deleted, or added.

Another Tool—Medicare Physician Fee Schedule Database (MPFSDB)

Many Medicare carriers provide on their Web site the Medicare Physician Fee Schedule Database (MPFSDB). This database includes information useful in determining Medicare allowables. But, just as important, it includes information about which surgical procedure codes can be billed with a bilateral modifier, which ones qualify for cosurgery, which codes are subject to multiple surgical procedure reductions (and which codes should not be billed with a -51 modifier), etc.

One Medicare carrier provided the following example where improper billing would result in less reimbursement than is appropriate:

> . . . We have been receiving a large number of claims where modifier "50" is being billed incorrectly. The following examples show the correct and incorrect methods of billing this modifier with CPT code 92235, Fluorescein angiography (includes multi-frame imaging) with interpretation and report, when it is rendered globally.

> **Correct Billing When Performed on Both Eyes**

> 06/01/2002 92235ZD50 (with Number of Service [NOS] 1)

> In this case, Medicare would allow 150% of 99235's allowance.

> **Incorrect Billing**

> 06/01/2002 92235ZD (with Number of Service [NOS] 1)

> 06/01/2002 92235ZD (with Number of Service [NOS] 1)

> In the incorrect example above, the second line would be denied as a duplicate. We would have no way of knowing if this service was actually rendered bilaterally or if the second line was merely a clerical error. Thus, one would only receive 100% of 99235's allowance unless the claim is refiled.

The point is that billing staff should be familiar with all the tools available for determining proper coding. While receiving less reimbursement than appropriate may not make a physician an audit target, it may make it more difficult to maintain a viable, high-quality practice.

Variations in Policies Among Payers

Other payers may have rules that differ from Medicare's. For example, one of the more difficult coding topics involves billing for two or more surgical procedures performed on the same day during the same operative session. Payers are not consistent in their approach to reimbursement for secondary procedures, nor do they necessarily follow Medicare's *Correct Coding Manual* in terms of codes that may be billed together.

Some insurers will pay 100% for each of two procedures performed in the same operative field, whereas others will pay the second procedure at 75%. Some will pay bilateral procedures at twice the unilateral level, but others cut allowances in half for the second procedure.
Some will pay for two procedures performed at separate anatomic/incision sites at 100%, but others reduce the second by 25% or 50%. Some insurers pay for the first procedure at 100%, the second at 50%, the third at 25%, and any others at 10% of allowances (the percentages vary depending on the payer). Some follow Medicare's rule applicable in 1992, 1993, and 1994 (ie, 100% for the first procedure, 50% for the second, and 25% for the third through fifth).

Payer policies vary dramatically (although this may change in the future).

This chapter has only touched on the subject of CPT®, focusing primarily on the importance of documentation and selecting the correct codes to minimize audit exposure. Most of the audits performed by Medicare carriers are initiated to determine if the services billed were actually performed and were medically necessary based on the information in medical records. There are many other services, modifiers, coding guidelines, and related topics than can be covered here. It is hoped that this brief discussion provided some tips to help physicians improve the effectiveness and efficiency of coding in their offices.

Most important, this discussion should illustrate the necessity of adequate training, self-audits, and other compliance efforts to ensure that physicians are selecting the proper codes and documenting records sufficiently. Ongoing training will improve compliance efforts and ensure that physicians receive appropriate reimbursement under a payer's billing and reimbursement system.

If non-physician staff are involved in coding, it is essential to make sure they understand the coding system and rules applicable to each physician's specialty. Frequent internal audits (ie, quality checks) will help ensure compliance.

Chapters 2 and 9 give additional information on CPT® coding. Chapter 2 provides many examples of coding practices that could be deemed fraudulent or abusive. Chapter 9 covers ways to avoid audits.

Endnotes

1. That is, you do not have to distinguish between a level 3 or level 4 visit, or if the patient is new or established, etc. However, ICD-9 coding can be just as important as under fee-for-service arrangements because of quality management concerns.

2. For most wound repairs, select codes on the basis of complexity and length of wound. Wounds are measured in centimeters (one may lose reimbursement if wounds are measured in inches rather than centimeters). If there are multiple wounds, add together the length of various wounds in same category (trunk, face, etc).

Chapter 11

ICD-9 Diagnosis Coding

CPT® codes explain what service you performed.
ICD-9 codes explain why you performed that service.

ICD-9 codes help establish the medical necessity for various services. As explained in Chapter 8, Medicare carriers and other payers often establish prepayment edits with ICD-9 codes that must be included on claims to achieve payment when certain services are billed.

Carriers often look first at ICD-9 codes when determining the medical necessity for many common services. Proper use of ICD-9 codes will prevent many problems and help physicians justify more intensive services when required by a patient's condition.

Unfortunately, ICD-9 codes can also be used inappropriately. One could "justify" payment for certain medical services by selecting diagnosis codes that might bypass computer edits even though the diagnosis code is not representative of the patient's condition or documentation in the medical record. Audits by Medicare carriers and others will reveal instances where diagnosis codes are not reflective of the patient's condition. Such improper use of diagnosis codes could constitute fraud or abuse.

A basic principle of ICD-9 coding is that one should select codes that are representative of the patient's condition as documented in the medical record and that indicate the medical necessity of the service billed on claim forms.

One can minimize fraud and abuse implications by selecting codes that are truly representative of the patient's condition as reflected by documentation in the medical record. Even if you "violate" some of the ICD-9 coding conventions—such as use of the fourth digit when codes with a fifth digit are available—the fraud and abuse implications are greatly reduced. Obviously, failure to adhere to these coding conventions may delay claims payment.

ICD-9 codes can also be used to some extent in monitoring quality of care. For example, quality management systems can use claims data to monitor treatment patterns and referral patterns by diagnosis. As another example, health plans may monitor primary care physicians with diabetic patients to ensure that patients are referred to an ophthalmologist at appropriate intervals. (Obviously, there are serious limitations to the use of diagnosis codes alone for quality management purposes.)

The *International Classification of Diseases, 9th Revision, Clinical Modifications* (ICD-9-CM) is published in three volumes: Volume I, Diseases: Tabular Listing; Volume II, Diseases, Alphabetic Listing; and Volume III, Procedures: Tabular and Alphabetic. Although volume III is not needed to bill for physician services under Medicare Part B, ICD-9 is often sold in three-volume sets.

In general, the ICD-9 coding system is easy to use. After a diagnosis is located in volume II (the alphabetic index), that code is referred to in volume I to see if further instructions apply. These instructions are in the form of notes suggesting the use of additional codes and conditions requiring codes found elsewhere.

Some people make ICD-9 coding for physician services more difficult than it really is. Most payers recognize that most physicians' staff cannot code diagnoses to the standard of hospital medical records personnel who have very specialized training in all aspects of diagnosis coding. Thus, physicians should concentrate on providing ICD-9 codes that match documentation in the medical record and that explain why a medical service was performed.

In addition to coding for the primary reason for the encounter, it is also important to provide ICD-9 codes for conditions that make the patient's condition more complicated and contribute to the need for more extensive examinations, treatments, and/or medical decision making.

Once commonly used codes are established for a practice, reference to books will be infrequent. A list of common codes should be included on superbills, in computer databases, or on charts posted at insurance staff desks. When an unusual diagnostic condition arises, physicians should document medical records with sufficient information for staff to locate codes easily.

Under the ICD-9 system, each disease entity is assigned a three-digit category (for example, 239 in the listing below). In most cases, a fourth digit has been added and should be used when available. Some codes have been expanded to include a fifth digit, which should also be used when claims are coded.

ICD-9 guidelines for outpatient services indicate that a code is invalid if it has not been coded to the full number of digits required for that code. Some of the most common errors occur with diabetes mellitus (250xx), which requires five digits, and osteoarthrosis (715xx), which also needs fifth-digit coding. On the other hand, some conditions, such as chronic airway obstruction (chronic obstructive pulmonary disease, ICD-9 code 496), have no fourth or fifth digits.

A complete listing of the three-digit disease categories is found in Appendix E, volume I, of the ICD-9 book.

The following is an example of entries in ICD-9-CM.

> 239   Neoplasms of unspecified nature
>
> > 239.0   Digestive system
> > 239.1   Respiratory system
> > 239.2   Bone, soft tissue, skin
> > 239.3   Breast
> > 239.4   Bladder

Thus, ICD-9 code 239.4 would justify a cystourethroscopy with biopsy (CPT® code 52204) but would not justify a mastectomy. Further, use of only the three-digit code 239 *could* cause the claim to be rejected pending additional information, since it is not specific enough to determine medical necessity for the service performed. Fourth and fifth digits should be used if provided in the code book.

The code(s) that best justifies the medical necessity for the service should be selected. If multiple CPT® codes are billed on the same claim form, an ICD-9 code should be selected that justifies each service performed. Medicare carriers often refer to this as *linking*, that is, matching a CPT® code with one or more ICD-9 codes that indicate the medical necessity for a service. For example, if a patient comes to the office for a follow-up visit for chronic ischemic heart disease (414.9) but also complains of a urinary infection (599.0):

- The office visit evaluation and management (E/M) service is coded with support by ICD-9 code 414.9 (and 599.0).

- The urinalysis (CPT® code 81000) is charged by means of ICD-9 code 599.0 for urinary tract infection.

As explained earlier, use of different, unrelated diagnoses codes for an E/M service and a minor surgical procedure on the same day will help avoid possible denials under Medicare's global surgery rules.

Modifier -25 is attached to the E/M code. The E/M encounter is coded with the appropriate diagnosis (one that primarily explains the E/M service). The procedure is coded with its corresponding diagnosis.

Diagnoses do not necessarily have to be unrelated if the physician performed a significant, separately identifiable E/M service in addition to a minor surgical procedure. However, it helps to support the -25 modifier when they are unrelated.

Physicians, when billing for their services under Part B Medicare, are allowed to code for problems, symptoms, and conditions such as coughing, wheezing, fever, neck pain, headaches, light flashes, and the like.[1] However, it is better to provide a final diagnosis if available. Codes that describe symptoms and signs, as opposed to diagnoses, should be provided for reporting purposes when a diagnosis has not been established. Many, but not all, symptoms and conditions are listed under ICD-9 codes 780.0 to 799.9. Of course, physicians must help hospitals choose a final diagnosis, because it is a requirement for payment to the hospital under Medicare's Part A diagnosis-related group system.

If the physician cannot diagnose pneumonia definitively when filing for physician services, he or she should code by using symptoms such as fever, chest pain, coughing, and the like. Surgeries should be supported by the diagnosis precipitating the operation unless the postoperative diagnosis is known to be different at the time the claim is submitted.

Again, actual code selection is not difficult for most medical conditions. The real art is knowing how to use ICD-9 codes to support or justify services rendered and to avoid denials. Another illustration of the importance of diagnostic coding is avoiding denials for unnecessary concurrent care. Below is an example:

> Assume a diabetic patient is admitted to the hospital with severe chest pain by a cardiologist. The patient's family physician must treat the diabetic condition with diet and insulin orders. If both physicians bill for daily hospital care by using the cardiac diagnosis, the one submitting claims first will be paid. The physician who waits may not be paid.

> However, if the cardiologist uses a diagnosis related to the heart condition and the family physician uses a diagnosis of diabetes, both should be paid notwithstanding the fact they are treating the patient concurrently.

The key to avoiding denials for "unnecessary" concurrent care is to code for the specific conditions you are treating. However, the claim form should not be loaded up with unrelated diagnoses.

Identifying new or multiple diagnoses will help justify multiple services as payers develop computer screens with service volumes. For example, a patient may present with blood in the urine. This diagnosis might justify a urinalysis and pelvic examination on one day and a cystoscopic examination on another day. If a biopsy indicates a malignant neoplasm of the lateral wall of the urinary bladder, 188.2 could be used to substantiate a laser cystourethroscopy at another time. However, a different diagnosis should be used only if it represents the patient's condition and is documented in the medical record.

Accurately Describing the Patient Encounter

Claims reviewers point to the importance of describing the patient encounter as completely as possible. The reasons services are performed can be described numerically via ICD-9 codes that explain the true context of the encounter, including symptoms and conditions that prompt a physician to order tests and services. For example:

> A 46-year-old man with a history of a myocardial infarction and a strong family history of diabetes presents with a sudden onset of chest pain so severe that he became sweaty and almost passed out (or he may have; he was not sure). He felt that he couldn't catch his breath. His physician orders an electrocardiogram, cardiac enzymes, glucose, glucose tolerance, and chemistry profile, and later schedules a treadmill test (the patient was sent because he had some definite costochondral tenderness). A claim was submitted for all services by means of ICD-9 code 733.6 for costochondritis.

This one diagnosis code might not justify all the services, and it does not accurately describe the patient's condition. The visit could have been coded as follows:

780.2	Syncope
786.50	Chest pain
780.8	Diaphoresis (profuse sweating)
412	History of myocardial infarction
V18.0	Family history of diabetes

Earlier, we advised against loading up claims with irrelevant diagnoses, but it sometimes helps to carry things a step farther than the obvious. For example, the diagnoses below might warrant a higher level of service than merely coding for a sore throat (assuming the patient also presents with these problems and they are documented in the medical record):

462   Sore throat
785.6   Enlarged lymph nodes (swollen glands)
780.6   Pyrexia of unknown origin (chills with fever)
780.7   Fatigue and malaise

CPT® guidelines indicate that examination of a patient with a sore throat would normally be coded as a relatively low-level E/M service. However, the additional diagnoses above might persuade a payer to allow a level 3 or level 4 visit code. Of course, the medical records should indicate that the physician performed aspects of the higher-level service.

Chronic or coexisting conditions that are considered during medical decision making should be reported to support higher-level services. Personal and family history may also be coded by means of V codes to support complex history taking.

Remember, you can often bill a level 2 hospital visit (99232) when the patient develops a minor complication that must be assessed during the encounter. Document nausea, dizziness, headaches, leg pain, etc, and be sure to communicate this to billing staff.

Coding Underlying Diseases

Underlying diseases are sometimes required to be coded along with the particular manifestation. The manifestations appear in italics in the alphabetic and tabular sections of the ICD-9-CM. The italics indicate that ICD-9 considers this diagnosis a manifestation of an underlying disease that should be coded first. For example, consider the ICD-9 listing below:

573.1   Hepatitis in viral diseases classified elsewhere

         Code first underlying disease as:
                  Coxsackie virus disease (074.8)
                  Cytomegalic inclusion virus disease (078.5)
                  Infectious mononucleosis (075)

The italicized words *Code first underlying disease as* mean that the physician must identify the cause of hepatitis. The cause should be listed on the claim form first and the manifestation as an additional code. Thus, in block 21 of the HCFA 1500 claim form (or equivalent field for electronic claims), "A075" is listed on one line by Number 1 and "573.1" by Number 2 (*note:* some coders consider it better to code 573.1 first in this example).

Understanding the Terminology

The abbreviation NEC means "not elsewhere classified." Codes with the description NEC would be used when more specific information is not available to the physician or ICD-9 classifications are not further subdivided.

The abbreviation NOS means "not otherwise specified." This abbreviation is the equivalent of "unspecified." For example, if the type of bacterial infection is not known at the time a claim is submitted, a code with NEC, unspecified, or NOS is used.

In some cases, a listing for an ICD-9 code has a note that uses the word "excludes", as demonstrated as follows:

> 454   Varicose Veins of Lower Extremities
>   **Excludes: that complicating pregnancy, childbirth or the puerperium (671.0)**
>   [boldface added]

In these cases, one would use the 454 series unless the varicose veins were a complication of pregnancy, childbirth, or the puerperium.

Special Coding Circumstances

Injuries

Injuries are described by diagnoses of fractures, contusions, dislocations, sprains, lacerations, burns, and the like. The code is found under the *type of injury* (fracture, laceration, etc) and then the *anatomic site* (hand, foot, etc). The most severe injury is coded as the principal diagnosis for multiple injuries. Fractures are coded as to type and whether closed or open. Coders usually select a "closed" diagnosis unless the physician indicates otherwise.

E Codes

Use of E codes as a primary diagnosis is not recommended in most cases. Most carriers will not recognize these codes as a primary diagnosis, and payment denial may result.[2]

E codes document the method of injury; E819 indicates a motor vehicle traffic accident of unspecified nature. E codes also cover poisonings, bites, drowning, chemical exposure, environmental exposure, and other such adverse occurrences.

Here is a coding example:

> A bicyclist receives an open wound to the elbow requiring sutures when his cycle is hit by a nearsighted dog. The physician who repairs the laceration could bill by means of the following diagnoses:

> 881.11   **Open wound to elbow, complicated** [boldface added]

> E826.1   Pedal cycle accident

In addition to explaining the patient's condition, ICD-9 codes such as these provide some useful information about the physician's practice. The more physicians know about their practices, the better equipped they will be to negotiate with payers and make informed decisions about their practices. Use of 10 to 15 carefully selected codes can greatly increase any physician's knowledge about his or her practice, regardless of specialty. A physician or practice manager can select these 10 to 15 E codes in a few minutes.

However, the high levels of specificity available through the ICD-9 system are not necessary for this purpose. NOS (not otherwise specified) codes are adequate for a physician collecting practice information. For example, an orthopedic practice may want to know how many patients are being treated as a result of cycling accidents. The appropriate E code is E826.1, and this includes all modes of bicycling accidents.

Information of this nature can help physicians develop patient education initiatives as well as provide guidance for the physician's own continuing education (there may be some excellent continuing medical education courses on cycling injuries physicians may want to attend if their practice handles a high volume of this injury).

Avoiding "Rule Out" or "Probable/Possible" Codes

"Rule out" codes are to be avoided if possible. In the urological example cited earlier, the hematuria diagnostic code should be used rather than a "rule out neoplasm" designator. If a physician orders magnetic resonance imaging for a patient with suspected multiple sclerosis, "rule out" codes should not be used, nor should multiple sclerosis be coded as an established condition. Appropriate symptoms, such as dizziness, blurred vision, muscular weakness, and the like, should be selected.

Some payers will deny claims supported only by "rule out" codes. It is also possible that these diagnoses could result in a patient having his or her insurance canceled, troubles with an employer, or family problems because of a *possible* diagnosis of cancer, diabetes, human immunodeficiency virus infection, and the like. Coding consultants recommend using ICD-9 codes for the symptoms that suggest the patient may have the condition.[3]

Some physicians will document "rule out" situations in the medical record, but instruct coding staff to use diagnosis codes for the documented signs and symptoms that cause the physician to suspect the condition may exist. This is acceptable.

V Codes

Follow-up visits for patients who have been treated for a malignancy can be justified by using V codes. Mammograms—where patients are at high risk—are coded as follows (for other than screening mammograms):

V16.3   For patients with family history of breast cancer

V10.3   For patients with personal history of breast cancer

V15.89   When specific reason patient is at high risk is not known (this and similar codes should be used judiciously, and denials are possible)

In addition to V codes, any specific findings from examinations or symptoms such as breast mass should be listed.

A V code is often the proper diagnosis code to bill for screening exams that are covered (with limitations) by Medicare and other payers—screening mammographies, colon cancer screening, Pap smears, and the like. Check billing guidelines for screening exams closely.

Patient Admitted for Surgery That Is Subsequently Canceled

When a patient is admitted for surgery that is subsequently canceled, the diagnosis for which the patient was admitted is listed first, and V64.0 to V64.3 ("Persons encountering health services for specific procedures, not carried out") is listed last.

Locating ICD-9 Codes

Usually it is easier to locate a code by looking in the index for the *condition*, not the site. For example, to locate a code for "breast lump," the physician would look under "lump," not under "breast." The site (breast) is listed under "lump."

No matter how well coders know the ICD-9 system and how hard physicians try to communicate diagnostic information to coders, sometimes it is necessary to look for a code that will justify medical necessity.

The following breakdown of the ICD-9 book will help in this respect:

001-139.8	Infectious and parasitic diseases
140-239.9	Neoplasms (cancerous tissues)
240-279.9	Endocrine, nutritional, metabolic, immunity
280-289.9	Blood and blood-forming organs
290-319	Mental disorders
320-389.9	Nervous system and sense organs
390-459.9	Circulatory system
460-519.9	Respiratory system
520-579.9	Digestive system
580-629.9	Genitourinary system
630-676.9	Pregnancy, childbirth, puerperium
680-709.9	Skin and subcutaneous tissue
710-739.9	Musculoskeletal system and connective tissue
740-759.9	Congenital anomalies
760-779.9	Conditions in the perinatal period
780-799.9	Symptoms, signs, and conditions
800-999.9	Injury and poisoning (fractures, dislocations, cuts, etc)
V Codes	Other factors influencing health status and contact with health services

Summary of ICD-9 Coding Tips

The tips that follow are a compilation of ICD-9 coding suggestions from a variety of Medicare carriers.

It is best to first identify the appropriate code by using the alphabetic list found in Volume 2 of the ICD-9-CM. However, you must look in Volume 1 of the ICD-9-CM to find the corresponding code because that is where you will find instructions that further clarify and specify the best code with which to document the patient's condition.

Note: Begin coding with Volume 2 (alphabetic list), but do not stop until you check Volume 1 (tabular list) for further clarification and specification. On the other hand, you should never begin coding with Volume 1, as this may lead to coding errors.

Choosing Diagnosis Codes

Physicians must use the appropriate ICD-9-CM code(s) ranging from 001.0 through V82.9 to identify diagnoses, symptoms, conditions, problems, complaints, or other reasons for the encounter with the patient. Medicare Part B does not recognize diagnosis codes beginning with "E" or "M." To ensure correct diagnosis coding, follow these guidelines:

- Code documented complaints, signs, symptoms, problems, and conditions that coexist at the time of the encounter and that require or affect patient care, treatment, or management. (*Note*: A maximum of four ICD-9 codes can be reported on Medicare claim forms.).

- Use the diagnoses codes that are most responsible for the service or procedure billed.

- Do not code conditions previously treated and no longer existing.

- It is acceptable to code chronic conditions as often as they relate to the patient encounters.

- Code to the highest degree of certainty for that encounter. Coding symptoms, signs, abnormal test results, or other reasons for the visit is appropriate when this is the level of certainty documented by the physician.

- Do not code diagnoses documented as "probable," "suspected," "questionable," or "rule out" as if they are confirmed diagnoses. Instead, use diagnosis codes that indicate the signs and symptoms that cause the physician to suspect a condition may exist.

- Code to the highest level of specificity. . . . Use three-digit codes only if there are no four- or five-digit codes within that code category. Use four-digit codes only if there are no five-digit codes for that category. Use five-digit codes when they exist in a code category. Sometimes fourth and fifth digits are not available. In these cases, do not add fourth and fifth digits to valid three-digit codes (ie, do not add zeroes to valid three-digit codes)[. . . . (Diabetes Mellitus) 250 requires 5 digits. The fourth digit must be 0 through 9; the fifth digit must be 0 through 3. (Osteoarthrosis and allied disorders) 715 requires 5 digits. The fourth digit must be 0, 1, 2, 3, 8, or 9; the fifth digit must be 0 through 9.]

- Each claim must contain at least one diagnosis code. Conversely, there can be no more than four diagnosis codes on a single Medicare claim.

- First list the code shown in the medical record to be chiefly responsible for the encounter. Next list up to three additional codes that describe any coexisting conditions. *Note:* Make sure to relate each service billed to the diagnosis code that represents the condition primarily responsible for that particular line item service.

Final Comments on ICD-9 Coding

We are in a new era of utilization and quality management by Medicare carriers. Private payers are also becoming involved at an increasing rate. While most private payers are not as particular as Medicare carriers, they are less prone to pay claims as submitted unless CPT® codes and ICD-9 codes make sense to their computer systems.

During the next few years, some payers will compare physicians' practice patterns to those of peers and, perhaps more ominously, to "established" norms. In the past few years, the CMS and Medicare carriers have enhanced their data processing systems to perform these comparisons and postpayment utilization review.

Managed care organizations will intensify quality management efforts. While there are limitations to ICD-9 coding in respect to quality management, it will be a factor in reviews until other aspects of medical records are automated (and that may take some time). Again, a physician cannot afford to be branded an overutilizer, provider of substandard care, and the like because of laxity in coding.

Right or wrong, ICD-9 coding may be a factor in a physician's rating in some health plans' quality management systems. Assigning an ICD-9 code that denotes the condition that was the focus of the patient encounter will help physicians maintain high-quality ratings.

There is a computer-based training course offered by CMS at
www.cms.hhs.gov/medlearn/. While this course is somewhat basic, it is a worthwhile
program for new staff members needing an introduction to ICD-9 coding.

ICD-10

ICD-9 was established in 1979. Advancements in knowledge and services since that
time have made a new revision necessary. The next level of classification system—
ICD-10—has been under development for several years by CMS/HCFA and the
World Health Organization.

The procedure coding section, ICD-10-PCS, was developed independently from the
disease index and tabular list of clinical modifications, ICD-10-CM. Both versions
have been expanded, and codes will contain more digits or characters than ICD-9.
ICD procedure coding will change from a numerical four-character system to an
alphanumerical seven-character code.

ICD-10 implementation is subject to regulations for national standards found in the
Health Insurance Portability and Accountability Act. The earliest estimated date for
mandatory use is not until 2005 (see below). Physicians should watch for announcements regarding ICD-10-CM and training materials.

If history is any indicator, CMS may plan early adoption of ICD-10, but it may be
years before claims with ICD-9 codes will be denied. However, this new coding system should be kept in mind when physicians make decisions about their practice.
For example, physicians purchasing a new computer system should make sure it will
handle ICD-10.

In the Summary Report of the April 18-19, 2002, ICD-9-CM Coordination and Maintenance Committee (under CMS), the following comments were made regarding ICD-10:

. . . Implementation of ICD-10-PCS was discussed in great detail at the May 17, 2001 C&M meeting. Organizations provided formal statements on their views as to whether or not ICD-10-PCS should be implemented. These formal statements are included in the Summary Report of the meeting and may be accessed at: www.hcfa.gov/medicare/icd9cm.htm. There was overwhelming support for moving forward with the implementation of ICD-10-PCS. However, there was also a great deal of support for implementing the diagnosis and procedure volumes at the same time. Therefore, CMS was urged to wait until ICD-10 diagnosis was completed by NCHS prior to proceeding with ICD-10-PCS.

The Health Insurance Portability and Accountability Act of 1996 (HIPAA), Public Law 104-191 established a formal process for naming national code set standards. In order to replace the current system, ICD-9-CM, with a new coding system, the HIPAA process must be followed. The next step in the process involves hearings by the National Committee on Vital and Health Statistics (NCVHS). This process began on April 9-10, 2002 with hearings before the NCVHS' Subcommittee on

Standards and Security. Reports of this committee can be found at: http://ncvhs.hhs.gov/.

There was general support for ICD-10-PCS along with recommendations from several organizations that ICD-10-PCS be implemented in 2005. . . .

Once the NCVHS concludes its hearings, it will make a recommendation to the Secretary of the Department of Health and Human Services (DHHS) as to whether ICD-10-PCS and ICD-10-CM should be named as national coding standards. After receiving the Committee's recommendation, the Secretary will decide if he will propose ICD-10-PCS and ICD-10-CM as national standards. Should he decide to propose them as standards, DHHS would publish a notice of proposed rulemaking setting out this proposal and requesting comments. Should the comments be favorable, then a final notice would be published naming the new coding standards. The public is advised to stay actively involved in this process by attending the public meetings and submitting any comments or recommendations.

Endnotes

1. Diagnosis coding for Part B physician services is different from that needed to justify the hospital's diagnosis-related group reimbursement. That is, physicians can use signs, symptoms, and conditions for their Part B services. Hospitals need a final diagnosis for their services under Part A.

2. E codes are required on some workers' compensation claims.

3. From the hospital's perspective, the coding rules are different—suspected, but uncertain, diagnoses are reported as if they are present for diagnosis-related group inpatient reimbursement purposes.

Chapter 12

Compliance Programs: A Way to Minimize Fraud and Abuse Liability

Compliance programs have received at lot of attention since the late 1990s. Although they are not mandated by law, there are a number of reasons for implementing an effective compliance program:

1 Effective compliance reviews and programs dramatically reduce the risk of violating fraud and abuse laws, including the relatively new offenses in the Health Insurance Portability and Accountability Act of 1996 (HIPAA) that apply to claims submitted to private or commercial insurance companies.[1]

2 It instills a corporate culture of compliance with the law that has the added benefit of preventing fraud and abuse from occurring (or catching them very early).

3 Although not guaranteed, it may serve as a mitigating factor under Federal Sentencing Guidelines—the potential fine may be lowered. (Eventually, reasonable compliance efforts—depending on characteristics of the health care organization—may become a standard of conduct expected of such organizations.)

4 It offers some protection to board members, officers, owners, and key managers by demonstrating that these corporate officials are taking appropriate action to identify and correct any misconduct.[2]

5 It establishes a formal structure to ensure that policy changes, new laws, and new billing guidelines will be addressed.

6 An effective program provides greater assurance of coding and billing accuracy.

7 An effective program is based on complying with documentation guidelines.

8   It may discourage or make it more difficult for employees and others to pursue *qui tam* suits.

9   It will help in dealing with a civil or criminal investigation, if one occurs, by establishing the degree of intent involved and defining each participant's responsibilities.

10   It could help the health care organization maintain—and actually improve—its image from a public relations standpoint.

11   Mandatory compliance programs are a part of most fraud settlements with the government.

12   It helps protect the organization from fines, penalties, exclusion, etc, that may severely damage its ability to survive. It may protect the careers of physicians who are "guilty by association."

13   An effective compliance program may reduce the audit risks retiring physicians or physicians leaving a practice for other reasons may face with respect to future payer recoupment efforts.

Compliance efforts, including audits, can produce a number of positive outcomes. The article below—which appeared in the *MAGNet*, a newsletter of the MAG Mutual Insurance Company (a company headquartered in Georgia and owned by its physician policyholders)—illustrates several positive outcomes of compliance activities.

Correct Coding Results In Compliance Improvements and Revenue Gains

It is nearly impossible to pick up a medical publication without reading about Medicare/Medicaid "fraud and abuse" and compliance. Often lost in the warnings of government audits and sanctions is the other side of the equation—proper coding does not necessarily mean revenue loss.

Consultants from MAG Mutual HealthCare Consultants, Inc.—a member of the MAG Mutual Group—worked with a large physician group concerned with the importance of maintaining compliance. As may occur under Medicare's complex billing guidelines, some overpayments were discovered during the review. But, the consultants also identified coding errors that resulted in significant underpayments to the group.

In this physician group, the computer system used for laboratory procedures interfaces with the billing software. The lab system's *internal lab codes* are specific to the group's testing protocols. Those internal lab codes, when entered by the laboratory department, are converted by the system into specific CPT codes for billing purposes.

After analyzing the monthly *CPT Productivity/Frequency Report* by physician specialty, it was apparent that some potential errors were occurring with lab codes for various blood indices. After discussions with the lab manager and a review of forms used to order lab tests, it was clear the problems represented both good and bad news for the physician group.

The bad news was that, some of the converted internal lab codes resulted in the Medicare carrier making overpayments to the group of some $8,000. As part of the group's compliance plan, the overpayments were refunded with an explanation of what was clearly a billing error.

The good news is that the highest volume tests were being billed under a CPT code which produced significantly less payment than the correct code. In this instance, the underpayments were close to $300,000.

What started as an internal audit as part of the group's formal compliance plan, produced significant additional revenue for the clinic. That revenue will reoccur each year.

And, just as importantly, the audit process caught what government investigators might consider an abusive billing practice before it got serious. This validated the group's compliance program as an effective process to detect, correct, and prevent inappropriate billing activities.

The physicians were pleased with the results and have requested that our consultants expand the project to other aspects of the group's billing operations. The client is on the road to compliance and achieving appropriate revenue for their services.

Reasonable and Effective Compliance Efforts

In our discussion of compliance programs, keep in mind that we are talking about effective programs. Compliance programs must exhibit characteristics of a reasonable program designed to identify, correct, and prevent instances of misconduct. While no plan is foolproof, effective compliance programs will help physicians identify problems early enough to allow for voluntary disclosure, and they demonstrate that any offenses are aberrational and that penalties should be minimal.

If a compliance program is implemented, it must also be *maintained* to be effective. A compliance program that exists in name only actually may document inappropriate intent and is potentially more damaging than not having any program.

In the context of this book, *compliance program* means compliance efforts related to reimbursement for patient services, referrals for tests and other services, and business arrangements that could be construed as kickbacks. Other laws and issues are applicable to medical practices that may be part of an extensive compliance plan but are not addressed here, such as the HIPAA provisions related to privacy and security of patient information; Clinical Laboratory Improvement Act; Occupational Health and Safety Administration; antitrust; employment and benefit laws; the Americans With Disabilities Act; standards of clinical practice; sexual harassment; moral issues; tax issues; building codes; credit and collection policies; and licensing requirements.

At this point the question becomes, what are reasonable compliance efforts? There are several documents that offer insight: the Office of Inspector General (OIG) *Compliance Program Guidance for Individual and Small Group Physician Practices* (released September 25, 2000); the OIG's *Draft Compliance Program Guidance for Individual and Small Group Physician Practices* (published in the June 12, 2000, *Federal Register*); the OIG's *Model Compliance Plan for Clinical Labs* (published in the March 3, 1997, *Federal Register*); the United States Sentencing Guidelines; the OIG's *Compliance Program Guidance for Hospitals* (released February 1998); *Solicitation of Information and Recommendations for Developing OIG Compliance Program Guidance for Individual Physicians and Small Group Practices* (September 8, 1999); *Compliance Program Guidance for Third-Party Medical Billing Companies* (December 18, 1998); *Federal Fraud Enforcement—Physician Compliance*, published by the American

Medical Association (September 25, 1997); and various OIG-mandated compliance plans imposed on medical practices as part of a settlement for alleged fraudulent activity.

On September 8, 1999, the OIG formally requested input for developing OIG compliance program guidance for individual physicians and small group practices. A draft of the guidelines was issued on June 7, 2000 (published in the *Federal Register* on June 12). Final guidelines were released by the OIG on September 25, 2000.

The excerpts below from the *Compliance Program Guidance for Individual and Small Group Physician Practices* indicate the OIG's attitude with respect to what a medical practice is expected to do. Larger groups should also note the comments below regarding the OIG's expectations.[3]

[Excerpt from the Introduction]

Through this document, the OIG provides its views on the fundamental components of physician practice compliance programs, as well as the principles that a physician practice might consider when developing and implementing a voluntary compliance program. While this document presents basic procedural and structural guidance for designing a voluntary compliance program, it is not in and of itself a compliance program. Indeed, as recognized by the OIG and the health care industry, there is no "one size fits all" compliance program, especially for physician practices. Rather, it is a set of guidelines that physician practices can consider if they choose to develop and implement a compliance program.

As with the OIG's previous guidance, these guidelines are not mandatory. Nor do they represent an all-inclusive document containing all components of a compliance program. Other OIG outreach efforts, as well as other Federal agency efforts to promote compliance, can also be used in developing a compliance program. However, as explained later, if a physician practice adopts a voluntary and active compliance program, it may well lead to benefits for the physician practice. . . .

Another section of the OIG's *Compliance Program Guidance* states:

[Excerpt from Section II. A.]

These seven components provide a solid basis upon which a physician practice can create a compliance program. The OIG acknowledges that full implementation of all components may not be feasible for all physician practices. Some physician practices may never fully implement all of the components. However, as a first step, physician practices can begin by adopting only those components which, based on a practice's specific history with billing problems and other compliance issues, are most likely to provide an identifiable benefit.

The extent of implementation will depend on the size and resources of the practice. Smaller physician practices may incorporate each of the components in a manner that best suits the practice. By contrast, larger physician practices often have the means to incorporate the components in a more systematic manner. For example, larger physician practices can use both this guidance and the Third-Party Medical Billing Compliance Program Guidance, which provides a more detailed compliance program structure, to create a compliance program unique to the practice.

The OIG recognizes that physician practices need to find the best way to achieve compliance for their given circumstances. Specifically, the OIG encourages physician practices to participate in other provider's compliance programs, such as the compliance programs of the hospitals or other settings in which the physicians practice. Physician Practice Management companies also may serve as a source of compliance program guidance. A physician practice's participation in such compliance programs could be a way, at least partly, to augment the practice's own compliance efforts.

The opportunities for collaborative compliance efforts could include participating in training and education programs or using another entity's policies and procedures as a template from which the physician practice creates its own version. The OIG encourages this type of collaborative effort, where the content is appropriate to the setting involved (i.e., the training is relevant to physician practices as well as the sponsoring provider), because it provides a means to promote the desired objective without imposing excessive burdens on the practice or requiring physicians to undertake duplicative action. However, to prevent possible anti-kickback or self-referral issues, the OIG recommends that physicians consider

limiting their participation in a sponsoring provider's compliance program to the areas of training and education or policies and procedures.

The key to avoiding possible conflicts is to ensure that the entity providing compliance services to a physician practice (its referral source) is not perceived as nor is it operating the practice compliance program at no charge. For example, if the sponsoring entity conducted claims review for the physician practice as part of a compliance program or provided compliance oversight without charging the practice fair market value for those services, the anti-kickback and Stark self-referral laws would be implicated. The payment of fair market value by referral sources for compliance services will generally address these concerns.

[The document goes on to describe the seven components in detail.]

Appendix C includes the complete text of the OIG's compliance guidance for small medical practices.

As mentioned earlier, the guidance documents for individual and small physician group practices, billing companies, hospitals, laboratories, and other entities discuss the seven essential elements at length. These guidance documents provide information to make informed decisions about the things medical practices should do with respect to compliance efforts.

The seven essential elements of a compliance program are presented below. The next chapter expands on these essential elements with specific references to medical practices.

Seven Basic Components of a Compliance Program

The OIG *Compliance Program Guidance for Individual and Small Group Physician Practices* provides a concise summary of the essential elements of a compliance program. It states the following:

A. The Seven Basic Components of a Voluntary Compliance Program

The OIG believes that a basic framework for any voluntary compliance program begins with a review of the seven basic components of an effective compliance program. The following list of components, as set forth in previous OIG compliance program guidances, can form the basis of a voluntary compliance program for a physician practice:

1. conducting internal monitoring and auditing through the performance of periodic audits;

2. implementing compliance and practice standards through the development of written standards and procedures;

3. designating a compliance officer or contact(s) to monitor compliance efforts and enforce practice standards;

4. conducting appropriate training and education on practice standards and procedures;

5. responding appropriately to detected violations through the investigation of allegations and the disclosure of incidents to appropriate Government entities;

6. developing open lines of communication, such as (a) discussions at staff meetings regarding how to avoid erroneous or fraudulent conduct and (b) community bulletin boards, to keep practice employees updated regarding compliance activities; and

7. enforcing disciplinary standards through well-publicized guidelines.

How much of the seven elements presented above can a medical practice reasonably be expected to adopt? While it is not possible to answer this with certainty without looking at a practice's particular situation, the comments below seem pertinent.

Technically, a practice does not have to implement a compliance plan because it is not mandated by law (except as part of settlement agreements). However, some level of compliance effort seems prudent in today's environment.

If a compliance plan is intended to afford the benefits available should a group become subject to a fraud investigation, then ideally, it should be designed to cover each of the identified elements. If that is not possible for a particular medical practice, physicians can still take reasonable steps that will help them minimize compliance risks by adopting a plan that demonstrates serious intent to prevent, detect, and correct inappropriate activity.

The text in the next two chapters includes recommendations by consultants and attorneys experienced in developing compliance programs for medical practices that are designed to prevent, detect, and correct inappropriate activity.

Chapter 14 specifically addresses recommendations for small group practices or solo practitioners. In small practices, some cost-effective compromises are usually necessary with respect to the compliance activities appropriate in larger entities.

Endnotes

1. In the past, it was not uncommon for some health care organizations to bill Medicare and Medicaid services differently from those covered by private or commercial insurers under the assumption that nongovernmental payers were less likely to pursue legal action for improper billing. In light of the Health Insurance Portability and Accountability Act and increased focus on fraud, billing operations should be reviewed to uncover any inappropriate billing policies based on the payer. Please note, however, that there are legitimate differences between billing guidelines for government programs and privately insured plans in certain situations.

2. Increasingly, these officials may be deemed responsible by the government, or even stockholders, for a failure to take appropriate action to identify and correct misconduct.

3. This document is reproduced in Appendix C and is available online at www.oig.hhs.gov/fraud/complianceguidance.html.

13

Developing a Compliance Program

According to the OIG's guidance, a physician compliance program is comprised of seven basic components. In introducing the steps for implementing a voluntary compliance program, the OIG's guidance states:

Steps for Implementing a Voluntary Compliance Program

As previously discussed, implementing a voluntary compliance program can be a multi-tiered process. Initial development of the compliance program can be focused on practice risk areas that have been problematic for the practice such as coding and billing. Within this area, the practice should examine its claims denial history or claims that have resulted in repeated overpayments, and identify and correct the most frequent sources of those denials or overpayments. A review of claim denials will help the practice scrutinize a significant risk area and improve its cash flow by submitting correct claims that will be paid the first time they are submitted. As this example illustrates, a compliance program for a physician practice often makes sound business sense.

The following is a suggested order of the steps a practice could take to begin the development of a compliance program. The steps outlined below articulate all seven components of a compliance program and there are numerous suggestions for implementation within each component. Physician practices should keep in mind, as stated earlier, that it is up to the practice to determine the manner in which and the extent to which the practice chooses to implement these voluntary measures.

Step One: Auditing and Monitoring

An ongoing evaluation process is important to a successful compliance program. This ongoing evaluation includes not only whether the physician practice's standards and procedures are in fact current and accurate, but also whether the compliance program is working, i.e., whether individuals are properly carrying out their responsibilities and claims are submitted appropriately.

Therefore, an audit is an excellent way for a physician practice to ascertain what, if any, problem areas exist and focus on the risk areas that are associated with those problems. There are two types of reviews that can be performed as part of this evaluation: (1) a standards and procedures review; and (2) a claims submission audit.

[At this point, the document goes on to describe the auditing and monitoring process.]

The final compliance program guidance lists seven *steps*—the first step being a compliance audit of the practice. All previous compliance program guidances, including the draft for small group practices, did not use the term steps. Instead, seven essential elements were discussed.

Auditing and Monitoring are critical to the success of any compliance program. However, some small group practices may find an extensive internal audit too overwhelming to even begin. The OIG has identified several mechanisms for small group practices to begin audit procedures. Auditing would occur very early in the process and on a frequent basis to ensure the continued effectiveness of compliance efforts.

Each of the seven steps/elements is discussed in the exact order they are presented in the OIG's guidance. As a practical matter, it may be best to appoint a Compliance Officer before beginning any real work with respect to a compliance program (even though the OIG lists appointment of a Compliance Officer as Step 3). Someone needs to be charged with the responsibility of developing, coordinating, monitoring, and ensuring the effectiveness of compliance activities.

For footnotes and additional discussion, refer to the complete text of the *OIG Compliance Program Guidance for Individual and Small Group Physician Practices* in Appendix C. It includes footnotes, many of which clarify and provide examples on the OIG's perspective.

The Seven Essential Elements

A. Auditing and Monitoring

An ongoing evaluation process is critical to the success of a compliance program. Although many monitoring techniques are available, one effective tool to promote and ensure compliance is the performance of regular, periodic compliance audits by internal or external auditors who have expertise in federal and state health care program requirements. The audits should focus on ensuring that CPT®/ICD-9 codes and medical necessity are supported by documentation in the medical record (and that such documentation is reflective of the patient encounter); the medical practice is complying with other billing rules, such as refunding of credit balances; compliance with antikickback and self-referral statutes and the like; the practice is adhering to the compliance plan; and the compliance plan is effective in minimizing improper activity.

The written plan should create an audit process that will:

- establish a standard audit process for initiating the program and as a guide for monitoring the progress of the compliance plan

- assess the practice's compliance efforts through regular audits

- test compliance with the practice's written policies and procedures and all applicable federal and state laws

- test compliance with payer billing policies and guidelines

- test agreement between codes used on billing forms (ie, CMS/HCFA 1500 or equivalent) and medical record documentation

- monitor the work of new employees

- respond to complaints from both employees and patients

- require a formal audit report to be submitted to the compliance officer and the governing body to ensure awareness of the results and any steps necessary to correct past problems and prevent them from recurring

The establishment of a standard audit process should address current activities that may contribute to noncompliance or that may need to be the focus of improvement. This audit should be designed so that the methodology for selecting and examining records may also be used during future periodic audits. In addition, this and subsequent audits should be used to measure the effectiveness of the practice's present educational or other compliance-related efforts.

An initial audit is often performed by an outside party with a high level of understanding about Medicare and Medicaid regulations and coding issues, but it can be performed by internal staff with similar skills. Often, the initial audit will include frequency distributions of ICD-9 codes and CPT® codes by category (evaluation and management, surgical, radiology, etc). In the future, significant deviations from the initial results should trigger a reasonable inquiry to determine the cause of the deviation.

The auditing and monitoring activities also require attention to compliance with rules and regulations not directly related to coding, including inappropriate self-referrals (under Stark I and II and some state laws); the antikickback statute; use of "incident to" services; and other matters. See element 7.

It should be mentioned that some attorneys advise their clients to conduct the initial audit beginning with services performed no earlier than the date the medical practice launches its formal compliance program. Their philosophy is that there is no benefit in going back into a period of time where the medical practice may not have been under a formal compliance program. This is a matter to discuss with your advisors—attorneys and consultants.

The *OIG Compliance Program Guidance for Individual and Small Group Physician Practices* states:

Step One: Auditing and Monitoring

An ongoing evaluation process is important to a successful compliance program. This ongoing evaluation includes not only whether the physician practice's standards and procedures are in fact current and accurate, but also whether the compliance program is working, i.e., whether individuals are properly carrying out their responsibilities and claims are submitted appropriately. Therefore, an audit is an excellent way for a physician practice to ascertain what, if any, problem areas exist and focus on the risk areas that are associated with those problems. There are two types of reviews that can be performed as part of this evaluation: (1) a standards and procedures review; and (2) a claims submission audit.

1. Standards and procedures

It is recommended that an individual(s) in the physician practice be charged with the responsibility of periodically reviewing the practice's standards and procedures to determine if they are current and complete. If the standards and procedures are found to be ineffective or outdated, they should be updated to reflect changes in Government regulations or compendiums generally relied upon by physicians and insurers (i.e., changes in Current Procedural Terminology (CPT) and ICD-9-CM codes).

2. Claims Submission Audit

In addition to the standards and procedures themselves, it is advisable that bills and medical records be reviewed for compliance with applicable coding, billing and documentation requirements. The individuals from the physician practice involved in these self-audits would ideally include the person in charge of billing (if the practice has such a person) and a medically trained person (e.g., registered nurse or preferably a physician (physicians can rotate in this position)). Each physician practice needs to decide for itself whether to review claims retrospectively or concurrently with the claims submission. In the Third-Party Medical Billing Compliance Program Guidance, the OIG recommended that a baseline, or "snapshot," be used to enable a practice to judge over time its progress in reducing or eliminating potential areas of vulnerability. This practice, known as "benchmarking," allows a practice to chart its compliance efforts by showing a reduction or increase in the number of claims paid and denied.

The practice's self-audits can be used to determine whether:

- bills are accurately coded and accurately reflect the services provided (as documented in the medical records);

- documentation is being completed correctly;

- services or items provided are reasonable and necessary; and

- any incentives for unnecessary services exist.

A baseline audit examines the claim development and submission process, from patient intake through claim submission and payment, and identifies elements within this process that may contribute to non-compliance or that may need to be the focus for improving execution. This audit will establish a consistent methodology for selecting and examining records, and this methodology will then serve as a basis for future audits.

There are many ways to conduct a baseline audit. The OIG recommends that claims/services that were submitted and paid during the initial three months after implementation of the education and training program be examined, so as to give the physician practice a benchmark against which to measure future compliance effectiveness.

Following the baseline audit, a general recommendation is that periodic audits be conducted at least once each year to ensure that the compliance program is being followed. Optimally, a randomly selected number of medical records could be reviewed to ensure that the coding was performed accurately. The OIG realizes that physician practices receive reimbursement from a number of different payors, and we would encourage a physician practice's auditing/monitoring process to consist of a review of claims from all Federal payors from which the practice receives reimbursement. Of course, the larger the sample size, the larger the comfort level the physician practice will have about the results. However, the OIG is aware that this may be burdensome for some physician practices, so, at a minimum, we would encourage the physician practice to conduct a review of claims that have been reimbursed by Federal health care programs.

If problems are identified, the physician practice will need to determine whether a focused review should be conducted on a more frequent basis. When audit results reveal areas needing additional information or education of employees and physicians, the physician practice will need to analyze whether these areas should be incorporated into the training and educational system.

There are many ways to identify the claims/services from which to draw the random sample of claims to be audited. One methodology is to choose a random sample of claims/services from either all of the claims/services a physician has received reimbursement for or all claims/services from a particular payor. Another method is to identify risk areas or potential billing vulnerabilities. The codes associated with these risk areas may become the universe of claims/services from which to select the sample. The OIG recommends that the physician practice evaluate claims/services selected to determine if the codes billed and reimbursed were accurately ordered, performed, and reasonable and necessary for the treatment of the patient.

One of the most important components of a successful compliance audit protocol is an appropriate response when the physician practice identifies a problem. This action should be taken as soon as possible after the date the problem is identified. The specific action a physician practice takes should depend on the circumstances of the situation. In some cases, the response can be as straight forward as generating a repayment with appropriate explanation to Medicare or the appropriate payor from which the overpayment was received. In others, the physician practice may want to consult with a coding/billing expert to determine the next best course of action. There is no boilerplate solution to how to handle problems that are identified.

It is a good business practice to create a system to address how physician practices will respond to and report potential problems. In addition, preserving information relating to identification of the problem is as important as preserving information that tracks the physician practice's reaction to, and solution for, the issue.

Internal audits of documentation and coding accuracy should not focus totally on E&M coding. Much of what one reads about auditing, documentation, and the like emphasizes E&M coding. But this is only one area of audit risk, and in some physician specialties E&M coding is a very small aspect of coding.

B. Written Policies and Standards Indicating a Strong Commitment to Compliance

A written compliance plan should ensure that everyone in the medical practice understands the obligation to comply with federal and state laws and standards that address areas of potential fraud or abuse, such as claims filing, inappropriate code "gaming," medical record documentation, and financial relationships with other health care providers.

In this section, the written policies and procedures should:

- clearly advise physicians and employees of the standards they are expected to follow and of the consequences of their failure to follow such standards

- include reference to applicable health care laws and regulations

- require the continuing development of written compliance policies and mandate distribution to, and training of, all individuals who are affected by those policies

- identify the person or persons responsible for overall management of the compliance program

The OIG *Compliance Program Guidance for Individual and Small Group Physician Practices* states:

Step Two: Establish Practice Standards and Procedures

After the internal audit identifies the practice's risk areas, the next step is to develop a method for dealing with those risk areas through the practice's standards and procedures. Written standards and procedures are a central component of any compliance program. Those standards and procedures help to reduce the prospect of erroneous claims and fraudulent activity by identifying risk areas for the practice and establishing tighter internal controls to counter those risks, while also helping to identify any aberrant billing practices. Many physician practices already have something similar to this called "practice standards" that include practice policy statements regarding patient care, personnel matters and practice standards and procedures on complying with Federal and State law.

The OIG believes that written standards and procedures can be helpful to all physician practices, regardless of size and capability. If a lack of resources to develop such standards and procedures is genuinely an issue, the OIG recommends that a physician practice focus first on those risk areas most likely to arise in its particular practice. Additionally, if the physician practice works with a physician practice management company (PPMC), independent practice association (IPA), physician-hospital organization, management services organization (MSO) or third-party billing company, the practice can incorporate the compliance standards and procedures of those entities, if appropriate, into its own standards and procedures. Many physician practices have found that the

adoption of a third party's compliance standards and procedures, as appropriate, has many benefits and the result is a consistent set of standards and procedures for a community of physicians as well as having just one entity that can then monitor and refine the process as needed. This sharing of compliance responsibilities assists physician practices in rural areas that do not have the staff to perform these functions, but do belong to a group that does have the resources. Physician practices using another entity's compliance materials will need to tailor those materials to the physician practice where they will be applied.

Physician practices that do not have standards or procedures in place can develop them by: (1) developing a written standards and procedures manual; and (2) updating clinical forms periodically to make sure they facilitate and encourage clear and complete documentation of patient care. A practice's standards could also identify the clinical protocol(s), pathway(s), and other treatment guidelines followed by the practice.

Creating a resource manual from publicly available information may be a cost-effective approach for developing additional standards and procedures. For example, the practice can develop a "binder" that contains the practice's written standards and procedures, relevant CMS/HCFA directives and carrier bulletins, and summaries of informative OIG documents (e.g., Special Fraud Alerts, Advisory Opinions, inspection and audit reports). If the practice chooses to adopt this idea, the binder should be updated as appropriate and located in a readily accessible location.

If updates to the standards and procedures are necessary, those updates should be communicated to employees to keep them informed regarding the practice's operations. New employees can be made aware of the standards and procedures when hired and can be trained on their contents as part of their orientation to the practice. The OIG recommends that the communication of updates and training of new employees occur as soon as possible after either the issuance of a new update or the hiring of a new employee.

1. Specific Risk Areas

The OIG recognizes that many physician practices may not have in place standards and procedures to prevent erroneous or fraudulent conduct in their practices. In order to develop standards and procedures, the physician practice may consider what types of fraud and abuse related topics need to be addressed based on its specific needs. One of the most important things in making that determination is a listing of risk areas where the practice may be vulnerable.

To assist physician practices in performing this initial assessment, the OIG has developed a list of four potential risk areas affecting physician practices. These risk areas include: (a) coding and billing; (b) reasonable and necessary services; (c) documentation; and (d) improper inducements, kickbacks and self-referrals. This list of risk areas is not exhaustive, or all-encompassing. Rather, it should be viewed as a starting point for an internal review of potential vulnerabilities within the physician practice. The objective of such an assessment is to ensure that key personnel in the physician practice are aware of these major risk areas and that steps are taken to minimize, to the extent possible, the types of problems identified. While there are many ways to accomplish this objective, clear written standards and procedures that are communicated to all employees are important to ensure the effectiveness of a compliance program. Specifically, the following are discussions of risk areas for physician practices:

a. Coding and Billing

A major part of any physician practice's compliance program is the identification of risk areas associated with coding and billing. The following risk areas associated with billing have been among the most frequent subjects of investigations and audits by the OIG:

- billing for items or services not rendered or not provided as claimed;

- submitting claims for equipment, medical supplies and services that are not reasonable and necessary;

- double billing resulting in duplicate payment;

- billing for non-covered services as if covered;

- knowing misuse of provider identification numbers, which results in improper billing;

- unbundling (billing for each component of the service instead of billing or using an all-inclusive code);

- failure to properly use coding modifiers;

- clustering; and

- upcoding the level of service provided.

The physician practice written standards and procedures concerning proper coding reflect the current reimbursement principles set forth in applicable statutes, regulations and Federal, State or private payor health care program requirements and should be developed in tandem with coding and billing standards used in the physician practice. Furthermore, written standards and procedures should ensure that coding and billing are based on medical record documentation. Particular attention should be paid to issues of appropriate diagnosis codes and individual Medicare Part B claims (including documentation guidelines for evaluation and management services). A physician practice can also institute a policy that the coder and/or physician review all rejected claims pertaining to diagnosis and procedure codes. This step can facilitate a reduction in similar errors.

b. Reasonable and Necessary Services

A practice's compliance program may provide guidance that claims are to be submitted only for services that the physician practice finds to be reasonable and necessary in the particular case. The OIG recognizes that physicians should be able to order any tests, including screening tests, they believe are appropriate for the treatment of their patients. However, a physician practice should be aware that Medicare will only pay for services that meet the Medicare definition of reasonable and necessary.

Medicare (and many insurance plans) may deny payment for a service that is not reasonable and necessary according to the Medicare reimbursement rules. Thus, when a physician provides services to a Medicare beneficiary, he or she should only bill those services that meet the Medicare standard of being reasonable and necessary for the diagnosis and treatment of a patient. A physician practice can bill in order to receive a denial for services, but only if the denial is needed for reimbursement from the secondary payor. Upon request, the physician practice should be able to provide documentation, such as a patient's medical records and physician's orders, to support the appropriateness of a service that the physician has provided.

c. Documentation

Timely, accurate and complete documentation is important to clinical patient care. This same documentation serves as a second function when a bill is submitted for payment, namely, as verification that the bill is accurate as submitted. Therefore, one of the most important physician practice compliance issues is the appropriate documentation of diagnosis and treatment. Physician documentation is necessary to determine the appropriate medical treatment for the patient and is the basis for coding and billing determinations. Thorough and accurate documentation also helps to ensure accurate recording and timely transmission of information.

i. Medical Record Documentation

In addition to facilitating high quality patient care, a properly documented medical record verifies and documents precisely what services were actually provided. The medical record may be used to validate: (a) the site of the service; (b) the appropriateness of the services provided; (c) the accuracy of the billing; and (d) the identity of the care giver (service provider). Examples of internal documentation guidelines a practice might use to ensure accurate medical record documentation include the following:

- The medical record is complete and legible;

- The documentation of each patient encounter includes the reason for the encounter; any relevant history; physical examination findings; prior diagnostic test results; assessment, clinical impression, or diagnosis; plan of care; and date and legible identity of the observer;

- If not documented, the rationale for ordering diagnostic and other ancillary services can be easily inferred by an independent reviewer or third party who has appropriate medical training;

- CPT and ICD-9-CM codes used for claims submission are supported by documentation and the medical record; and

- Appropriate health risk factors are identified. The patient's progress, his or her response to, and any changes in, treatment, and any revision in diagnosis is documented.

The CPT and ICD-9-CM codes reported on the health insurance claims form should be supported by documentation in the medical record and the medical chart should contain all necessary information.

Additionally, CMS and the local carriers should be able to determine the person who provided the services. These issues can be the root of investigations of inappropriate or erroneous conduct, and have been identified by CMS and the OIG as a leading cause of improper payments.

One method for improving quality in documentation is for a physician practice to compare the practice's claim denial rate to the rates of other practices in the same specialty to the extent that the practice can obtain that information from the carrier. Physician coding and diagnosis distribution can be compared for each physician within the same specialty to identify variances.

ii. CMS/HCFA 1500 Form

Another documentation area for physician practices to monitor closely is the proper completion of the CMS/HCFA 1500 form. The following practices will help ensure that the form has been properly completed:

- link the diagnosis code with the reason for the visit or service;

- use modifiers appropriately;

- provide Medicare with all information about a beneficiary's other insurance coverage under the Medicare Secondary Payor (MSP) policy, if the practice is aware of a beneficiary's additional coverage.

d. Improper Inducements, Kickbacks and Self-Referrals

A physician practice would be well advised to have standards and procedures that encourage compliance with the anti-kickback statute and the physician self-referral law. Remuneration for referrals is illegal because it can distort medical decision-making, cause overutilization of services or supplies, increase costs to Federal health care programs, and result in unfair competition by shutting out competitors who are unwilling to pay for referrals. Remuneration for referrals can also affect the quality of patient care by encouraging physicians to order services or supplies based on profit rather than the patients' best medical interests.

In particular, arrangements with hospitals, hospices, nursing facilities, home health agencies, durable medical equipment suppliers, pharmaceutical manufacturers and vendors are areas of potential concern. In general the anti-kickback statute prohibits knowingly and willfully giving or receiving anything of value to induce referrals of Federal health care program business. It is generally recommended that all business arrangements wherein physician practices refer business to, or order services or items from, an outside entity should be on a fair market value basis. Whenever a physician practice intends to enter into a business arrangement that involves making referrals, the arrangement should be reviewed by legal counsel familiar with the anti-kickback statute and physician self-referral statute.

In addition to developing standards and procedures to address arrangements with other health care providers and suppliers, physician practices should also consider implementing measures to avoid offering inappropriate inducements to patients. Examples of such inducements include routinely waiving coinsurance or deductible amounts without a good faith determination that the patient is in financial need or failing to make reasonable efforts to collect the cost-sharing amount.

Possible risk factors relating to this risk area that could be addressed in the practice's standards and procedures include:

- financial arrangements with outside entities to whom the practice may refer Federal health care program business;

- joint ventures with entities supplying goods or services to the physician practice or its patients;

- consulting contracts or medical directorships;

- office and equipment leases with entities to which the physician refers; and

- soliciting, accepting or offering any gift or gratuity of more than nominal value to or from those who may benefit from a physician practice's referral of Federal health care program business.

In order to keep current with this area of the law, a physician practice may obtain copies, available on the OIG web site or in hard copy from the OIG, of all relevant OIG Special Fraud Alerts and Advisory Opinions that address the application of the anti-kickback and physician self-referral laws to ensure that the standards and procedures reflect current positions and opinions.

2. Retention of Records

In light of the documentation requirements faced by physician practices, it would be to the practice's benefit if its standards and procedures contained a section on the retention of compliance, business and medical records. These records primarily include documents relating to patient care and the practice's business activities. A physician practice's designated compliance contact could keep an updated binder or record of these documents, including information relating to compliance activities. The primary compliance documents that a

practice would want to retain are those that relate to educational activities, internal investigations and internal audit results. We suggest that particular attention should be paid to documenting investigations of potential violations uncovered by the compliance program and the resulting remedial action. Although there is no requirement that the practice retain its compliance records, having all the relevant documentation relating to the practice's compliance efforts or handling of a particular problem can benefit the practice should it ever be questioned regarding those activities.

Physician practices that implement a compliance program might also want to provide for the development and implementation of a records retention system. This system would establish standards and procedures regarding the creation, distribution, retention, and destruction of documents. If the practice decides to design a record system, privacy concerns and Federal or State regulatory requirements should be taken into consideration.

While conducting its compliance activities, as well as its daily operations, a physician practice would be well advised, to the extent it is possible, to document its efforts to comply with applicable Federal health care program requirements. For example, if a physician practice requests advice from a Government agency (including a Medicare carrier) charged with administering a Federal health care program, it is to the benefit of the practice to document and retain a record of the request and any written or oral response (or nonresponse). This step is extremely important if the practice intends to rely on that response to guide it in future decisions, actions, or claim reimbursement requests or appeals.

In short, it is in the best interest of all physician practices, regardless of size, to have procedures to create and retain appropriate documentation. The following record retention guidelines are suggested:

- The length of time that a practice's records are to be retained can be specified in the physician practice's standards and procedures (Federal and State statutes should be consulted for specific time frames, if applicable);

- Medical records (if in the possession of the physician practice) need to be secured against loss, destruction, unauthorized access, unauthorized reproduction, corruption, or damage; and

- Standards and procedures can stipulate the disposition of medical records in the event the practice is sold or closed.

C. Designation of a Compliance Officer or Contact

As mentioned earlier, a strong argument can be made for making this step the first action taken in implementing a compliance program. Someone needs to be assigned the responsibility for ensuring that compliance efforts are carried out and effective. In larger groups, there may be a full-time compliance officer. In smaller practices, the responsibilities may be assigned to an individual performing other duties or to several individuals. The compliance officer functions could even be handled by a committee. While it may be necessary to appoint a physician or office manager in a small or solo practice, consultants usually advise designating someone whose income is not directly tied to billing results.

To the extent possible, the written plan should make it clear that the designated compliance officer/contact(s) should:

- be a person with good oral and written communiction skills, experience in billing and coding, demonstrated attention to detail, and of high integrity

- be able to influence behavior and organizational activities, ie, an individual who has substantial control over the medical practice or a substantial role in setting policy for the practice

- know and understand all aspects of the compliance plan and periodically revise the plan to reflect changes in the organization, new laws, new billing guidelines, and the like

- consult with counsel and/or advisors about interpretations of the plan

- with help from counsel and/or advisors, monitor all developments and changes in laws and regulations that may affect a medical practice and communicate those changes to the appropriate staff

- coordinate periodic audits and internal investigations within the medical practice

- respond to compliance-related inquiries or complaints presented by employees and others and ensure that employees report any suspected fraudulent or abusive activity without fear of retaliation

- facilitate communication about compliance issues between professional and support personnel

- have access to all documents, billing forms, medical records, etc, that may be necessary to fulfill responsibilities

- report periodically to the compliance committee, board of directors, and upper-level management as to progress related to the compliance program, status of investigations into all complaints and compliance issues, training programs, recommendations to reduce compliance risks, recommended revisions to the plan, and the like

- ensure that any consultants, billing services, and independent contractors working with the medical practice are aware of and abide by the compliance program and standards of conduct

- have sufficient funding and support to fulfill responsibilities

The OIG *Compliance Program Guidance for Individual and Small Group Physician Practices* states:

Step Three: Designation of a Compliance Officer/Contact(s)

After the audits have been completed and the risk areas identified, ideally one member of the physician practice staff needs to accept the responsibility of developing a corrective action plan, if necessary, and oversee the practice's adherence to that plan. This person can either be in charge of all compliance activities for the practice or play a limited role merely to resolve the current issue. In a formalized institutional compliance program there is a compliance officer who is responsible for overseeing the implementation and day-to-day operations of the compliance program. However, the resource constraints of physician practices make it so that it is often impossible to designate one person to be in charge of compliance functions.

It is acceptable for a physician practice to designate more than one employee with compliance monitoring responsibility. In lieu of having a designated compliance officer, the physician practice could instead describe in its standards and procedures the compliance functions for which designated employees, known as "compliance contacts," would be responsible. For example, one employee could be responsible for preparing written standards and procedures, while another could be responsible for conducting or arranging for periodic audits and ensuring that billing questions are answered. Therefore, the compliance-related responsibilities of the designated person or persons may be only a portion of his or her duties.

Another possibility is that one individual could serve as compliance officer for more than one entity. In situations where staffing limitations mandate that the practice cannot afford to designate a person(s) to oversee compliance activities, the practice could outsource all or part of the functions of a compliance officer to a third party, such as a consultant, PPMC, MSO, IPA or third-party billing company. However, if this role is outsourced, it is

beneficial for the compliance officer to have sufficient interaction with the physician practice to be able to effectively understand the inner workings of the practice. For example, consultants that are not in close geographic proximity to a practice may not be effective compliance officers for the practice.

One suggestion for how to maintain continual interaction is for the practice to designate someone to serve as a liaison with the outsourced compliance officer. This would help ensure a strong tie between the compliance officer and the practice's daily operations. Outsourced compliance officers, who spend most of their time off-site, have certain limitations that a physician practice should consider before making such a critical decision. These limitations can include lack of understanding as to the inner workings of the practice, accessibility and possible conflicts of interest when one compliance officer is serving several practices.

If the physician practice decides to designate a particular person(s) to oversee all compliance activities, not just those in conjunction with the audit-related issue, the following is a list of suggested duties that the practice may want to assign to that person(s):

1. overseeing and monitoring the implementation of the compliance program;

2. establishing methods, such as periodic audits, to improve the practice's efficiency and quality of services, and to reduce the practice's vulnerability to fraud and abuse;

3. periodically revising the compliance program in light of changes in the needs of the practice or changes in the law and in the standards and procedures of Government and private payor health plans;

4. developing, coordinating and participating in a training program that focuses on the components of the compliance program, and seeks to ensure that training materials are appropriate;

5. ensuring that the HHS-OIG's List of Excluded Individuals and Entities, and the General Services Administration's (GSA's) List of Parties Debarred from Federal Programs have been checked with respect to all employees, medical staff and independent contractors; and

6. investigating any report or allegation concerning possible unethical or improper business practices, and monitoring subsequent corrective action and/or compliance.

Each physician practice needs to assess its own practice situation and determine what best suits that practice in terms of compliance oversight.

D. Conducting Effective Training and Education

It is essential that the compliance plan include periodic training and retraining of physicians, managers, employees, and others associated with the medical practice. Training should be applicable to all employees, and it should be designed to meet specific needs with respect to the employee's position, key aspects of the organization's compliance program, applicable state and federal laws, billing and documentation guidelines, and the like.

The written plan may require participation in an effective education and training program that would include:

- an explanation of the compliance plan and the role of each employee in the compliance plan

- extensive education specific to those working in areas where application of the health care fraud and abuse laws frequently occur; eg, physicians need to understand medical record documentation requirements, and both physicians and billing staff need to understand that billing forms must be based on documentation in the medical record

- arrangements for training in such areas such as CPT® coding, diagnostic coding, Medicare/Medicaid rules and regulations, Stark I and II, the antikickback statute, the False Claims Act, Medicare exclusions and civil monetary penalties, and the Health Insurance Portability and Accountability Act of 1996 (HIPAA) (see Chapter 3)

- a requirement for continuous distribution throughout the year of memoranda about program changes and legislation impacting each employee's specific responsibilities

- for new employees, an orientation program emphasizing the practice's commitment to ethics and the compliance program

The written plan should require maintenance of a log or file of all training programs and those in attendance, training memorandums, etc.

Although the OIG has conceded that a physician's office is less complicated than a large integrated corporate provider, it still highly recommends annual training for all employees. The OIG also suggests training for any new hires added to the practice in a given year and the distribution of "timely updates" of legal developments (as they occur) to all employees. This should be viewed as a minimum standard that the physician may want to exceed.

It is also a good idea to discuss compliance issues periodically in staff meetings, during employee performance evaluations, etc. These instances are a good time to remind employees of the importance of compliance.

The OIG *Compliance Program Guidance for Individual and Small Group Physician Practices* states:

Step Four: Conducting Appropriate Training and Education

Education is an important part of any compliance program and is the logical next step after problems have been identified and the practice has designated a person to oversee educational training. Ideally, education programs will be tailored to the physician practice's needs, specialty and size and will include both compliance and specific training.

There are three basic steps for setting up educational objectives:

1. determining who needs training (both in coding and billing and in compliance);

2. determining the type of training that best suits the practice's needs (e.g., seminars, in-service training, self-study or other programs); and

3. determining when and how often education is needed and how much each person should receive.

Training may be accomplished through a variety of means, including in-person training sessions (i.e., either on site or at outside seminars), distribution of newsletters, or even a readily accessible office bulletin board. Regardless of the training modality used, a physician practice should ensure that the necessary education is communicated effectively and that the practice's employees come away from the training with a better understanding of the issues covered.

1. Compliance Training

Under the direction of the designated compliance officer/contact, both initial and recurrent training in compliance is advisable, both with respect to the compliance program itself and applicable statutes and regulations. Suggestions for items to include in compliance training are: the operation and importance of the compliance program; the consequences of violating the standards and procedures set forth in the program; and the role of each employee in the operation of the compliance program.

There are two goals a practice should strive for when conducting compliance training: (1) all employees will receive training on how to perform their jobs in compliance with the standards of the practice and any applicable regulations; and (2) each employee will understand that compliance is a condition of continued employment. Compliance training focuses on explaining why the practice is developing and establishing a compliance program. The training should emphasize that following the standards and procedures will not get a practice employee in trouble, but violating the standards and procedures may subject the employee to disciplinary measures. It is advisable that new employees be trained on the compliance program as soon as possible after their start date and employees should receive refresher training on an annual basis or as appropriate.

2. Coding and Billing Training

Coding and billing training on the Federal health care program requirements may be necessary for certain members of the physician practice staff depending on their respective responsibilities. The OIG understands that most physician practices do not employ a professional coder and that the physician is often primarily responsible for all coding and billing. However, it is in the practice's best interest to ensure that individuals who are directly involved with billing, coding or other aspects of the Federal health care programs receive extensive education specific to that individual's responsibilities. Some examples of items that could be covered in coding and billing training include:

- coding requirements;

- claim development and submission processes;

- signing a form for a physician without the physician's authorization;

- proper documentation of services rendered;

- proper billing standards and procedures and submission of accurate bills for services or items rendered to Federal health care program beneficiaries; and

- the legal sanctions for submitting deliberately false or reckless billings.

3. Format of the Training Program

Training may be conducted either in-house or by an outside source. Training at outside seminars, instead of internal programs and in-service sessions, may be an effective way to achieve the practice's training goals. In fact, many community colleges offer certificate or associate degree programs in billing and coding, and professional associations provide various kinds of continuing education and certification programs. Many carriers also offer billing training.

The physician practice may work with its third-party billing company, if one is used, to ensure that documentation is of a level that is adequate for the billing company to submit accurate claims on behalf of the physician practice. If it is not, these problem areas should also be covered in the training. In addition to the billing training, it is advisable for physician practices to maintain updated ICD-9, HCPCS and CPT manuals (in addition to the carrier bulletins construing those sources) and make them available to all employees involved in the billing process. Physician practices can also provide a source of continuous updates on current billing standards and procedures by making publications or Government documents that describe current billing policies available to its employees.

Physician practices do not have to provide separate education and training programs for the compliance and coding and billing training. All in-service training and continuing education can integrate compliance issues, as well as other core values adopted by the practice, such as quality improvement and improved patient service, into their curriculum.

4. Continuing Education on Compliance Issues

There is no set formula for determining how often training sessions should occur. The OIG recommends that there be at least an annual training program for all individuals involved in the coding and billing aspects of the practice. Ideally, new billing and coding employees will be trained as soon as possible after assuming their duties and will work under an experienced employee until their training has been completed.

E. Responding to Detected Offenses, Internal Investigation, and Corrective Action

Compliance programs should require that when the chief compliance officer or others involved in management become aware of potential violations or misconduct, they promptly investigate the matter to determine whether a material violation has occurred. If a violation has occurred, management should take steps to rectify it, report it to the government if necessary, and make any appropriate repayments to the government.

As a response to a compliance issue, the written plan should require an internal investigation, which might include:

- confidential employee interviews

- a coding and billing review

- a review of some or all of the following items:

    all contracts with physicians or the medical practice (including medical director agreements, space leases, and equipment leases)

    all contracts with independent contractor suppliers of professional services (such as therapy services, nursing services, and services of professional aides and assistants)

    explanations of benefits

    all written employment agreements and written policies for physician compensation (the method used to compensate physicians for diagnostic tests they order are an issue under Stark II)

    all agreements to provide physician services to purchasers of such services (such as nursing homes, hospitals, and other entities)

    all managed care contracts

    all agreements with consultants and advisors and any reports produced by those consultants and providers (if these agreements are not in writing, then a list of the agreements and the amount paid to the consultants)

    all contracts for billing services

    documents related to any investigations, lawsuits, administrative proceedings, or Medicare or Medicaid overpayment requests, whether threatened or pending

    documents related to any acquisitions or sales of the medical practice

On completion of the investigation, the written plan should require the medical practice to:

- take immediate corrective action to cure any problem and implement steps to prevent it from happening again

- when appropriate, make restitution, but only after considering the events that prompted the overpayment and knowing the proper way to make restitution

- confer with counsel to decide if disclosure of compliance information should be made to the appropriate authorities

- initiate disciplinary action that may be appropriate

- prepare a report to the compliance officer, management, and the governing body that outlines the alleged misconduct, subsequent finding, and corrective action taken and/or planned.

The *OIG Compliance Program Guidance for Individual and Small Group Physician Practices* states:

Step Five: Responding to Detected Offenses and Developing Corrective Action Initiatives

When a practice determines it has detected a possible violation, the next step is to develop a corrective action plan and determine how to respond to the problem. Violations of a physician practice's compliance program, significant failures to comply with applicable Federal or State law, and other types of misconduct threaten a practice's status as a reliable, honest, and trustworthy provider of health care. Consequently, upon receipt of reports or reasonable indications of suspected noncompliance, it is important that the compliance contact or other practice employee look into the allegations to determine whether a significant violation of applicable law or the requirements of the compliance program has indeed occurred, and, if so, take decisive steps to correct the problem. As appropriate, such steps may involve a corrective action plan, the return of any overpayments, a report to the Government, and/or a referral to law enforcement authorities.

One suggestion is that the practice, in developing its compliance program, develop its own set of monitors and warning indicators. These might include: significant changes in the number and/or types of claim rejections and/or reductions; correspondence from the carriers and insurers challenging the medical necessity or validity of claims; illogical patterns or unusual changes in the pattern of CPT-4, HCPCS or ICD-9 code utilization; and high volumes of unusual charge or payment adjustment transactions. If any of these warning indicators become apparent, then it is recommended that the practice follow up on the issues. Subsequently, as appropriate, the compliance procedures of the practice may need to be changed to prevent the problem from recurring.

For potential criminal violations, a physician practice would be well advised in its compliance program procedures to include steps for prompt referral or disclosure to an appropriate Government authority or law enforcement agency. In regard to overpayment issues, it is advised that the physician practice take appropriate corrective action, including prompt identification and repayment of any overpayment to the affected payor.

It is also recommended that the compliance program provide for a full internal assessment of all reports of detected violations. If the physician practice ignores reports of possible fraudulent activity, it is undermining the very purpose it hoped to achieve by implementing a compliance program.

It is advised that the compliance program standards and procedures include provisions to ensure that a violation is not compounded once discovered. In instances involving individual misconduct, the standards and procedures might also advise as to whether the individuals involved in the violation either be retrained, disciplined, or, if appropriate, terminated. The physician practice may also prevent the compounding of the violation by conducting a review of all confirmed violations, and, if appropriate, self-reporting the violations to the applicable authority.

The physician practice may consider the fact that if a violation occurred and was not detected, its compliance program may require modification. Physician practices that detect violations could analyze the situation to determine whether a flaw in their compliance program failed to anticipate the detected problem, or whether the compliance program's procedures failed to prevent the violation. In any event, it is prudent, even absent the detection of any violations, for physician practices to periodically review and modify their compliance programs.

F. Effective Lines of Communications, Including Access to the Compliance Officer

An open line of communication among the compliance officer, physicians, and support staff is critical to the successful implementation and operation of a compliance program. If fraud and abuse are going to be reduced, there should be a policy with an open door, anonymity, and no retribution available to all employees to encourage communication. Investigating concerns can clarify the gray areas of interpretation of Medicare and Medicaid guidelines and regulations, but in all cases, the medical practice should encourage employees not to guess, but to ask if there is confusion or a question. Where appropriate, awards for reporting violations should be available.

The written plan should establish methods that would ensure:

- effective communications within the medical practice among the compliance officer, physicians, support staff, consultants, billing companies, and others involved

- a process to facilitate reporting of questions, complaints, or suspected violations to the compliance officer

- that employees and others who may utilize the reporting process have confidence that confidentiality will be maintained, that there will be no retaliation, and that the complaint will be investigated

Note: Many who have implemented compliance plans within physician offices acknowledge the difficulty of ensuring confidentiality. Instead, they set confidentiality as an objective but do not guarantee it, especially in smaller groups.

Also notice that the OIG's *Compliance Guidance* does not require establishment of a hotline to report concerns anonymously. The *OIG Compliance Program Guidance for Individual and Small Group Physician Practice* states:

Step Six: Developing Open Lines of Communication

In order to prevent problems from occurring and to have a frank discussion of why the problem happened in the first place, physician practices need to have open lines of communication. Especially in a smaller practice, an open line of communication is an integral part of implementing a compliance program. Guidance previously issued by the OIG has encouraged the use of several forms of communication between the compliance officer/committee and provider personnel, many of which focus on formal processes and are more costly to implement (e.g., hotlines and e-mail). However, the OIG recognizes that the nature of some physician practices is not as con-ducive to implementing these types of measures. The nature of a small physician practice dictates that such communication and information exchanges need to be conducted through a less formalized process than that which has been envisioned by prior OIG guidance.

In the small physician practice setting, the communication element may be met by implementing a clear "open door" policy between the physicians and compliance personnel and practice employees. This policy can be implemented in conjunction with less formal communication techniques, such as conspicuous notices posted in common areas and/or the development and placement of a compliance bulletin board where everyone in the practice can receive up-to-date compliance information.

A compliance program's system for meaningful and open communication can include the following:

- the requirement that employees report conduct that a reasonable person would, in good faith, believe to be erroneous or fraudulent;

- the creation of a user-friendly process (such as an anonymous drop box for larger practices) for effectively reporting erroneous or fraudulent conduct;

- provisions in the standards and procedures that state that a failure to report erroneous or fraudulent conduct is a violation of the compliance program;

- the development of a simple and readily accessible procedure to process reports of erroneous or fraudulent conduct;

- if a billing company is used, communication to and from the billing company's compliance officer/contact and other responsible staff to coordinate billing and compliance activities of the practice and the billing company, respectively. Communication can include, as appropriate, lists of reported or identified concerns, initiation and the results of internal assessments, training needs, regulatory changes, and other operational and compliance matters;

- the utilization of a process that maintains the anonymity of the persons involved in the reported possible erroneous or fraudulent conduct and the person reporting the concern; and

- provisions in the standards and procedures that there will be no retribution for reporting conduct that a reasonable person acting in good faith would have believed to be erroneous or fraudulent.

The OIG recognizes that protecting anonymity may not be feasible for small physician practices. However, the OIG believes all practice employees, when seeking answers to questions or reporting potential instances of erroneous or fraudulent conduct, should know to whom to turn for assistance in these matters and should be able to do so without fear of retribution. While the physician practice may strive to maintain the anonymity of an employee's identity, it also needs to make clear that there may be a point at which the individual's identity may become known or may have to be revealed in certain instances.

G. Enforcement of Standards Through Well-Publicized Disciplinary Guidelines

A viable compliance program must include the initiation of corrective and/or disciplinary action against individuals who have failed to comply with the organization's compliance policies and/or federal or state laws or who have otherwise engaged in wrongdoing that has the potential of impairing the organization's status as a reliable, honest, and trustworthy entity.

The written compliance plan should include:

- a policy statement setting forth the degrees of disciplinary actions that may be imposed for failing to comply with the company's code of conduct, company policies, and the law

- a policy indicating that disciplinary action may be appropriate where a responsible employee's failure to detect a violation is attributable to his or her negligence or reckless conduct

- a policy that disciplinary action will be taken on a fair and equitable basis and that variations in the form of discipline for individuals similarly situated will be limited

- a requirement that disciplinary policies be communicated in the compliance educational process for new as well as current employees

- a requirement that managers sign an annual acknowledgment that they have reviewed the plan, complied with the plan, and properly instructed employees they supervise as to their responsibilities under the plan

- a system of record keeping on all internal disciplinary actions

- a prohibition on the employment of individuals who have been convicted of a criminal offense related to health care or who are listed by a federal agency as excluded or otherwise ineligible for participation in federally funded health care programs

- a requirement that a reasonable background check will be made for new employees who have discretionary authority to make decisions that may involve compliance issues

The OIG *Compliance Program Guidance for Individual and Small Group Physician Practice* states:

Step Seven: Enforcing Disciplinary Standards Through Well-Publicized Guidelines

Finally, the last step that a physician practice may wish to take is to incorporate measures into its practice to ensure that practice employees understand the consequences if they behave in a non-compliant manner. An effective physician practice compliance program includes procedures for enforcing and disciplining individuals who violate the practice's compliance or other practice standards. Enforcement and disciplinary provisions are necessary to add credibility and integrity to a compliance program.

The OIG recommends that a physician practice's enforcement and disciplinary mechanisms ensure that violations of the practice's compliance policies will result in consistent and appropriate sanctions, including the possibility of termination, against the offending individual. At the same time, it is advisable that the practice's enforcement and disciplinary procedures be flexible enough to account for mitigating or aggravating circumstances. The procedures might also stipulate that individuals who fail to detect or report violations of the compliance program may also be subject to discipline. Disciplinary actions could include: warnings (oral); reprimands (written); probation; demotion; temporary suspension; termination; restitution of damages; and referral for criminal prosecution. Inclusion of disciplinary guidelines in in-house training and procedure manuals is sufficient to meet the "well publicized" standard of this element.

It is suggested that any communication resulting in the finding of non-compliant conduct be documented in the compliance files by including the date of incident, name of the reporting party, name of the person responsible for taking action, and the follow-up action taken. Another suggestion is for physician practices to conduct checks to make sure all current and potential practice employees are not listed on the OIG or GSA lists of individuals excluded from participation in Federal health care or Government procurement programs.

Performing an Internal Audit

One of the first steps in the establishment of an effective compliance program is an intense audit and investigation to assess activities that represent high risk. Generally, we recommend that these audits be conducted by an independent party experienced in fraud and abuse; however, physicians can conduct these assessments themselves if they are objective and thorough. The audit should be structured to include four components:

- A coding and billing review

- A legal analysis

- Confidential employee interviews

- A review of the organization's documents and records

Coding and Billing Review

This review is usually best performed by an outside party with a high level of understanding of Medicare regulations and related coding issues. The objective of the review is to determine:

- if correct CPT® codes, modifiers, place of service codes, and the like are being used

- if those codes are supported both by documentation within a patient's chart and by appropriate diagnostic codes[1]

- if applicable Health Care Financing Administration guidelines—such as those for evaluation and management codes, use of the -25 modifier, and billing by teaching physicians for resident services—are being followed

- how effective the organization's current internal controls are in identifying and correcting misconduct (this is usually a by-product of the first three items)

Once coding and billing methods that need corrective action have been identified, the next step should include one or more of the following options:

- To train—and retrain—physicians and billing department staff to use proper coding techniques

- To train top administrative staff to understand these same techniques

- To develop and implement methods for capturing all charges

- To create uniformity within the organization's system for coding physician services

- To provide periodic training sessions to ensure that all recommendations are being followed

Legal Analysis

Legal guidance is needed from an expert well versed in health care law and related regulations to make sure a health care organization is not in violation of such familiar legislation as the antikickback statute, Stark laws, HIPAA, False Claims Act, and other applicable standards. (See the section below regarding review of records and documents.)

Confidential Employee Interviews

When an investigation, initial audit, or annual assessment is performed, it is usually desirable to interview employees. During an initial audit, key employees' knowledge with respect to compliance issues and training needs should be assessed. Interviews should also attempt to determine compliance concerns that may need to be investigated and corrected.

Before an interview is conducted, it is very important to explain to the employee why these questions are being asked—"It is part of the medical practice's voluntary effort to ensure compliance, and the medical practice's physicians and managers encourage employees to give honest answers (without fear of reprisal)."

Sometimes it helps to start the interview by asking: "Have you ever been through a compliance review? What have you been told about this audit?" The reason for the review should then be explained in response to the employee's level of understanding. It should be stressed that the physicians and managers are doing this voluntarily and that they are committed to ensuring that things are done properly. Stress that the responses are confidential. It also helps to say, "Before we get started, do you have any questions of me?"

Sometimes, it may be desirable to have the practice's attorney review the questions or assist or conduct the interview.

When an investigation into a compliance incident report or audit finding is performed, the appropriate questions will depend on the circumstances. If it is possible that one or more of the employees has been *knowingly* involved in fraudulent activity, it may be desirable to have the practice's attorney review the questions or even conduct the interview. Physicians should not make any promises that they cannot keep if fraud is involved.

The interviewing of employees should be aimed not only at gaining an understanding of accounting procedures, paper flow, and other billing activities, but also toward ferreting out any unethical or illegal activity that is occurring within an organization. The interviewer should not avoid the hard questions. It is better to know now what has occurred or is occurring than to learn of transgressions later, after they have been continuing for some time or are discovered by an administrative or criminal investigation.

At a minimum, the following questions should be asked when an audit is conducted:

- Have you heard any rumors or reports of unethical or illegal conduct by other employees, physicians, managers, or others?

- Have you noticed any conduct by any employees, physicians, managers, or others that you believe was illegal or unethical?

- Have you been asked to take part in conduct that you believe was illegal or unethical?

- Are there any other concerns related to compliance that you would like to discuss?

  It should be made clear that the interview is confidential, but that the information may be disclosed to the organization's management by the interviewer without revealing the employee's name. Also, the employee should be instructed not to disclose any part of the discussion to other parties.

  Before the interviews are conducted, employees should be provided an explanation of what is occurring and why. They should understand that the health care organization is formalizing its compliance efforts.

  Finally, when the interview questions have been asked, employees should be given a card with a telephone number or address where they can communicate any concerns—anonymously if they desire—that were not discussed in the interviews (or to report anything they thought of later). A complete record of concerns expressed in these interviews and follow-up activities should be maintained by the compliance officer.

Review of Records and Documents

The last component of an internal audit should be a thorough review of the organization's records (not medical records, which are part of the coding review component), including, but not limited to:

- policies and procedures related to compliance issues

- corporate documents relating to the business and tax structure of the organization

- all contracts with physicians (including medical director agreements, space leases, equipment leases, and all other agreements between the organization and physicians)

- all contracts with independent contractor suppliers of professional services (such as therapy services, nursing services, and all professional aides and assistants)

- all contracts between the entity and insiders within the organization, including officers, directors, and key employees (if these agreements are not in writing, then the organization should prepare brief descriptions of the verbal agreements and the amount of consideration paid)

- a representative sample of Medicare notices of reimbursement (explanations of benefits) issued during the past 5 years (as well as those of other payers)

- documentation regarding all licensure and accreditation surveys conducted within the past 5 years, including all lists of deficiencies and plans of correction

- all written employment agreements

- all agreements to provide the organization's services to purchasers of services (such as nursing homes, hospitals, and other entities)

- all managed care contracts

- all agreements with consultants and advisors and any documentation produced by those consultants and advisors (if these agreements are not in writing, then a list of the agreements and the amount paid to the consultants for the past 5 years should be compiled)

- all contracts for billing services

- complete documentation regarding the bad-debt collection process, including the policies and procedures for the collection process and communication sent to the entity's accounts

- documents related to any investigations, lawsuits, and administrative proceedings, whether threatened or pending

- documents related to acquisitions or sales

- corporate, board, and committee minutes

A health care organization should perform a compliance evaluation of any medical practice it plans to acquire or merge with. Medical practices should carefully consider the organizations with which they do business.

Making the Internal Audit Report a Privileged Document

The results of the internal audit should be reduced to a written report. However, such a report can be a "smoking gun" to the OIG or the FBI during an investigation. This document can be legally withheld from review if the attorney-client privilege can be utilized. Generally, to do this:

1   Have the entity's attorney request the audit and make it clear the intent of the audit is to assist the attorney in providing legal advice.

2   Have the attorney hire the outside party that will conduct the audit and emphasize that the audit is intended to help the attorney in preparing legal advice, and that the final audit report will be the property of the attorney.

3   Have the attorney present and actively participate in all significant meetings, such as the final presentation of audit findings.

4   Have the audit report marked "attorney-client privileged" and distributed only to those needing to know its content, such as staff personnel directly responsible for implementing compliance efforts.

We will discuss the issue of attorney-client privilege in greater detail later, because it is not always as simple as presented here.

Writing the Compliance Plan

A written compliance program should be developed.[2] The formality of any compliance program should vary with a health care organization's size, with larger ones typically requiring more formal programs. The following are examples of documents that should be maintained in a formal compliance plan:

1   Code of conduct

2   Reporting mechanism for compliance concerns or complaints

3   Policies related to, and documentation of, training and education programs, topics covered, and attendees

4   Compliance officer (or equivalent) duties and responsibilities

5   All policies and procedures related to billing and coding activities

6   Log of compliance incident reports, results of investigations, and corrective action

7   Audit and monitoring reports

8   Minutes of compliance committee meetings

9   Listing of board of director actions related to compliance issues

10 Contracts with compliance implications

11 Disciplinary actions

12 Other topics

Every health care compliance program should include a written code of conduct, containing specific ethical standards and policies.

The governing body and upper-level management should formally adopt the code of conduct and communicate their commitment and expectations to all employees by making presentations at training sessions and orientation programs, and by distributing written communications periodically. Managers should communicate their commitment and expectations to the employees reporting to them. Managers should understand their responsibilities with respect to the compliance plan and disciplinary actions that may apply should they fail to fulfill these responsibilities. Annually, managers should sign an acknowledgment that they have reviewed the compliance plan, complied with the plan, and properly instructed employees they supervise as to their responsibilities under the plan.

This code of conduct should clearly advise employees of the standards they are expected to follow and of the consequences for their failure to follow such standards. The code of conduct should include all applicable health care laws and regulations, as well as other common laws typically covered in codes of conduct, such as securities law, employment law, antitrust law, conflicts of interest, discrimination, business ethics, corporate political activity, and environmental law.

The code of conduct should clearly state that employees and others:

- are expected to cooperate with government officials in the event of an investigation

- are not to hide, destroy, alter, delay, or otherwise tamper with documents or other evidence either as a result of a request for information or in anticipation of such a request

- must not exert influence on any other employee (or former employee) to keep them from responding appropriately to an investigation

- are not to contact any beneficiary or insured whose records may be part of an investigation

- should report questioning by government officials to the corporate compliance officer should the investigation not be general knowledge

- will not be disciplined solely for telling the truth to the best of their knowledge

The code of conduct should be distributed to all officers, directors, and employees. These individuals should be required to sign an acknowledgment that they have received, read, understood, and agree to abide by the code of conduct.[3]

Training Programs

Frequent training programs and seminars are key components to ensuring compliance and should be tailored to employees' jobs and roles in a medical practice or other health care organization. Recommended areas of training include CPT® coding, diagnostic coding, documentation guidelines, Medicare rules and regulations, employees' responsibilities in the event of an investigation, how to report a compliance incident, Stark I and II, the antikickback statute, the False Claims Act, HIPAA, civil exclusions, civil monetary penalties, and fraud and abuse, including the statutes concerning mail fraud, wire fraud, conspiracy to commit an offense against the United States, false claims against the United States, and false statements to an agency of the United States.[4]

Training programs should be designed so that employees are not subjected to complex discussions on issues that do not affect them—such as someone in housekeeping attending a program on antitrust, kickbacks, and CPT® coding. Make sure employees and agents can understand your compliance program.

In addition to the formal training programs, memoranda regarding specific statutes applicable to certain employees may be distributed throughout the year. Creative ways of ensuring that training information is effectively disseminated to employees include newsletters, pay stub messages, posters, public recognition of employees who demonstrate a commitment to ethical conduct, consideration of employee ethics in performance evaluations, and continual messages to employees that emphasize the health care organization's dedication to a compliance program. For new employees, the medical practice or health care organization should conduct a comprehensive orientation regarding the company's commitment to ethics, the code of conduct, and the compliance program.

It is clear that the government will not recognize compliance programs that are merely a sham, not effective, or ill prepared. The compliance program must represent reasonable efforts to identify, correct, and prevent misconduct. In fact, a poorly designed compliance program might do more harm than good by providing a false sense of security and by inadvertently acting as a statement of ill intent.

Identifying a Compliance Officer or the Equivalent

To administer a compliance program, the practice should designate an individual or individuals responsible for overseeing the compliance program.

The decision of whom to appoint as compliance officer(s) should depend on an organization's size and culture. Regardless of whether it is a single individual, a committee, legal counsel, or a consultant, the duties of an organization's compliance officer include knowing and understanding all aspects of the compliance plan, ensuring that delegations of responsibility under the compliance program are made in writing to, and understood by, individuals believed to be of high integrity, consulting with counsel for interpretations regarding requirements under the plan, and amending the plan to make it more effective. The compliance officer should also work with counsel to monitor all developments and changes in relevant state and federal laws and regulations that may affect the organization.

The compliance officer(s) should be identified in writing to all employees, preferably as part of the code of conduct. Employees should be trained in the mechanics for reporting suspected violations of the code of conduct and illegal activity to the compliance officer.

Efforts must be made to ensure that the compliance officer operates without fear of retribution when taking action or reporting activities that might reflect negatively on upper-level management. Ways to achieve some degree of autonomy include requiring an affirmative vote of the board of directors to discipline or terminate the compliance officer, or offering an employment contract that provides appropriate protections.

Compliance Officer for a Small Medical Practice

A common question asked by smaller medical practices is, "How can we afford a compliance officer?" The OIG *Compliance Program Guidance for Individual and Small Group Physician Practices* provides some comfort in that it is clear the person(s) responsible for administering a compliance program can do other things. In fact, the OIG's *Compliance Program Guidance* talks about "compliance contacts" as an alternative for small medical practices. The OIG's *Compliance Program Guidance* also discusses an "open door" among physicians, compliance personnel, and other practice employees.

The key is to focus on finding affordable ways of fulfilling the compliance officer's responsibilities. A large practice may be able to afford a full-time compliance officer. In fact, a full-time compliance officer and support staff may be the only way a large group can fulfill compliance responsibilities.

A smaller practice may be able to fulfill the key responsibilities in other ways. One approach is to use practice management consultants and/or attorneys experienced in compliance issues to perform many of the duties and responsibilities.

Another approach would be designation of an office manager, another employee, or a physician who fully understands the duties and responsibilities implicit in the concept of a compliance officer to handle the functions. The key is for the compliance officer to accomplish the responsibilities.

These responsibilities may be augmented by help from other staff, an attorney, and/or a practice management consultant. The compliance plan—taken as a whole—should demonstrate a concerted effort and commitment to compliance and an effective approach to ensuring compliance.

Review the OIG's comments regarding compliance officers in small group practices under Step 3 of the Seven Basic Elements of a Compliance Plan.

Summary of Compliance Officer Duties and Responsibilities

- Develop, implement, and maintain the organization's formal, written compliance plan. The plan should be reviewed and updated at least semiannually.

- Develop, review, and maintain all compliance policies, procedures, standards of conduct, and employee compliance handbooks.

- Ensure the effectiveness of the organization's compliance efforts.

- Maintain a reporting system that encourages employees and others to submit any compliance concerns through telephone hotlines or similar mechanism. Compliance incident reports should be cataloged (ie, logged and given a number) so that actions can be tracked and reported. To ensure that all compliance incident reports are addressed, the compliance officer should maintain a list of incident reports that have not been resolved. Employees should be periodically reminded of the incident reporting system.

- Ensure that all compliance incident reports are properly investigated (this may require legal counsel or a consultant's opinion) and that appropriate action is taken *and documented thoroughly*. The compliance officer will communicate in writing the results and proposed action to the compliance committee, governing body, and upper-level management.

- Identify areas that represent a high risk with respect to compliance issues, perform appropriate audits, and recommend and/or take corrective action.

- Document the monitoring of the compliance program to ensure it is effective, including periodic employee interviews, internal audits, investigation of concerns, recommendations regarding identified compliance issues, and program refinements.

- Develop training programs to keep employees aware of their responsibilities and policies and procedures applicable to their jobs. When appropriate, develop specific training programs for departments, specified activities, etc.

- Maintain records of attendance at training programs and ensure that employees have attended all required training sessions, including an annual review and update.

- Develop new employee orientation programs emphasizing compliance responsibilities, the compliance plan, and how their job fits into the system.

- Issue meaningful, periodic reports to upper-level management and governing body (see next section).

- Maintain certifications or acknowledgments that employees have read and understand the organization's compliance plan.

- Recommend appropriate disciplinary action for employees who violate the code of conduct; however, it is management's and/or the governing body's responsibility to approve such action.

- Maintain documentation of all meetings, discussions, actions taken, etc, with respect to compliance issues.

- *Keep compliance efforts going.* Compliance is a long-term commitment.

Periodic Reports to Management and Governing Body

The compliance officer should issue monthly (more often if required) reports to upper-level management; quarterly reports to the board of directors; and a detailed annual assessment of how well the plan is accomplishing its goals and objectives.[5]

These reports should include:

- compliance issues that have occurred since the last report and actions taken

- significant revisions or updates proposed to the compliance plan, code of conduct, policies and procedures, and standards

- proposed or enacted legislation or regulations that significantly impact the organization with recommendations for ensuring compliance

- the status of any internal investigations into compliance incident reports and periodic audits[6]

- any disciplinary actions taken or proposed under the compliance plan

- recommendations for improving compliance efforts

Compliance Committee

Most large organizations should consider establishing a compliance committee composed of the compliance officer and key management personnel, including the president or chief executive officer, the corporation's attorney, representatives of the governing body (which would include physicians in a medical practice), and other key personnel. Sometimes, compliance responsibilities are absorbed by an existing committee; however, compliance is an issue that deserves its own committee—or at the very least, subcommittee status. Even in a committee structure, there must be an identified compliance officer.

The OIG's *Model Compliance Plan for Medical Billing Companies* said the following regarding compliance committees:

> The OIG recommends, where feasible,[7] that a compliance committee be established to advise the compliance officer and assist in the implementation of the compliance program.[8] When assembling a team of people to serve as the billing company's compliance committee, the company should include individuals with a variety of skills. Appropriate members of the compliance committee include the director of billing and the director of coding. The OIG strongly recommends that the compliance officer manage the compliance committee. Once a billing company chooses the people that will accept the responsibilities vested in members of the compliance committee, the billing company must train these individuals on the policies and procedures of the compliance program. . . .

Encouraging Expression of Compliance Concerns

To ensure that the health care organization creates an atmosphere amenable to employees coming forward with suspected violations, it is preferable to allow employees to report potential violations confidentially either in person, in writing, or via telephone. It should also be stressed that:

- no violation reported by an employee in good faith will be the sole reason for subjecting an employee to discipline

- the organization will, to the extent appropriate and possible, endeavor to conceal the identity of anyone reporting a possible violation

- the failure to report a known or suspected violation will be grounds for discipline

Making Compliance Part of Every Employee's Job Duties

A health care organization should not only rely on reports of possible violations but should also actively monitor and audit the conduct of employees. Management should make it clear that the compliance program is taken seriously, that all steps will be taken to ensure that it is followed, and that an employee's compliance performance will be considered in his or her evaluation.

Keeping Compliance Efforts Going

For a compliance program to be deemed effective, it is imperative that a health care organization exercise due diligence in seeking to prevent and detect fraudulent conduct by its employees and other agents. At a minimum, due diligence requires:

- a health care organization to establish compliance standards and procedures that, if followed by its employees and other agents, will reduce the prospect of criminal conduct

- specific individual(s) with high-level positions to be assigned overall responsibility to oversee compliance with relevant standards and procedures

- a health care organization to use due care not to delegate substantial discretionary authority to individuals whom the organization knows, or should have known through the exercise of due diligence, have a propensity to engage in illegal activities

- a health care organization to take steps to effectively communicate its standards and procedures to all employees and other agents, eg, by requiring participation in training programs or by disseminating publications that clearly explain what is required

- a health care organization to take reasonable steps to achieve compliance with its standards, eg, by having in place, utilizing, and monitoring auditing systems reasonably designed to detect criminal conduct by its employees and other agents, and by having in place and publicizing a reporting system whereby employees and other agents could report criminal conduct by others within the organization without fear of retribution

- the standards to be *consistently enforced* through appropriate and consistent disciplinary mechanisms, including, as appropriate, discipline of individuals responsible for the failure to detect an offense (adequate discipline of individuals responsible for an offense is a necessary component of enforcement; however, the form of discipline that is appropriate will be case specific)

- that, after an offense has been detected, an organization take all reasonable steps to respond appropriately to the offense and to prevent further similar offenses—including any necessary modifications to its program to prevent and detect violations.

Taking an Active Role

By taking an active role as just outlined, medical practices should be able to detect and cure any compliance deficiencies for reporting physician services and, in turn, be prepared for any visits by the OIG or FBI. In the event of an investigation, a creditable compliance program may make a difference between being sanctioned and not being sanctioned; between a long, drawn-out inquiry and a short investigation; and between a large and a small civil penalty.

Reevaluate the Program

It is essential that an organization continually reevaluate and adjust its compliance program to ensure that its goals are achieved. There are many reasons for reevaluations: personnel changes, new laws, new interpretation of laws, new billing guidelines, loss of momentum such that it is necessary to reaffirm commitment to the program, etc.

There is often a lot of enthusiasm when a compliance program begins. Unfortunately, this enthusiasm may wane over time, particularly if no significant events are identified for months and months. This period may be when a practice becomes most vulnerable to problems—both those related to fraud and abuse, and those related to effective business operations such as collections, insurance follow-up, and the like. At a minimum, stick with established audit routines to ensure compliance efforts are working.

Attorney-Client Privilege

In some cases, the government could subpoena information obtained through internal audits and investigations. As a general rule, a health care corporate entity has no right to protect such information except, perhaps, where it is protected by the attorney-client privilege or a related doctrine. Even where this privilege exists, the underlying documents—medical records, receipts, etc—are not protected.

While courts have varied in their interpretation of the attorney-client privilege in these instances, the chance of protecting information increases when the health care entity specifically requests an attorney to offer legal advice regarding steps that should be taken to implement and maintain an effective compliance program or what actions should be taken with respect to specific compliance issues. Thus, the attorney should be asked to render legal advice and, in the course of rendering such advice, the attorney should request reports from accountants or consultants. Further, the attorney-client privilege must not have been waived (by allowing the accountant's or consultant's opinion, prepared at the attorney's request, to be viewed by anyone who does not share a common interest with the corporate client or who does not have a "need to know").

Courts may not recognize this privilege when it is clear that the attorney's role is primarily to try to protect adverse facts from discovery in legal proceedings. In fact, simply transferring potentially incriminating internal documents to an attorney does not invoke the attorney-client privilege. Of course, the attorney-client privilege does not apply if the attorney's opinion is requested to assist the health care entity in conducting illegal activities.

Some attorneys discuss what might be called a self-evaluation or self-assessment privilege that might protect internal investigations that are independent of the attorney-client privilege. Others argue that a work product doctrine might be used to protect a consultant's opinion.

In summary, there are enough legal issues related to the protection of information gained through an internal investigation that it is impossible to state with certainty what degree of protection exists. An effective compliance plan will include internal investigations based on monitoring results and reports of compliance concerns, and these investigations may be conducted by or for the practice's attorney. The physician and the attorney should discuss the best way to maximize any potential protection that may apply.

Voluntary Disclosure

Another difficult question is whether a medical practice should make voluntary disclosure when a violation is identified. The American Medical Association provides particularly valuable insight into this issue in *Federal Fraud Enforcement—Physician Compliance* (published September 25, 1997):

> One of the more difficult questions that an organization may face is whether it should voluntarily disclose compliance problems to regulatory authorities. . . . Voluntary disclosure of compliance problems does not provide any automatic protections or guarantees of leniency. The fact that an organization maintains a compliance plan does not

restructure the organization as an investigatory arm of the OIG, and disclosure is not mandated.

. . . In the event that an internal investigation discovers that a material violation has occurred, it sometimes may be advisable to report the matter to the federal government. However, such a decision needs to be discussed with counsel. If the organization, with advice from counsel, believes that failure to disclose will call into question the veracity of the plan and limit the reduced culpability protections that the plan is designed to afford, disclosure may be appropriate.

In 1998, the OIG issued the following provider self-disclosure protocol:

[*Federal Register*, October 30, 1998, Volume 63 (Notices), pages 58399-58403; from the *Federal Register* Online via GPO Access (wais.access.gpo.gov)] [DOCID:fr30oc98-95]

DEPARTMENT OF HEALTH AND HUMAN SERVICES
Office of Inspector General

Publication of the OIG's Provider Self-Disclosure Protocol

AGENCY: Office of Inspector General (OIG), HHS.
ACTION: Notice.

SUMMARY: This Federal Register notice sets forth the OIG's recently-issued Provider Self-Disclosure Protocol. This Self-Disclosure Protocol offers health care providers specific steps, including a detailed audit methodology, that may be undertaken if they wish to work openly and cooperatively with the OIG to efficiently quantify a particular problem and, ultimately, promote a higher level of ethical and lawful conduct throughout the health care industry.

FOR FURTHER INFORMATION CONTACT: Ted Acosta, Office of Counsel to the Inspector General, (202) 619-2078.

SUPPLEMENTARY INFORMATION: The OIG has long stressed the role of the health care industry in combating health care fraud, and believes that health care providers can play a cooperative role in identifying and voluntarily disclosing program abuses. The OIG's use of voluntary self-disclosure programs, for example, is premised on a belief that health care providers must be willing to police themselves, correct underlying problems and work with the Government to resolve these matters. Based on insights gained from a pilot program undertaken as part

of Operation Restore Trust, discussions with the provider community and the growing need for an effective disclosure mechanism, the OIG has now developed a more open-ended process, or protocol, for making a disclosure and allowing a health care provider to cooperative work with the OIG. Unlike the previous voluntary disclosure pilot programs, this self-disclosure protocol gives detailed guidance to the provider on what information is appropriate to include as part of an investigative report and how to conduct an audit of the matter, while setting no limitations on the conditions under which a health care provider may disclose information to the OIG.

A reprint of the OIG's Provider Self-Disclosure Protocol follows.

Provider Self-Disclosure Protocol

I. Introduction

The Office of Inspector General (OIG) of the United States Department of Health and Human Services (HHS) relies heavily upon the health care industry to help identify and resolve matters that adversely affect the Federal health care programs (as defined in 42 U.S.C. 1320a-7b(f)). The OIG believes that, as participants in the Federal health care programs, health care providers have an ethical and legal duty to ensure the integrity of their dealings with these programs. This duty includes an obligation to take measures, such as instituting a compliance program, to detect and prevent fraudulent, abusive and wasteful activities. It also encompasses the need to implement specific procedures and mechanisms to examine and resolve instances of non-compliance with program requirements. Whether as a result of voluntary self-assessment or in response to external forces, health care providers must be prepared to investigate such instances, assess the potential losses suffered by the Federal health care programs, and make full disclosure to the appropriate authorities. To encourage providers to make voluntary disclosures, the OIG issues this Provider Self-Disclosure Protocol (Protocol).

The concept of voluntary self-disclosure is not new to the OIG. For many years, the OIG has worked informally with providers and suppliers that came forward to cooperate with OIG to resolve billing, marketing or quality of care problems. In 1995, as part of the Operation Restore Trust (ORT) initiative, HHS and the Department of Justice (DOJ) announced a pilot voluntary disclosure program, which embraced OIG's longstanding policy favoring voluntary self-disclosure. The demonstration program was developed in coordination with representatives of the OIG, DOJ, various United States Attorneys' Offices, the Federal Bureau of Investigation and the Centers for Medicare and Medicaid Services CMS. The pilot program was limited to five States (New York, Florida, Illinois, Texas and California) and four different types of providers (home health agencies, skilled nursing facilities, durable medical equipment suppliers, and hospice providers). It gave those qualifying entities a formal mechanism for disclosing and seeking the resolution of matters relating to the Medicare and Medicaid programs. In 1997, the pilot voluntary disclosure program was concluded. While there was limited participation in the pilot, the OIG gained valuable insight into the variables influencing the decision to make a disclosure to the Government.

The OIG believes it must continue encouraging the health care industry to conduct voluntary self-evaluations and providing viable opportunities for self-disclosure. By establishing this Protocol, the OIG renews its commitment to promote an environment of openness and cooperation. The Protocol has no rigid requirements or limitations.

Rather, it provides the OIG's views on what are the appropriate elements of an effective investigative and audit working plan to address instances of noncompliance. Providers that follow the Protocol expedite the OIG's verification process and thus diminish the time it takes before the matter can be formally resolved. Failure to conform to each element of the Protocol is not necessarily fatal to the provider's disclosure, but will likely delay the resolution of the matter.

The OIG's principal purpose in producing the Protocol is to provide guidance to health care providers that decide voluntarily to disclose irregularities in their dealings with the Federal health care programs.

Because a provider's disclosure can involve anything from a simple error to outright fraud, the OIG cannot reasonably make firm commitments as to how a particular disclosure will be resolved or the specific benefit that will enure to the disclosing entity. In our experience, however, opening lines of communication with, and making full disclosure to, the investigative agency at an early stage generally benefits the individual or company. In short, the Protocol can help a health care provider initiate with the OIG a dialogue directed at resolving its potential liabilities. [boldface added]

The decision to follow the OIG's suggested Protocol rests exclusively with the provider. While the OIG can offer only limited guidance on what is inherently a case-specific judgement, there are several considerations that should influence the decision. First, a provider that uncovers an ongoing fraud scheme within its organization immediately should contact the OIG, but should not follow the Protocol's suggested steps to investigate or quantify the scope of the problem. If the provider follows the Protocol in this type of situation without prior consultation with the OIG, there is a substantial risk that the Government's subsequent investigation will be compromised.

Second, the OIG anticipates that a provider will apply the Protocol's suggested steps only after an initial assessment substantiates there is a problem with non-compliance with program requirements. The initial identification of potential risk areas should be less intensive and need not conform to the Protocol's suggested procedures. Similarly, when the OIG conducts a national review of a particular billing practice, providers should consider the option of conducting a limited assessment of the practice under OIG review, rather than incur the expense of a comprehensive audit. In such cases, an audit that conforms to the Protocol's guidelines may be appropriate only in instances where a preliminary assessment suggests the provider has in fact engaged in the practices under OIG scrutiny.

II. The Provider Self-Disclosure Protocol

Unlike the earlier pilot program, there are no pre-disclosure requirements, applications for admission or preliminary qualifying characteristics that must be met. The Provider Self-Disclosure Protocol is open to all health care providers, whether individuals or entities, and is not limited to any particular industry, medical specialty or type of service. While no written agreement setting out the terms of the self-assessment will be required, the OIG expects the commitment of the health care provider to disclose specific information and engage in specific self-evaluative steps relating to the disclosed matter. In contrast to the pilot disclosure program, the fact that a disclosing health care provider is already subject to Government inquiry (including investigations, audits or routine oversight activities) will not automatically preclude a disclosure. The disclosure, however, must be made in good faith. The OIG will not continue to work with a provider that attempts to circumvent an ongoing inquiry or fails to fully cooperate in the self-disclosure process. In short, the OIG will continue its practice of working with providers that are the subject of an investigation or audit, provided that the collaboration does not interfere with the efficient and effective resolution of the inquiry.

The Provider Self-Disclosure Protocol is intended to facilitate the resolution of only matters that, in the provider's reasonable assessment, are potentially violative of Federal criminal, civil or administrative laws. Matters exclusively involving overpayments or errors that do not suggest that violations of law have occurred should be brought directly to the attention of the entity (e.g., a contractor such as a carrier or an intermediary) that processes claims and issues payment on behalf of the Government agency responsible for the particular Federal health care program (e.g., CMS/HCFA for matters involving Medicare). The program contractors are responsible for processing the refund and will review the circumstances surrounding the initial overpayment. If the contractor concludes that the overpayment raises concerns about the integrity of the provider, the matter may be referred to the OIG. Accordingly, the provider's initial decision of where to refer a matter involving non-compliance with program requirements should be made carefully.

The OIG is not bound by any findings made by the disclosing provider under the Provider Self-Disclosure Protocol and is not obligated to resolve the matter in any particular manner. Nevertheless, the OIG will work closely with providers that structure their disclosures in accordance with the Provider Self-Disclosure Protocol in an effort to coordinate any investigatory steps or other activities necessary to reach an effective and prompt resolution. It is important to note that, upon review of the provider's disclosure submission and/or reports, the OIG may conclude that the disclosed matter warrants a referral to DOJ for consideration under its civil and/or criminal authorities. Alternatively, the provider may request the participation of a representative of DOJ or a local United States Attorney's Office in settlement discussions in order to resolve potential liability under the False Claims Act or other laws. In either case, the OIG will report on the provider's involvement and level of cooperation throughout the disclosure process to any other Government agencies affected by the disclosed matter.

III. Voluntary Disclosure Submission

The disclosing provider will be expected to make a submission as follows.

A. Effective Disclosure

The disclosure must be made in writing and must be submitted to the Assistant Inspector General for Investigative Operations, Office of Inspector General, Department of Health and Human Services, 330 Independence Avenue, SW, Cohen Building, Room 5409, Washington, DC 20201. Submissions by telecopier, facsimile or other electronic media will not be accepted.

B. Basic Information

The submission should include the following—

1. The name, address, provider identification number(s) and tax identification number(s) of the disclosing health care provider. If the provider is an entity that is owned, controlled or is otherwise part of a system or network, include a description or diagram describing the pertinent relationships and the names and addresses of any related entities, as well as any affected corporate divisions, departments or branches. Additionally, provide the name and address of the disclosing entity's designated representative for purposes of the voluntary disclosure.

2. Indicate whether the provider has knowledge that the matter is under current inquiry by a Government agency or contractor. If the provider has knowledge of a pending inquiry, identify any such Government entity or individual representatives involved. The provider must also disclose whether it is under investigation or other inquiry for any other matters relating to a Federal health care program and provide similar information relating to those other matters.

3. A full description of the nature of the matter being disclosed, including the type of claim, transaction or other conduct giving rise to the matter, the names of entities and individuals believed to be implicated and an explanation of their roles in the matter, and the relevant periods involved.

4. The type of health care provider implicated and any provider billing numbers associated with the matter disclosed. Include the Federal health care programs affected, including Government contractors such as carriers, intermediaries and other third-party payers.

5. The reasons why the disclosing provider believes that a violation of Federal criminal, civil or administrative law may have occurred.

6. A certification by the health care provider or, in the case of an entity, an authorized representative on behalf of the disclosing entity stating that, to the best of the individual's knowledge, the submission contains truthful information and is based on a good faith effort to bring the matter to the Government's attention for the purpose of resolving any potential liabilities to the Government.

C. Substantive Information

As part of its participation in the disclosure process, the disclosing health care provider will be expected to conduct an internal investigation and a self-assessment, and then report its findings to the OIG. The internal review may occur after the initial disclosure of the matter. The OIG will generally agree, for a reasonable period of time, to forego an investigation of the matter if the provider agrees that it will conduct the review in accordance with the Internal Investigation Guidelines and the Self-Assessment Guidelines set forth below.

IV. Internal Investigation Guidelines

All disclosures to the OIG under the Provider Self-Disclosure Protocol should include a report based on an internal investigation conducted by the health care provider. While a provider is free to discuss its preliminary findings with the OIG prior to completion of its investigation, the matter cannot be resolved until a comprehensive assessment has been completed pursuant to the following guidelines:

A. Nature and Extent of the Improper or Illegal Practice

A voluntary disclosure report should demonstrate that a full examination of the practice has been conducted. The report should contain a written narrative that—

1. Identifies the potential causes of the incident or practice (e.g., intentional conduct, lack of internal controls, circumvention of corporate procedures or Government regulations);

2. Describes the incident or practice in detail, including how the incident or practice arose and continued;

3. Identifies the division, departments, branches or related entities involved and/or affected;

4. Identifies the impact on, and risks to, health, safety, or quality of care posed by the matter disclosed,

with sufficient information to allow the OIG to assess the immediacy of the impact and risks, the steps that should be taken to address them, as well as the measures taken by the disclosing entity;

5. Delineates the period during which the incident or practice occurred;

6. Identifies the corporate officials, employees or agents who knew of, encouraged, or participated in, the incident or practice and any individuals who may have been involved in detecting the matter;

7. Identifies the corporate officials, employees or agents who should have known of, but failed to detect, the incident or practice based on their job responsibilities; and

8. Estimates the monetary impact of the incident or practice upon the Federal health care programs, pursuant to the Self-Assessment Guidelines below.

B. Discovery and Response to the Matter

The internal investigation report should relate the circumstances under which the disclosed matter was discovered and fully document the measures taken upon discovery to address the problem and prevent future abuses. In this regard, the report should—

1. Describe how the incident or practice was identified, and the origin of the information that led to its discovery.

2. Describe the entity's efforts to investigate and document the incident or practice (e.g., use of internal or external legal, audit or consultative resources).

3. Describe in detail the chronology of the investigative steps taken in connection with the entity's internal inquiry into the disclosed matter including the following—

(a) A list of all individuals interviewed, including each individual's business address and telephone number, and their positions and titles in the relevant entities during both the relevant period and at the time the disclosure is being made. For all individuals interviewed, provide the dates of those interviews and the subject matter of each interview, as well as summaries of the interview. The health care provider will be responsible for advising the individual to be interviewed that the information the individual provides may, in turn, be provided to the OIG. Additionally, include a list of those individuals who refused to be interviewed and provide the reasons cited;

(b) A description of files, documents, and records reviewed with sufficient particularity to allow their retrieval, if necessary; and

(c) A summary of auditing activity undertaken and a summary of the documents relied upon in support of the estimation of losses. These documents and information must accompany the report, unless the calculation of losses is undertaken pursuant to the Self-Assessment Guidelines, which contain specific reporting requirements.

4. Describe the actions by the health care provider to stop the inappropriate conduct.

5. Describe any related health care businesses affected by the inappropriate conduct in which the health care provider is involved, all efforts by the health care provider to prevent a recurrence of the incident or practice in the affected division as well as in any related health care entities (e.g., new accounting or internal control procedures, increased internal audit efforts, increased supervision by higher management or through training).

6. Describe any disciplinary action taken against corporate officials, employees and agents as a result of the disclosed matter.

7. Describe appropriate notices, if applicable, provided to other Government agencies, (e.g., Securities and Exchange Commission and Internal Revenue Service) in connection with the disclosed matter.

C.

The internal investigation report must include a certification by the health care provider, or in the case of an entity an authorized representative on behalf of the disclosing health care provider, indicating that, to the best of the individual's knowledge, the internal investigation report contains truthful information and is based on a good faith effort to assist the OIG in its inquiry and verification of the disclosed matter.

V. Self-Assessment Guidelines

To estimate the monetary impact of the disclosed matter, the provider also should conduct an internal financial assessment and prepare a report of its findings. This self-assessment may be performed at the same time as the internal investigation, or commenced after the scope of the non-compliance with program requirements has been established. In either case, the OIG will verify a provider's calculation of Federal health care program losses and it is strongly recommended that, at a minimum, the review conform to the following guidelines.

A. Approach

The self-assessment should consist of a review of either—(1) all of the claims affected by the disclosed matter for the relevant period; or (2) a statistically valid sample of the claims that can be projected to the population of claims affected by the matter for the relevant period. This determination should be based on the size of the population believed to be implicated, the variance of characteristics to be reviewed, the cost of the self-assessment, the available resources, the estimated duration of the review, and other factors as appropriate.

B. Basic Information

Regardless of which of these two approaches is used, the disclosing provider should submit to the OIG a work plan describing the self-assessment process. The OIG will review the proposal and, where appropriate, provide comments on the plan in a timely manner. At its option, the OIG may choose to carry out any necessary activities at any stage of the review to verify that the process is undertaken correctly and to validate the review findings. While the OIG is not obligated to accept the results of a provider's self-assessment, findings based upon procedures which conform to the Protocol will be given substantial weight in determining any program overpayments. In addition, the OIG will use the validated provider self-assessment report in preparing a recommendation to DOJ for resolution of the provider's False Claims Act or other liability. Among the issues that should be addressed in the plan are the following—

1. Review Objective—There should be a statement clearly articulating the objective of the review and the review procedure or combination of procedures applied to achieve the objective.

2. Review Population—The plan should identify the population, which is the group about which information is needed. In addition, there should be an explanation of the methodology used to develop the population and the basis for this determination.

3. Sources of Data—The plan should provide a full description of the source of the information upon which the review will be based, including the legal or other standards to be applied, the sources of payment data and the documents that will be relied upon (e.g., employment contracts, rental agreements, etc.).

4. Personnel Qualifications—The plan should identify the names and titles of those individuals involved in any aspect of the self-assessment, including statisticians, accountants, auditors, consultants and medical reviewers, and describe their qualifications.

C. Sample Elements

If the provider, in consultation with the OIG, determines that the financial review will be based upon a sample, the work plan should also include the sampling plan as follows—

1. Sampling Unit—The plan should define the sampling unit, which is any of the designated elements that comprise the population of interest.

2. Sampling Frame—The plan should identify the sampling frame, which is the totality of the sampling units from which the sample will be selected. In addition, the plan should document how the audit population differs from the sampling frame and what effect this difference has on conclusions reached as a result of the audit.

3. Sample Size—The size of the sample must be determined through the use of a probe sample. Accordingly, the plan should include a description of both the probe sample and the full sample. At a minimum, the full sample must be designed to generate an estimate with a ninety (90) percent level of confidence and a precision of twenty-five (25) percent. The probe sample must contain at least thirty (30) sample units and cannot be used as part of the full sample.

4. Random Numbers—Both the probe sample and the sample must be selected through random numbers. The source of the random numbers used must be shown in the sampling plans. The OIG strongly recommends the use of its Office of Audit Services' Statistical Sampling Software, also known as "RAT-STATS," which is currently available free of charge through the internet at http://oig.hhs.gov/organization/OAS/ratstat.html.

5. Sample Design—Unless the disclosing provider demonstrates the need to use a different sample design, the self-assessment should use simple random sampling. If necessitated, the provider may use stratified or multistage sampling. Details about the strata, stages and clusters should be included in the description of the audit plan.

6. Estimate of Review Time per Sample Item—The plan should estimate the time expended to locate the sample items and the staff hours expended to review a sample item.

7. Characteristics Measure by the Sample—The sampling plan should identify the characteristics used for testing each sample item. For example, in a sample drawn to estimate the value of overpayments due to duplicate payments, the characteristics under consideration are the conditions that must exist for a sample item to be a duplicate. The amount of the duplicate payment is the measurement of the overpayment.

    The sampling plan must also contain the decision rules for determining whether a sample item entirely meets the criterion for having characteristics or only partially meets the criterion.

8. Missing Sample Items—The sampling plan must include a discussion of how missing sample items were handled and the rationale.

9. Other Evidence—Although sample results should stand on their own in terms of validity, sample results may be combined with other evidence in arriving at specific conclusions. If appropriate, indicate what other substantiating or corroborating evidence was developed.

10. Estimation Methodology—Because the general purpose of the review is to estimate the monetary losses to the Federal health care programs, the methodology to be used must be variables sampling using the difference estimator. To estimate the amount implicated in the disclosed matter, the provider must use the mean point estimate. The statistical estimates must be reported using a ninety (90) percent confidence level. The use of RAT-STATS to calculate the estimates is strongly recommended.

11. Reporting Results—The sampling plan should indicate how the results will be reported at the conclusion of the review. In preparing the report, enough details must be provided to clearly indicate what estimates are reported.

D. Certification

Upon completion of the self-assessment, the disclosing health care provider, or in the case of an entity its authorized representative, must submit to the OIG a certification stating that, to the best of the individual's knowledge, the report contains truthful information and is based on a good faith effort to assist OIG in its inquiry and verification of the disclosed matter.

VI. OIG's Verification

Upon receipt of a health care provider's disclosure submission, the OIG will begin its verification of the disclosure information. The extent of the OIG's verification effort will depend, in large part, upon the quality and thoroughness of the internal investigative and self-assessment reports. Matters uncovered during the verification process, which are outside of the scope of the matter disclosed to the OIG, may be treated as new matters outside the Provider Self-Disclosure Protocol.

To facilitate the OIG's verification and validation processes, the OIG must have access to all audit work papers and other supporting documents without the assertion of privileges or limitations on the information produced. In the normal course of verification, the OIG will not request production of written communications subject to the attorney-client privilege. There may be documents or other materials, however, that may be covered by the work product doctrine, but which the OIG believes are critical to resolving the disclosure. The OIG is prepared to discuss with provider's counsel ways to gain access to the underlying information without the need to waive the protections provided by an appropriately asserted claim of privilege.

VII. Payments

Because of the need to verify the information provided by a disclosing health provider, the OIG will not accept payments of presumed overpayments determined by the health care provider prior to the completion of the OIG's inquiry. However, the provider is encouraged to place the overpayment amount in an interest-bearing escrow account to minimize further losses. While the matter is under OIG inquiry, the disclosing provider must refrain from making payment relating to the disclosed matter to the Federal health care programs or their contractors without the OIG's prior consent. If the OIG consents, the disclosing provider will be required to agree in writing that the acceptance of the payment does not constitute the Government's agreement as to the amount of losses suffered by the programs as a result of the disclosed matter, and does not affect in any manner the Government's ability to pursue criminal, civil or administrative remedies or to obtain additional fines, damages or penalties for the matters disclosed.

VIII. Cooperation and Removal from the Provider Self-Disclosure Protocol

The disclosing entity's diligent and good faith cooperation throughout the entire process is essential. Accordingly, the OIG expects to receive documents and information from the entity that relate to the disclosed matter without the need to resort to compulsory methods.

If a provider fails to work in good faith with the OIG to resolve the disclosed matter, that lack of cooperation will be considered an aggravating factor when the OIG assesses the appropriate resolution of the matter. Similarly, the intentional submission of false or otherwise untruthful information, as well as the intentional omission of relevant information, will be referred to DOJ or other Federal agencies and could, in itself, result in criminal and/or civil sanctions, as well as exclusion from participation in the Federal health care programs.

Dated: October 21, 1998.
June Gibbs Brown,
Inspector General.

Cooperation With Investigations

Medical practices should adopt a policy that all physicians, support staff, and others are expected to cooperate in any investigation conducted by government enforcement agencies. Similarly, cooperation should be required for internal investigations whether conducted by the practice's staff or an outside firm.

It should be expressly stated that it is considered a violation of the compliance plan to hide, alter, destroy, or otherwise modify or withhold documents subject to an investigation.

If anyone is approached by a government enforcement agency, or receives a request for information or subpoena as part of an investigation, he or she should *immediately* report the matter to the compliance officer. Such investigations should be coordinated by the practice's attorney.

Similarly, physicians and staff should be required to report to the compliance officer instances in which they are approached by any individual, known or unknown, who asks compliance-related questions. Employees should be told that if the medical practice conducts an investigation to assess a compliance concern or the success of compliance efforts, they will be formally introduced to any outside auditors.

Endnotes

1. Often physicians are in the best position to designate what services were provided and what diagnoses apply. Ideally, physicians would select CPT® and ICD-9 codes from superbills or encounter forms that are easy to use. Adequate training should be provided to simplify this activity.

    Those health care organizations that rely on coding staff to sift through operative notes and other medical records to select billing codes are asking for problems (and it is terribly inefficient). However, if physicians are too resistant to assuming the selection of CPT® and/or ICD-9 codes, designate a special place in the medical records where physicians record a narrative description of the procedures performed (ie, a description useful in helping staff select CPT® codes) and the reasons for the services performed (ie, information useful in aiding staff in selecting ICD-9 diagnosis codes). Physicians should be trained to become somewhat familiar with CPT® and ICD-9 terminology so that they can dictate descriptions that facilitate code selection by coding staff.

2. This document would be shared with OIG or FBI to demonstrate compliance efforts if necessary.

3. To prevent any compliance documents, including the code of conduct, from being characterized by a prosecutor or a plaintiff as a minimum standard maintained by an organization, be sure to include explicit language stating that the compliance program and code of conduct are intended to exceed the minimum standards of the law.

4. Some organizations may incorporate these aspects of compliance along with other areas, such as sexual harassment, the Americans with Disabilities Act, equal employment opportunity laws, etc.

5. If the organization has a compliance committee, reports should be provided depending on the frequency of meetings. The committee should make periodic reports to the governing body.

6. To ensure that all compliance incident reports are addressed, the compliance officer should maintain a special list of incident reports that have not been resolved.

7. The OIG recognizes that smaller physician practices may not be able to establish a compliance committee. In those situations, the compliance officer should fulfill the responsibilities of the compliance committee.

8. The compliance committee benefits from having the perspectives of individuals with varying responsibilities in the organization, such as operations, finance, audit, human resources, utilization review, medicine, coding, and legal, as well as employees and managers of key operating units. These individuals should have the requisite seniority and comprehensive experience within their respective departments to implement any necessary changes in the company's policies and procedures.

14

Compliance Efforts in Smaller Medical Practices

Medical practices are well advised to implement a formal compliance program, as discussed in the previous chapter. Obviously, a smaller practice would not have as extensive a plan as a larger practice, but the plans would be similar in that they both must address all of the elements of an effective compliance plan.

Since the primary goal of these formal plans is to ensure compliance, practices should adopt efforts that help them accomplish this goal.

Some suggestions for improving compliance follow (also see Appendix C, the *OIG Compliance Program Guidance for Individual and Small Group Physician Practices*).

Suggestions for Improving Compliance

The suggestions in this section were compiled by consultants experienced in medical office practices.

- Physicians should select CPT® codes from a carefully designed superbill or encounter form (do not limit your selection of office visit codes to certain levels). You should select ICD-9 codes as well; however, it is relatively easy for staff to find appropriate codes if you are careful to include narrative diagnostic information in a designated place in the medical record.

- Learn the coding and billing rules applicable to the services your practice provides.

- Be aware of any differences with respect to billing guidelines among Medicare, Medicaid, and nongovernmental payers.

- Understand the types of fraud or abuse that could occur in your practice or other associated health care organizations (do not overlook antikickback laws, prohibitions on self-referrals, and the like).

- Be cautious if someone offers you "special" discounts, free (or less than market value) services, cash, etc, to make referrals or order services.

- Make sure to read every bulletin published by your Medicare carrier and other payers. Learn their publication schedule—monthly, every 2 months, quarterly, etc. If you miss one, make sure you request a copy. Collect all articles or notices related to your services. Make sure you are in compliance. Check Internet sites for carrier newsletters. There is a new site—www.lmrp.net—that HCFA is planning to update quarterly with local medical review policies from carriers nationwide.

- Managed care plans typically have what they call a *provider manual*. Make sure you obtain, read, understand, and update these manuals. Periodically, make sure you are complying with each manual's requirements.

- Perform self-audits as discussed earlier in this book by periodically comparing a sample of billing claim forms to documentation in your medical records. Make sure the documentation supports the CPT® and ICD-9 codes billed. Make sure the codes billed on claim forms correspond to those physicians checked on superbills or encounter forms.

  There are numerous audit tips in other sections of this book. Here are a few more ideas:

- Actual copies or overheads of insufficient documentation or incorrect code selection make good teaching tools. One can sit down with those involved, show what was billed or documented, and then show what should have been billed.

- Sometimes, it is advisable to select a random sample from a specific category of services rather than simply relying on a sample from *all* services. For example, if a Medicare carrier just published documentation requirements for billing an encounter *incident to* a physician's service where a patient sees a Physician Assistant (PA), it's a good idea to select at least 30 charts for a few quarters to see if documentation meets those guidelines. Again, if documentation is lacking, develop a corrective action plan and monitor it until you are sure it is working.

- Be sure to include hospital, emergency department, nursing home, etc, records in your internal audits. It used to be that Medicare carriers would write a letter to a physician's office asking them to submit 15 or so designated charts for review. Increasingly, carriers are sending auditors into hospitals and nursing homes to review records. In these cases, physicians don't know an audit occurred until they receive an overpayment request. The point is, make sure documentation in hospitals, emergency departments, nursing homes, etc, meets the requirements.

- A report available from most practice management computer systems—*CPT®
  Productivity/Frequency Report by Physician Specialty*—is an invaluable tool for spotting
  potential coding problems. Similarly, review Explanations of Benefits looking for
  denials, requests for additional information, unusual coding patterns, etc. Also, look
  at claims (or parts of claims) that were written-off. Check correspondence sent to
  payers in response to a request for additional information. Talk to coding staff.
  Stay involved.

- Take advantage of the information available on the Internet—www.lmrp.net;
  www.hcfa.gov/medlearn; www.oig.hhs.gov; your carrier's Web site; etc.

- Look at a sample explanation of benefits. Where claims were denied for insufficient
  information or otherwise, look at how your staff followed up on the denial. If the
  claim was eventually paid, was the additional information provided to the payer
  consistent with medical record documentation? If the claim was not followed up,
  you may need to reevaluate your billing and collection system. In fact, one effective
  review technique is to thumb through several weeks' worth of explanations of benefits to spot unusual trends, denials, unfamiliar codes, and other unusual items.

- If possible, get an outside firm to review the appropriateness of your billing operations and other arrangements covered by fraud and abuse laws.

- Discuss with your attorney, accountant, and/or management consultant any ideas
  they may have to improve your compliance efforts.

- In adding a new physician or employee to your practice, discuss compliance issues. If
  you are merging with other physicians or buying a practice, perform a compliance
  audit before you establish terms of the merger or purchase. Make sure the purchase
  or merger agreement addresses how recoupments for services rendered prior to the
  purchase or merger will be handled.

- If you are entering an established practice, it is a good idea to discuss their compliance philosophy, programs, and efforts.

- If you are referring patients to entities with which you have an interest, make sure
  you are not violating federal or state self-referral laws.

- Get a copy of Medicare's *Correct Coding Initiative*, read it, and keep it up to date (the
  coding edits are updated quarterly).

- Watch specialty society publications that may discuss audit targets or coding issues
  in your specialty.

- If you have a good practice management computer system, produce a monthly CPT®
  and ICD-9 code utilization report by physician. This report will show how many
  evaluation and management services at various levels, surgical procedures, and other
  services were billed. Also, look at the frequency of modifiers such as -25.

  Look for patterns that are not easily explained. If you are in a group, compare your
  utilization to others of a similar specialty. Investigate any discrepancies. Do not easily succumb to the "my patients are sicker" syndrome if you appear at the upper end
  of utilization reports.

- Talk with your colleagues in other parts of the country to determine if they are aware of anything you need to monitor.

- Keep a file of billing disputes and inquiries. Periodically, review this file to ensure that the inquiries were handled appropriately. Make sure that your staff treats all patient complaints seriously. Dissatisfied patients can certainly complain to Medicare carriers or to managed care plans, or even call one of the attorneys who advertise in the newspaper for those who may have been a victim of health care fraud.

- Question anything that looks suspicious. For example, if you start receiving lab reports that include tests you did not order, investigate the circumstances. Sometimes, labs will add tests to "profiles" that may not have been ordered by the physician.

- Do not erase or obliterate entries in the medical record. If it is necessary to make a change, line through any incorrect portion so that the original entry can be read, and write in the correct entry. Date the corrected entry on the date the correction is made. Initial the correction.

- Make sure that you have established a system to safeguard records. In the event of an audit, it is very difficult and highly suspicious to substantiate services if you cannot locate records.

- Provide everyone in your practice a written code of conduct statement that outlines your commitment to compliance. Encourage employees to bring to your attention any concerns they have. The statement should clearly indicate that appropriate disciplinary action will be taken for those who knowingly participate in fraudulent or abusive billing activities, or for those who are in a position responsible for detecting potential misconduct.

- Make sure the code of conduct and the practice's compliance activities are discussed during orientation programs for new employees.

- Hold periodic meetings with your staff to discuss compliance issues and concerns. Ask participants to relate any unusual billing activities that may have occurred since your last meeting, such as denials, requests for additional information, a payer changing the code(s) you billed, payments greater than expected, or duplicate payments. Go over Medicare and other payers' bulletins with respect to billing guidelines impacting your practice. Do not keep putting off these meetings.

- When there is an action to be taken, specifically assign the responsibility to someone. Otherwise, things may not get done because people think someone else is responsible or will handle the activity. Follow up to make sure critical activities are performed.

- Be careful to avoid jokes or other actions that an employee could misinterpret as a lack of commitment to compliance or an inducement to commit fraud or abuse or to tamper with records to conceal misconduct.

- Perform an adequate background check on all potential employees, including checking the OIG Web site www.oig.hhs.gov/fraud/exclusions/listofexcluded.html. Where possible, it is also advisable to perform background checks on companies that your practice uses for billing, computer maintenance, collections, practice management, and the like.

- Keep provider identification numbers as confidential as possible.

- You should inform your Medicare carrier and other payers if you close your practice, move, etc. This will help prevent someone else from using your identification numbers.

- If you have a "problem" employee—one who is in a position to commit fraudulent or abusive activities, destroy or alter records, and the like—you should carefully consider whether you should discipline, terminate, transfer, or take other appropriate action. A problem employee is a "ticking time bomb," who may manufacture fraudulent situations, file frivolous suits, or make frivolous accusations when he or she is finally disciplined. The point is, do not delay taking appropriate action with respect to a problem employee. Within the constraints of proper employee management considerations, do not leave a disgruntled employee in a position where he or she could perpetrate fraudulent activity.

- Make sure employees know that their participation in fraudulent or abusive activities may be grounds for discipline, including immediate dismissal.

- If you have to terminate an employee, it may be a good idea to ask the person to leave immediately on notification if he or she is in a position to sabotage records or take other inappropriate actions related to billing functions. You might also discuss with your attorney what can be done should an employee threaten a frivolous suit or other action.

- Try to be consistent in the way you handle employee concerns about potentially fraudulent or abusive actions. Investigate them, take appropriate corrective action, and communicate the results to the employee who identified the concern. The point here is that you should demonstrate through your actions that you will take appropriate steps to resolve issues brought to your attention.

- Make sure your staff attends as many training sessions as possible. They probably cannot attend too many. Physicians should try to attend these as well.

- Make sure you monitor your billing service if you use one. Ask them to identify the compliance efforts they take. Do they have an effective compliance program and are they adhering to it? Ask for a copy of their plan. Are you comfortable that they are knowledgeable with respect to compliance issues? Make it clear that you want them to tell you of any concerns they have. Saving on a billing service's charges is not worthwhile if the savings come from scrimping on training, hiring inexperienced staff, or improperly coding claims to get them through a payer's computer edits. Consider audit procedures just like those you would perform if billing were performed by your staff.

  You may even want to perform a periodic audit of their billing activities. In fact, you should look at a billing service just as you would if the activities were performed by your staff.

- Make sure you keep originals of all records and that your billing company provides you with EOBs and other billing documents. Billing companies are a valuable service to many physicians, but every consultant can recite horror stories of a billing service going out of business after the illness of a principal or due to financial or other problems. Sometimes physicians lose most of what they need to collect receivables, or contest unfavorable audit results.

- If you are subjected to an investigation, call your attorney. Do not say anything to your employees that could be construed as obstructing justice.

- Review all requests for records or supporting documentation from payers or enforcement agencies before they leave your office. Make sure the records support the services billed. If not, see if there are other relevant facts in the patient's chart that should be forwarded with notes for the requested date of service.

- Do not routinely waive insurance copayments or deductibles.

- Look back at Chapter 9 on how to minimize the risk of an audit.

- Read the *OIG Compliance Program Guidance for Individual and Small Group Physician Practices* and watch for release of the final guidance.

Policy Statement Illustration

The next pages provide an illustration of a letter to employees—including physicians—and a fraud and abuse policy statement for smaller medical groups. It is important to develop (and abide by) a philosophy statement that serves as the foundation for an effective compliance program. Many other activities are part of a compliance program, but this will provide a start toward implementing an effective plan. Again, please realize that a partially implemented plan is not a compliance program.

The illustration assumes that the letter and policy statement are presented at a series of meetings to cover all employees. Also, it assumes that supervisors and managers were presented the details of the compliance program earlier so that they can talk further with employees about the details.

Physicians who choose to adopt this illustration in their practice will have to modify it to apply to their specific situation. They also will need to have it reviewed by their attorney to ensure that it does not conflict with other policies in their group, state laws, and the like, and that it is, in all respects, appropriate for their purposes. They will need to implement the other components of a compliance plan as discussed in the previous chapter.

Remember, the items illustrated do not approach the intensity of the formal compliance program guidances released by the government. These actions do not guarantee leniency in the event of an investigation. The examples are designed to reflect relatively simply actions a small medical practice can take to help avoid compliance violations. Physicians should discuss the need for other actions with their attorney and practice advisors.

Illustration: Sample Introductory Letter

Trout Valley Medical
1000 Riverside Dr.
June 30, 1997

Dear Employees:

I am sure all of you have seen media reports regarding health care fraud and abuse. Some health care organizations have seriously compromised their ability to survive because they have not taken appropriate efforts to ensure compliance. Our practice has a commitment to our patients and employees which mandates that we take every reasonable effort to ensure that we are in compliance with all applicable local, state, and federal laws, including fraud and abuse laws.

While we believe our record clearly indicates we have always complied with the many and complex fraud and abuse laws, Trout Valley's Board of Directors has taken another step to enhance our ongoing efforts to ensure compliance in the future. On June 22, 1997, we adopted a formal Fraud and Abuse Compliance Plan to prevent problems from occurring. To prevent problems or in the event a problem does occur, the Compliance Program is designed to identify the issue and set into motion a series of corrective actions.

As part of this program, the Board of Directors established a Fraud and Abuse Compliance Committee. Members of the Committee include myself (as Compliance Officer and chairperson), Dr Parsons, Dr White, Mrs York (Group Administrator), Mr Byrd (Billing Office Director) and our attorney, Mr Clark. We have also charged Mrs York with specific responsibilities related to compliance issues. Dr Parsons has agreed to work with Mrs York on compliance-related matters. We have sought the assistance of our attorney and practice management consultants.

We have adopted the attached Policy Statement. While we realize that this policy statement may be perceived by some employees as heavy-handed, it is for all of our benefit. Today, no medical group can afford not to take every reasonable effort to ensure compliance with fraud and abuse laws. We have a commitment to our patients and our employees **that** requires us to maintain a strong, viable medical practice. We can only do this if we all work together to ensure that we comply with laws related to fraud and abuse, no matter how complex the rules may be, and no matter how difficult it is. You will be asked to sign a form that indicates you read, understand, and agree to comply with the Code of Conduct and the Compliance Plan.

As you will see, a cornerstone of our compliance efforts is that we encourage you to report any compliance concerns you may have. The Policy describes a reporting system that should allow one to communicate any concerns they may have. Please be assured that we will not take any disciplinary action against anyone solely because they submit a compliance concern. We need your input and we have to work together.

We will be performing an intense audit of our current billing practices and other activities. Part of that audit will include interviews with employees—including physicians—who have jobs with duties and responsibilities that could impact our compliance efforts. Mrs York will notify you if you are scheduled for one of these interviews. If not scheduled, you may request an interview if desired by contacting Mrs York or another member of the Compliance Committee. Please be assured that your comments will be kept confidential.

Should you have any questions regarding the compliance program, you may talk directly to Mrs York, Dr Parsons, or me. You may also raise any questions at any time, including staff meetings.

I think most of you will see the benefit of and welcome implementation of this program. It will ensure the viability of our practice so that we continue our mission to provide quality medical services to our patients. We appreciate your continued efforts in ensuring that we comply with applicable federal and state law, and the program requirements of federal, state, and private health care plans.

Sincerely,
Roger M. Crosby, MD

Illustration: Sample Policy Statement

Policy Statement
Fraud and Abuse Compliance Program
Adopted June 22, 1997

Trout Valley Medical Group has been, and continues to be, committed to creating an environment which ensures full compliance with all federal, state, and local laws. Implementation of Trout Valley's formal Fraud and Abuse Compliance Program is another step we are taking to achieve this goal. In the event an instance of noncompliance should still occur, the program is designed to detect and correct it in a timely manner.

Trout Valley Medical Group will conduct periodic audits—including employee interviews—to ensure ongoing compliance. Should any instance of noncompliance be identified through audits, or our employee reporting program discussed below, a corrective action plan will be developed to resolve the issue in a timely manner. We will continue to perform periodic reassessments to ensure ongoing compliance.

A cornerstone of Trout Valley's compliance efforts is that we encourage and demand that all compliance issues be raised, investigated, and promptly resolved. When reported as instructed below, concerns will be investigated in a timely manner. If desired, those reporting compliance concerns will receive a report of any investigation and corrective action. Trout Valley Medical Group will not take any disciplinary action against anyone solely because they have submitted a Compliance Incident Report or otherwise expressed a concern.

Any employee or member of Trout Valley Medical Group who participates in an activity that does not comply with federal and state laws or special payer guidelines may be subject to disciplinary action, including termination from employment. Appropriate disciplinary action will depend upon: (a) the nature of the activity; (b) whether the employee could reasonably be expected to identify the activity as noncompliant; (c) whether the employee was in a position to take appropriate corrective action; and/or (d) whether the employee was unduly influenced to participate in the activity. As a general rule, we believe there are adequate mechanisms for reporting a suspected noncompliant activity that (c) and (d) will seldom, if ever, apply.

Trout Valley is also committed to ensuring that all physicians and employees receive training appropriate for their job duties and responsibilities. Departmental supervisors are responsible for ensuring that employees receive appropriate training, including training related to Trout Valley's Fraud and Abuse Compliance Program.

The Compliance Program adopted by the Board of Directors requires your supervisor to report any employee's compliance concerns directly to the Compliance Officer, the Chairperson of Trout Valley's Compliance Committee—currently Dr Crosby—regardless of whether your supervisor believes the concern has merit. If, however, you are not comfortable submitting a report directly to your supervisor, you may communicate your concern verbally or in writing to Dr Crosby. Should you wish to remain anonymous you may send your concern in writing to Dr Crosby, Trout Valley Medical Group, 1000 Riverside Drive. Mark the envelope Confidential. Alternatively, you may submit any concerns through the Compliance Drop Box located in the break area.

Should you not be comfortable reporting your concern to your supervisor or Dr Crosby, you may communicate your concern verbally or in writing to Trout Valley's attorney—Mr Gene Clark. His telephone number is 999 456-7890. His address is 985 Sunset Boulevard. You may communicate your concern anonymously if you wish.

All employees, including management and physicians, receive Performance Evaluations at designated intervals. These Performance Evaluations will include assessment of each employee's successes and failures with respect to their duties and responsibilities under our compliance program.

Should you have any questions regarding this Policy Statement, you may talk directly with your supervisor or Dr Crosby. You may also raise any questions at monthly employee meetings.

Actions of the Office of Inspector General

Below are additional examples of criminal and civil actions cited in reports published by the Office of Inspector General (OIG), Department of Health and Human Services, for the period March 1995 through March 2002. Again, these pages do not provide examples or descriptions of all types of fraudulent or abusive behavior, nor do they provide examples of more prevalent repayment requests from audits by Medicare carriers.

- A cardiologist was fined about $80,000 and ordered to make repayments for echocardiography billed as if he performed both the technical and professional component when, in fact, he had not.

- The successor entity of a physician partnership, which primarily provided medical services to nursing home patients, agreed to pay $1.4 million for allegedly submitting false claims to Medicare. The successor entity also agreed to comply with a 5-year corporate integrity agreement.

- A physician was sentenced to 18 months and fined $40,000 **for accepting about $50,000 in kickbacks** over a two-year period for referring patients to an area cardiologist. [boldface added]

- A physician was sentenced to 5 years probation, ten months home confinement, and ordered to make restitution of $117,900 for billing acupuncture performed by an acupuncturist next door. **The osteopath used physical therapy codes because acupuncture is not a covered service under Medicare.** The osteopath also had to surrender his medical license. (In a similar case, a physician was convicted for billing acupuncture using neuromuscular testing and treatment codes.) [boldface added]

- The operator of a medical center, a receptionist, two patient "recruiters," and a physician were sentenced and ordered to pay restitution for procuring seniors to the center for a battery of tests billable to Medicare/caid. Although tests were deemed needed, the physician signed charts without seeing the patients. The "recruiters" were paid $30 to $150 per patient they attracted.

- A cardiologist agreed to pay the government $1.5 million to settle allegations of submitting false claims to Medicare. A *qui tam* suit initiated this investigation into the billing practices of the medical practice and the cardiologist. Based on a review by the carrier, a peer review organization nurse and an independent expert cardiologist, the government found that between 1993 and 1998, the practice submitted, or caused to be submitted, improper Medicare claims for services provided to patients by the cardiologist. The claims contained numerous instances of upcoding for evaluation and management services; of double billing for certain services; and of billing medically unnecessary cardiology-related tests, procedures, and office visits. In addition, the medical practice also agreed to enter into a 6-year comprehensive corporate integrity agreement.

- A mental health practice agreed to pay the government $850,000 to settle allegations of improper billing practices. From 1995 through 1999, the mental health practice used medical codes that improperly characterized services as being incident to services provided by a psychiatrist. The practice also used inappropriate medical codes in order to receive a higher rate of reimbursement. Finally, the practice failed to use a modifier to indicate that services were rendered by a social worker and should, therefore, be paid at the rate appropriate for that type of provider. As part of the settlement, the practice also entered into a corporate integrity agreement with OIG.

- An operator of physician clinics agreed to pay the government $344,764 to settle allegations of submitting false claims to Medicare. The entity employed physicians, physician's assistants, and nurse practitioners to visit patients in various nursing homes. Through an internal audit, the clinic operator determined that the services of the nurse practitioners and physician's assistants were inappropriately billed under a physician's provider number. This improper billing practice led the clinic operator to receive higher reimbursement from Medicare than it should have. Moreover, the conduct violated Medicare's "incident to" billing rules requiring, in part, the direct supervision of physicians when services are provided by nonphysician personnel. As part of the settlement agreement, the clinic operator entered into a 5-year corporate integrity agreement with OIG.

- A northern school of medicine agreed to pay the government approximately $2.3 million to resolve allegations of improperly billing Medicare. The school obtained excess Medicare funds based on claims for professional services rendered to Medicare beneficiaries that were not documented or not in compliance with Medicare's coding and reimbursement rules. As part of the settlement, the school entered into a 5-year, institutional compliance agreement requiring the facility to maintain a compliance committee and to perform an annual review of its billing for professional services.

- A physician, who had been excluded for 10 years, settled his liability under the CMPL, by paying $30,000. The physician had submitted claims to the Medicare program while excluded from program participation.

- A Midwestern hospital and an entity supplying physicians and billing services for those physicians' services at the hospital, agreed to pay the government $330,000 to settle a False Claims Act lawsuit against them. The government alleged that the defendants improperly billed 200 specific Medicaid claims for prenatal and newborn delivery services by misidentifying the provider of the service. The government also alleged that unsupervised residents, interns, and/or nurses actually provided these services. The defendants improperly billed these services under the individual provider number of an attending physician of the month, whether or not he or she actually provided the service. In addition to the total settlement amount, OIG also imposed comprehensive, 5-year corporate integrity agreements on both defendants.

- The government entered into a settlement agreement with a clinical laboratory, a physician, and another individual to resolve allegations that the laboratory submitted false claims to Medicare. As part of the settlement, the laboratory agreed to pay $1.2 million to resolve its civil and administrative liabilities for the improper conduct and to enter into a comprehensive, 5-year corporate integrity agreement with OIG. The clinical laboratory allegedly submitted false claims by billing for tests to identify a certain bacteria after a preliminary test showed no bacteria present and by unbundling certain urinalysis tests. The physician involved in the settlement owns the laboratory, and the other individual was the laboratory manager during the time period at issue.

- The United States entered into a global settlement with a large provider of kidney dialysis services and several of its subsidiaries, in which the provider agreed to pay approximately $486 million to settle allegations from a multi *qui tam* investigation. As part of the civil settlement agreement for credit balances, the company paid directly to CMS/HCFA $11 million for overpayments, which were previously reported to the FIs but never recouped. The allegations included the following: billing of unnecessary end stage renal disease (ESRD) laboratory tests and the paying of kickbacks to induce the ordering of such unnecessary tests; billing for noncovered intradialytic parenteral nutrition (IDPN) services, falsifying documents to obtain payment, and the paying of kickbacks in the form of "hang fees" and other forms of remuneration to induce the ordering of unnecessary IDPN services; failing to report "credit balances" and/or "unreconciled payments" and/or converting such monies to income rather than returning the monies to the federal health care programs; and billing for certain unnecessary diagnostic tests performed under clinical studies. As part of the settlement agreement, the provider agreed to adhere to an 8-year corporate integrity agreement. In addition, three of its subsidiaries pled guilty to criminal offenses, and agreed to permanent exclusion from the federal health care programs. This settlement represents the largest Medicare fraud settlement ever reached and is the result of a joint effort by OIG investigators and auditors along with other law enforcement agencies. There was also an agreement to resolve a large volume of IDPN claims through the end of 1999. In exchange for the provider surrendering its right to seek payment and pursue appeals for these 33 claims (which the provider asserted were worth about $196 million), HCFA agreed to pay or "credit" the provider about $59 million.

- A licensed physician was sentenced in a northern state to 4 months imprisonment, 4 months home confinement, 4 years supervised probation, and payment of $10,200 in fines. He also forfeited $60,000 to the government. From May 1995 through December 1997, the physician solicited and received kickbacks in exchange for patient referrals for DME. Through this illegal kickback scheme, he received approximately $78,130 in payments, which he failed to report as income on his 1995 tax return.

- An ophthalmologist was sentenced to 10 years and ordered to make restitution of $16.2 million on 132 counts of **mail fraud, false statements, false claims, and illegal money transfers**. The head of the ophthalmologist's "community relations staff" was paid a bonus for each patient undergoing cataract surgery after eye screening at nursing homes and senior centers. Reportedly, the ophthalmologist made false statements in patients' medical records to "justify" cataract, eyelid, laser, and other procedures. [boldface added]

- A 50-bed psychiatric hospital agreed to pay over $550,000 to settle allegations it filed false Medicaid claims as a result of a joint investigation [federal and state]. The hospital inflated the time its psychiatrists spent with patients by 35 to 60 minutes. The hospital also allegedly billed for some psychiatric services that were never delivered. Under the settlement, the companies also entered into an agreement to assure proper Medicaid training of employees and to audit all Medicaid billings for the next 5 years.

- A physician agreed to pay $300,000 in civil damages and penalties for defrauding Medicare, Medicaid, CHAMPUS, and the Railroad Retirement Board. **The physician billed for laboratory services that were unnecessary or not performed, and double-billed by fragmenting and unbundling services.** He was convicted earlier of Medicaid fraud in state court and pled guilty to mail fraud and money laundering in federal court. In the plea, he agreed to cooperate with the government in exchange for dismissal of charges under pretrial agreements against his corporation and his sister, a corporation employee. [boldface added]

- A physician and three others were sentenced following guilty pleas to health care fraud, mail fraud, and conspiracy. The physician was sentenced to 35 months imprisonment, 3 years probation, and payment of $470,710 in restitution. One individual was sentenced to 6 months home detention, 5 years probation, and payment of $30,000 in restitution. The second individual was sentenced to 10 months home detention, 5 years probation, and payment of $30,000 in restitution; and the third was sentenced to 5 years probation, 500 hours of community service, and payment of $10,000 in restitution. The defendants were owners and operators of clinics. The clinics provided noncovered services such as acupuncture, nutrition counseling, and massage therapy but billed Medicare and other insurers for physician office visits.

- A psychiatrist and his wife paid a $500,000 settlement for defrauding Medicare and Medicaid of $300,000 by billing for more therapy units than provided to beneficiaries, billing for unsupervised treatments, and billing for therapy not provided. The psychiatrist also attempted to dispose of records to prevent the government from seizing them.

- Two podiatrists were fined for **billing "excisions" when, in fact, they only performed routine foot care,** which is not covered by Medicare.[1] [boldface added]

- An OB/GYN agreed to pay $98,000 to settle allegations of false claims filed with Medicare and other government programs for Pap smears not provided, routine OB care billed as *emergency* visits, some services that had already been paid to the hospital, and services to his parents (services to relatives are not reimbursable under Medicare).

- A physician agreed to pay $43,700 for Medicare claims filed under his provider number, but performed by an unlicensed physical therapist. The therapist received 80% of reimbursements, the physician retained 20%. The physician also surrendered his license.

- The owner of a rehabilitation and wellness clinic was sentenced to 24 months confinement and payment of $186,622 in restitution. A registered nurse employed by the clinic was also sentenced to 21 months confinement and payment of $124,000 in restitution. The defendants defrauded Medicare and Medicaid by billing physical therapy and psychological services provided by unsupervised, unlicensed clinic employees as though directly supervised by a physician. To perpetrate the scheme, the defendants used a physician's signature stamp and photocopies of a physician's signature on patient evaluation and prescription forms.

- In the Midwest, a mental health center agreed to pay the government $106,574 to resolve allegations of paying kickbacks to a psychiatric clinic in order to induce Medicaid, psychiatric, inpatient referrals to the center. The government alleged that between 1987 and 1993, the center paid over $2,000 a month as a charitable contribution to a nonprofit entity, which was in turn paid over to an outpatient mental health facility. These payments were allegedly made to induce the referral of Medicaid patients from this facility to the center. The center is no longer enrolled as a Medicaid provider, and the individuals involved are no longer associated with the center.

- In a southern state, an individual was sentenced to 2 years probation, a $2,000 fine, and payment of $863 in back taxes to the Internal Revenue Service for failure to file an individual income tax return for 1994. He is the fifteenth individual sentenced in connection with an investigation involving numerous impotence clinics in the state that allegedly billed Medicare and CHAMPUS (now TRICARE) for medically unnecessary services. The investigation determined that numerous individuals, owning numerous diagnostic companies, paid illegal kickbacks to the owners of these impotence clinics during 1994 and 1995. At that time, the individual sentenced worked as a salesman for a diagnostic company owner. As part of his duties, the individual paid kickbacks to impotence clinic owners in exchange for Medicare patient referrals.

- The owner/operator of a medical staffing agency was excluded from program participation for 3 years. The individual fraudulently created and altered background check reports to show clear criminal records for employees contracted out by his agency. He was also forging nursing and certified nursing assistant licenses. He pled guilty to one count of second-degree forgery, was sentenced to 2 years probation, and ordered to pay restitution in the amount of $25,000.

- A diagnostic services clinic in a southern state was excluded for 20 years due to its ownership by an individual convicted of money laundering. The entity was involved in a scheme to create 11 clinics and bill for nonrendered services for current and former Medicaid recipients, both living and deceased. The fraudulent claims falsely identified names and provider numbers of physicians who were not affiliated with the clinics. This resulted in a combined loss to the Medicaid program in excess of $900,000. The convicted individual was sentenced to 45 months incarceration and ordered to pay restitution and fines of close to $800,000, and excluded by OIG for 20 years.

- A physician was excluded indefinitely because her license to practice medicine or provide health care in that state was suspended for reasons bearing on her professional competence. The physician prescribed drugs to her family and failed to keep any medical records regarding those treatments.

- A physician was sentenced to payment of $39,560 in restitution, $50,100 in fines, and 3 years supervised probation for mail fraud. According to the terms of his probation, the physician cannot engage in, or associate in any way with, the practice of medicine for a period of 3 years. The physician submitted false claims to Medicare for services not rendered and double billed workers' compensation and private insurance companies for the same services rendered to the same patients. Previously, he entered into a civil settlement in which he agreed to pay $700,000 and to be excluded for a period of 5 years. The physician also resigned from employment at a local hospital.

- A physician's medical billing clerk was sentenced to 5 months imprisonment and 2 years probation for submitting false claims to a private health insurance company. The billing clerk previously pled guilty to health care fraud. In addition to her prison sentence, the judge ordered her to pay $88,922 in restitution to the private insurer.

- As the result of an OIG investigation and audit, one of the largest operators of hospitals in rural areas and small cities agreed to pay the government $31.8 million for allegedly submitting false claims to Medicare, Medicaid, and TRICARE. The nationwide settlement resolved allegations of upcoding diagnostic codes for inpatient hospital discharges through which the company received increased reimbursement amounts at 36 of its hospitals. The OIG investigation revealed that the company initiated an aggressive coding procedure referred to as the optimization program. The program encouraged the chain's hospitals to meet very high, and often unrealistic, coding volume goals, which led to excessive rates of reimbursement by

Medicare, Medicaid, and TRICARE. The investigation further determined that the inappropriate coding occurred based on improper guidance and instruction provided by officials from the company's headquarters. As part of the settlement, the company also entered into a corporate integrity agreement with OIG.

- A physician was excluded from program participation for a minimum of 10 years after pleading guilty to two charges of mail fraud. The physician submitted claims to Medicare and Medicaid for psychiatric services that were not provided. The court placed the physician on supervised probation for 4 years and home confinement for 1 year. The individual was also ordered to pay fines and restitution totaling $500,200.

- Between October 1, 1999, and March 31, 2000, OIG collected $643,500 in settlement amounts from 24 hospitals and physicians. The following is a sampling of the alleged violations involved in the FY 2000 Patient Anti-Dumping Statute settlements from this reporting period. A small Midwestern psychiatric hospital paid $30,000 to settle allegations that it failed to provide appropriate medical screenings and transfers for two patients. One of the patients had a clear emergency medical condition, but was not screened or treated because he was not able to come up with a $2,000 down payment for medical services. A small hospital settled allegations that it failed to provide appropriate medical screening examinations in a number of cases where only the patients' vital signs were taken before they were discharged. The patients' primary care providers had been called for payment authorization, and such authorization was denied. One patient had been kicked in the face and presented with jaw pain, missing teeth, and bleeding; another patient was having difficulty breathing and sleeping, and had been vomiting. The hospital settled for $60,000.

- After a hearing, an administrative law judge imposed a $25,000 CMP on a hospital that refused to accept the appropriate transfer of a patient who had been critically injured in an automobile accident and required emergency vascular surgery. The transferring hospital did not have the specialized capabilities or facilities that were required to treat the life-threatening injury to the patient's abdominal aorta. After numerous calls to hospital emergency rooms and physicians, the patient was transferred to a hospital where surgery was performed in an attempt to save his life. The patient, however, died from his injuries and their aftereffects. The Oklahoma hospital has filed an appeal with the Departmental Appeals Board.

- An academic medical center that employs physician faculty to supervise medical residents and interns agreed to pay to the United States $1.5 million to resolve its civil liability. The claims alleged that the physicians failed to appropriately document their presence during the provision of professional services by residents. The entity also submitted claims for physician services when physicians were not present. In addition, the entity submitted claims for upcoded services. As part of the settlement agreement, the entity entered into a 5-year corporate integrity agreement.

- In order to resolve allegations that it failed to provide appropriate medical screenings for several individuals, a western hospital paid $67,000 in penalties. In one case, a patient was asked to pay for services prior to being treated. In others, managed care companies denied payment authorization and/or patients were instructed to see their doctors or go to a clinic instead of being seen at the hospital. Patients presented to the hospital with conditions including multiple dog bites and pneumonia.

- A small hospital settled an allegation that it failed to provide a 1-year-old patient a medical screening examination by paying $15,000. The infant presented with a high fever and earache, and exhibited extreme discomfort when held. Two days later she was diagnosed at another hospital with bacterial meningitis. She is permanently deaf.

- An emergency physician agreed to pay $6,000 as he allegedly inappropriately transferred a patient with a suspected intercranial bleed. Although the physician provided the patient with a screening examination after being informed the patient's MCO had denied treatment, the patient was nonetheless inappropriately transferred in an unstable condition.

- A southern hospital settled, for $35,000, an allegation that it failed to medically screen a patient with new onset of diabetes mellitus. The hospital allegedly refused treatment when the patient indicated he could not make a requested deposit and, instead, referred him to a clinic or the health department for treatment the next day. Upon leaving that hospital, however, the patient immediately presented to another hospital where he was admitted and discharged 3 days later.

- A western hospital paid $125,000 to settle allegations that it failed to provide several patients with appropriate medical screening examinations. The patients' MCOs denied payment authorization for treatment. In one instance, a patient presented to the emergency room complaining that he could not move the right side of his face. Another instance concerned a 5-year-old who presented with a stomachache of several days duration. The next day a pediatrician saw this child and immediately sent him to surgery for a ruptured appendix. Also, in another instance, a pregnant patient who had sharp abdominal pain went by car to another facility, without being medically screened, apparently because of insurance concerns.

- A health care corporation and a hospital agreed to pay the government a total of $726,063 to settle allegations of improprieties occurring in the hospital's psychiatric programs. The hospital contracted this corporation as a health care consultant to manage the hospital's psychiatric unit. Investigation showed that from July 1994 through April 1997, the corporation inappropriately admitted patients to the hospital; that patients at the facility stayed longer than medically necessary; and that the corporation and the hospital failed to provide adequate treatment plans for patients enrolled in the facility's partial hospitalization program.

- A consent judgment was entered against a physician and the largest, independent physiological laboratory, holding them jointly and severally liable for payment of $170,500 to the government. This settlement resolved the civil aspect of the case and occurred in conjunction with a guilty plea to a criminal false claims violation. Based on this guilty plea, the physician was sentenced to 4 months imprisonment and 3 years probation. Through his laboratory, the physician improperly billed for pulse oximetry tests not performed, stress tests when pulse oximetry tests were performed, and home evaluation and management visits not performed. As part of the global settlement, the physician agreed to a 7-year exclusion as well. Also in connection with this case, a second individual pled guilty to theft of public monies for billing Medicare for pulse oximetry tests not performed. This individual, who previously sold the laboratory to the physician, was sentenced to 2 years probation.

- A kidney clinic and physician agreed to pay the government $90,000 to resolve allegations of improper billing for dialysis treatments. During the period from 1987 through 1992, the clinic and physician allegedly billed Medicare for patients who were no shows and for patients who appeared but could not receive their scheduled treatment due to medical complications. The clinic also entered into a comprehensive, 3-year corporate integrity agreement with OIG.

- A podiatrist, who received kickbacks from a DME supplier in exchange for ordering lymphedema pumps for program beneficiaries, agreed to a 3-year exclusion and paid $30,000 in penalties to resolve the allegations. The podiatrist prescribed pumps that were expensive and not medically necessary for treatment of the beneficiaries' conditions.

- In Pennsylvania, a component of a university health system agreed to pay the federal government $30 million in *settlement of* charges of defrauding the Medicare program. According to the OIG, an audit and investigation revealed that *false* Medicare bills were submitted for physician services. Many of the claims improperly reported the level of care provided or falsely reported the involvement of attending physicians, in addition to residents, rendering the service. The resulting overpayment was approximately $10 million. The civil settlement also requires that the component institute a compliance program to assure correct billing practices in the future. [As this book goes to press, there are reports that some of the adverse audit findings regarding upcoding of levels of service (ie, evaluation and management codes) may be modified because HCFA and Medicare carriers did not issue definitive billing guidelines until several years after the services were rendered.] [italics added]

- An ophthalmologist was sentenced to 4 years in custody, 3 years supervised release, and a $75,000 fine for conspiring to submit false claims to Medicare. In accordance with his plea agreement, the ophthalmologist also previously repaid the government $8.55 million, representing the second largest single provider recovery in the United States and the largest in the Eastern District of New York. He was also permanently excluded from participating in the Medicare program. Investigation by OIG into the ophthalmologist's activities revealed that he performed cataract surgeries on patients who did not have cataracts and performed glaucoma laser procedures on patients who did not have glaucoma. He also billed for other ophthalmological procedures that were either not performed or were not medically necessary. As a result of the investigation, the state licensing office revoked his license to practice medicine.

- A recently retired psychiatrist agreed to pay the government $194,766 to settle allegations of submitting improper claims to Medicaid. The psychiatrist treated patients in area nursing homes. Between January 1993 and May 1998, he billed his services using a procedure code for a 50-minute visit when he actually spent an average of 2 to 3 minutes with these patients.

- A physician was sentenced to 18 months incarceration, 2 years supervised probation, and a $5,000 fine for obstruction of justice (witness tampering). The doctor's conviction stemmed from an investigation into a DME fraud scheme involving sales representatives working in Puerto Rico for a Pennsylvania DME company. The sales representatives were convicted of mail fraud for changing orders for wound care surgical dressings that were then billed to Medicare. One of the sales representatives admitted to paying the doctor kickbacks for referring wound care patients for the company's surgical supplies. After denying to federal agents that he received kickbacks for patient referrals, the doctor willfully attempted to coerce a witness to lie about paying him kickbacks.

- A corporation agreed to pay $2.1 million to settle the civil aspects of a scheme to defraud Medicare. **The corporation used its subsidiaries in two states to bill carriers in each other's areas to obtain the best reimbursement for x-ray and electrocardiographic services.** Approximately 6,000 false claims were submitted in violation of point-of-service regulations. One subsidiary's president and vice president agreed to plead guilty to criminal charges for their involvement in the scheme. [boldface added]

- Five nursing homes in two states agreed to pay nearly $2.9 million to resolve their civil liability for complicity in the submission of false claims to the Medicare program as a result of a joint audit and investigation. The nursing homes entered into contracts with a billing agent, under the terms of which the agent reviewed medical records and then billed Medicare for so called "lost charges." These charges were for medical supplies for which the nursing homes had initially not filed claims. **The billing agent induced Medicare to pay these claims by putting false diagnoses on the claims forms.** In fact, the supplies that were billed were not reimbursable by Medicare. Under the contracts, the nursing homes kept 50 percent of all reimbursement by Medicare. As part of the settlements, the nursing homes were required to enter into compliance plans designed to ensure the accuracy and validity of future billings and cost reports. [boldface added]

- An emergency physician agreed to pay $22,500 for an allegation that he failed to provide an appropriate medical screening examination and treatment for a woman who came to the emergency room with an ectopic pregnancy.

- A hospital paid nearly $1.3 million to resolve its civil liability for allegedly submitting false claims to the Medicare and Medicaid programs. The hospital submitted claims for experimental cardiac devices that had not received final approval by the Food and Drug Administration, in contravention of Medicare rules and policies.

- A medical center agreed to pay $1.7 million to settle allegations of Medicare and Medicaid fraud. The hospital submitted duplicate and multiple billings for venipuncture (blood specimen collection) and claims for venipunctures when other, nonreimbursable services were actually provided. **The claims were submitted through a computerized billing system designed by consultants who are also under investigation.** Estimated damages amounted to $390,000. The hospital has agreed to an independent audit of other billings, back to 1989, and to reporting any improper payments. In addition, it will set up a compliance program to educate employees on accurate and valid filing of claims with government programs. [boldface added]

- A nursing home failed to disclose that rent payments were made to a related party. If these costs had been allowed, the home would have received *more than it* was entitled to receive. Civil monetary penalties were pursued because of the nursing home's repeated attempts to mislead the government, even though no actual overpayment was made because the intermediary made the proper audit adjustments (prior to payment). [italics added]

- In a western state, a superior court judge turned down a proposal that a convicted ophthalmologist be permitted to spend a year performing eye surgery in an impoverished country, and ordered him to begin serving his 16-month prison sentence. In December 1991, the ophthalmologist was convicted in State court on 36 counts of grand theft for billing Medicare for services he did not perform. His scheme involved intentionally causing astigmatism by sewing a stitch too tightly in patients undergoing cataract surgery.

  When the patients returned complaining of vision problems, he cut the stitch and normal vision returned. The stitch-cutting was billed to Medicare as a $2,000 corneal transplant. During a 4-year period, he billed Medicare more than $1.3 million for over 680 eye operations. In a rare prison sentencing of a physician in State court for Medicare fraud, he also was fined $350,000, assessed a penalty of $280,000.

- The government settled a civil False Claims Act case as part of a global resolution to a matter involving an osteopathic physician allegedly involved in several fraudulent schemes concerning nursing home patients. Through these schemes, the osteopath allegedly submitted false claims to Medicare for services furnished to residents in nursing homes that were either upcoded or never provided. As part of the settlement agreement, he agreed to pay the federal government $2 million and the state $47,751. The osteopath also allegedly accepted kickbacks for referring residents (ineligible for hospice services) of nursing homes he owned to a hospice for which he was the medical director.

- A cardiologist paid $30,000 and entered into a 3-year physician integrity agreement to resolve OIG's CMP law case against him for payment of kickbacks. The cardiologist made a series of small payments to an internist to induce the internist to refer his patients, including Medicare beneficiaries, to the cardiologist for diagnostic testing. The OIG initiated the action based upon its CMP authority for remuneration offered, paid, solicited, or received after August 5, 1997.

- A physician agreed to pay $20,000 for an allegation that he failed to stabilize an individual who had an unstable emergency medical condition. Hours after being discharged from the emergency room, the patient presented to another hospital where he was admitted and treated for 10 days.

- Five physician groups in multiple jurisdictions settled allegations arising from a *qui tam* law suit, which revealed that they employed a billing agency that submitted upcoded emergency room services to Medicare, Medicaid, TRICARE, and FEHBP on their behalf. Under the terms of the settlement agreement, the physician groups have agreed to pay a combined total of $581,303. In addition, one of the physician groups entered into a corporate integrity agreement.

- In a western state, the estate of a deceased physician entered into a settlement agreement with the government to resolve his civil liability for improper Medicare claims submitted from July 1996 through December 1996. The government will recover $403,838 from the estate. The physician, who owned three medical clinics, died in a car accident in March 1999. The estate is resolving his liability for billing Medicare for procedures and services not authorized, not medically necessary, not rendered, or upcoded. The estate also agreed to waive $43,838 in withheld Medicare funds.

- Two physicians agreed to pay a combined amount of $182,986 to resolve their respective liabilities under the False Claims Act, CMP law, and OIG's exclusion authority. The physicians were alleged to have admitted Medicare beneficiaries to a hospital when hospitalization was not medically necessary. Both physicians have agreed to be permanently excluded from participating in any federal health care programs.

- A former anesthesiologist and an anesthesia practice agreed to pay the government $79,000 to resolve their civil liability under the False Claims Act and the CMP law. Between 1993 and 1996, the former anesthesiologist submitted improper claims to Medicare, Medicaid, and TRICARE for anesthesia services that did not meet the minimum criteria for the categories of service billed. In several instances, the anesthesiologist billed for services performed by certified registered nurse anesthetists (CRNAs) as though he personally provided the service. In other instances, the anesthesiologist was not even in the hospital at the time the CRNA rendered the service. Additionally, in 1997 the anesthesiologist submitted claims to Medicare, Medicaid, and TRICARE for services provided by physicians who were paid by the hospital. As part of the settlement, the anesthesiologist must annually certify that he is not involved in the submission of claims to federal health care programs.

- A physician, who also owned and operated a clinic, was sentenced to 5 years in prison and ordered to pay $2.87 million in restitution. The physician was convicted of multiple felony counts, including mail fraud, wire fraud, bankruptcy fraud, and making false statements. Evidence proved the physician deliberately misdiagnosed patients as suffering from a rare vascular disease that requires patients to obtain expensive pumps, braces, and other medical devices. The physician was also convicted of making false statements when he filed for bankruptcy in 1996.

- An OB-GYN practice and several individual physicians paid $109,900 to resolve their civil monetary penalty liability for violations of the physician self-referral (Stark) statute and the kickback provisions of the Civil Monetary Penalties Law. From 1997 through 2000, the physicians had a financial relationship with a mobile ultrasound company from which they received referral fees—ostensibly in the form of rent—in return for referring Medicare beneficiaries to the company for ultrasound studies and diagnostic testing.

- A physiatrist was sentenced to 5 years probation and payment of approximately $1.4 million in total restitution to the Medicare program and the Medicaid program for his scheme to bill for services not rendered. From 1993 to 1995, the physiatrist provided services at four nursing homes and had a private practice. During that time, he obtained the patient rosters at the nursing homes and systematically billed Medicare and Medicaid for a battery of tests he did not perform on residents. He also billed in this manner for patients of his private practice. The investigation revealed that thousands of the tests and procedures he billed, and received reimbursement for, were neither performed nor ordered by the attending physicians.

- As the result of a joint undercover investigation by OIG and the Federal Bureau of Investigation, five persons involved in a Medicare and Medicaid fraud scheme were sentenced to between 21 and 51 months in jail. Four, including the owner of two vascular testing clinics and a DME company as well as three of her employees, were ordered to make restitution totaling more than $2 million to Medicare and $243,500 to Medicaid. The four had paid individuals to submit to an extensive battery of diagnostic tests, which were placed in Medicare and Medicaid patient files and for which they filed for more than $4 million in claims. They also paid a carrier contract employee to pass on to them carrier records. The contract employee was sentenced to 12 months in jail.

- A state-owned hospital in Iowa agreed to repay Medicare $521,170 for overbilling for services. During a separate anesthesiology investigation, an allegation was made that the hospital was billing for ventilation management although this service should have been included in the global fee. Investigation showed that the hospital was billing for ventilation management for all intensive care patients, regardless of whether they received this service. **The hospital claimed to have understood from the carrier's medical director that it could bill for Medicare and private insurers in the *same fashion*.** [boldface added]

- The former owner of an ambulance company was sentenced to a year and a day in federal prison and 2 years supervised probation for Medicare and Medicaid fraud. Over a 2-year period, the woman and her husband defrauded the programs of $370,000 in false billings. They submitted bills for ambulance trips for dialysis patients that they claimed were not ambulatory, but surveillance cameras caught several of the patients walking to and from the ambulances with little or no assistance. Because of the couple's financial condition, the woman was ordered to pay restitution of only $926 and a special assessment of $250. Her husband pled guilty earlier and was sentenced to 3 years probation and ordered to pay $113 in court costs. The ambulance company has gone out of business.

- A laboratory owner was sentenced to 3 months in prison, followed by 90 days in home confinement and 3 years supervised probation for fraudulent Medicare billing. The man operated a mobile clinic, which offered free screenings for senior citizens. He or one of his employees would obtain their Medicare numbers and bill the program for unnecessary tests or tests not performed. He was ordered to pay restitution of $265,110.

- A dentist was sentenced to 1–2 years confinement on 15 counts of selling controlled drugs to patients. He was fined $2,500 on each count, for a total fine of $37,500. The confinement period was suspended to time served and he was put on indefinite probation not to exceed 5 years. This case was developed from Project Pharm-Div, a joint OIG and city police department undercover operation. The project is aimed at identifying and prosecuting individuals involved in the abuse of pharmaceutical drugs, fraud against Medicare and Medicaid, and various frauds involving the misuse of Social Security numbers. To date, 16 individuals and entities have been prosecuted in federal or state courts as a result of the project in this city.

- A physician was sentenced on the basis of a negotiated plea whereby he had agreed to cooperate with the government in exchange for dismissal of charges under pretrial diversions for his sister/employee, and for his corporation. During a 4-year period, he billed Medicare more than $1.5 million and was paid $560,000, over 60 percent of which was for laboratory services supposedly performed in-house. **A carrier utilization review showed he billed as much as 600 percent more than his peers in some areas. He was accused of billing Medicare, the Civilian Health Medical Program of the Uniformed Services (CHAMPUS), and private insurers for laboratory services not performed or not medically necessary, double billing, and money laundering.** His sister had been charged with offering a witness a bribe for refusing to cooperate with an OIG agent. He was sentenced to 1 year of confinement, 3 months to be served in prison, 3 months in a halfway house, and 6 months in monitored home confinement, after which he will serve 3 years probation. He was ordered to make restitution of $37,000. The sentence was reduced because of his substantial assistance to the government. Negotiations are continuing toward a settlement of pending civil damages. [boldface added]

- A pharmacy and its former office manager were sentenced for Medicare and Medicaid fraud. The pharmacy was ordered to make restitution of $22,700, while the office manager had to pay $25,000 plus $500 in court costs. He was also sentenced to 1 year in prison. **They had billed for urinary incontinence and decubitus ulcer kits, which were neither related to the patients' conditions nor medically necessary. They also billed for greater quantities than delivered.** The office manager was suspended from program participation in 1988 for 5 years because of a racketeering charge involving illegal drugs, and he was office manager of the pharmacy while under suspension. He has since set up several new businesses. [boldface added]

- The owner/operator of a retail optical store was sentenced for submitting false Medicare claims. From January 1989 until June 1993, Medicare paid him $237,000, of which $180,000 was overpayment. **He billed for eyeglasses not provided or misrepresented services to receive payment when none would have been allowed.** He also discussed kickback arrangements with another optical dealer. When confronted by agents, he made a complete written statement admitting his fraudulent activities. He was sentenced to 6 months probation and ordered to repay $24,000. A civil prosecution is underway for the remainder of the fraudulent amount. [boldface added]

- The twelfth and final person was sentenced in a scheme in which Traveler's Insurance employees issued Medicare checks to friends who forged and cashed them. The woman was sentenced to 4 months home confinement and 3 years probation. She was ordered to pay a $2,000 fine, a $150 special assessment, and restitution of $11,101 for the two Medicare checks she cashed. Those previously sentenced in the case included two Traveler's employees, a top manager of an international beverage company, a former deputy sheriff, and the chief buyer for a drugstore chain. The embezzlement involved 56 Medicare checks totaling $250,000.

- A woman was sentenced after pleading guilty to making false statements to Medicaid. As office manager for an optical store, **the woman altered patient records and physicians' prescriptions to charge Medicaid for tinted, ultraviolet, and scratch-resistant lenses that were not medically necessary.** She also failed to honor the company's warranty policy, charging Medicaid for replacement glasses when something went wrong with a pair of eyeglasses. She was sentenced to 18 months probation and 180 hours of community service, with a fine of $50. The optical company repaid $27,900 to Medicaid rather than risk civil action. [boldface added]

- A medical center and its former employee agreed to settle their liabilities for submitting claims for services that were not rendered, not medically necessary, or insufficiently documented during June 1994 through August 1995. The employee, the hospital's psychiatrist, had caused the filing of the claims. Their agreements, including penalties, totaled $647,000 of which $347,000 went to Medicaid, $289,065 to Medicare, and $10,935 to the Civilian Health and Medical Plan of the Uniformed Services (CHAMPUS).

- After a cancer center requested assistance in determining whether it had processed radiation oncology billing errors, a review showed it had been overpaid $655,570 by Medicare and $173,350 by Medicaid. **The center improperly billed the technical components for radiation oncology services to hospital inpatients that had already been billed by the hospital.** Investigation showed the billings were errors and not fraudulent. The center agreed to pay $831,500 to the Medicare trust fund. [boldface added]

- A nationally known provider of ultrasound and imaging diagnostic tests agreed to pay $4.2 million to settle allegations it entered an illegal arrangement with doctors throughout the United States. The laboratory marketed its services to doctors who were not trained to interpret test results, telling them they could bill for the professional component of the tests. When a doctor ordered an imaging test from the laboratory, it billed Medicare for the technical component. It then sent the test to a specialist for interpretation, who did not bill Medicare but charged the referring doctor a low flat rate. The doctor then billed Medicare for the professional component and got the difference between the specialist's fee and the Medicare-allowed amount. As a result, the laboratory received a total of $2.1 million in Medicare payments to which it was not entitled.

- A laboratory and its owner agreed to settle civil allegations that they submitted false claims totaling more than $1.6 million for transtelephonic EKGs. The services were supposedly provided to nursing home patients in Illinois, Indiana, Michigan, Tennessee, Kentucky, and North and South Carolina. The services were either medically unnecessary or never rendered. The owner had dissipated a large part of his assets, and therefore the amount of settlement was only $200,000, including $12,000 in EKG equipment. The owner agreed to a lifetime program exclusion.

- A physician owner of a laboratory entered a civil settlement agreement to pay the government $500,000 for submitting false Medicare claims. The physician performed various non-invasive tests on large groups of Medicare beneficiaries living in senior citizen apartment complexes. He billed Medicare for tests that were medically unnecessary and were not ordered by the patients' attending physicians.

- The owner of two home health agencies (HHAs) was sentenced for making false statements in a Medicare cost report. Her family wrote off personal expenses in the cost reports. She then funneled the proceeds through the two HHAs and eventually into the family's personal bank account. She was sentenced to 42 months in prison and 3 years probation, ordered to make restitution totaling more than $2.26 million, and fined $111,540. She was further ordered to make immediate payment of more than $66,370, which was the profit from sale of her residence, and to forfeit two parcels of property, estimated as worth $300,000, to be paid to the department. The HHAs were placed on 5 years probation. Charges against her husband and son were dropped.

- A psychiatrist was sentenced after being convicted of Medicare/Medicaid fraud. He was sentenced to 87 months incarceration, 36 months of supervised release, and 400 hours of post-release community service. His medical group's former business manager was sentenced to 33 months incarceration and 36 months supervised release. The defendants conspired to defraud Medicare, Medicaid, and CHAMPUS by filing claims for services not rendered as claimed or not covered by the programs. Between 1992 and 1996, the government paid the group more than $5.2 million.

- A woman was sentenced to 3 years probation and restitution of $400 for violating the Medicare antikickback statute. The woman owned and operated a company in south Florida, which referred Medicare beneficiaries to several psychiatric hospitals in central Florida, as well as other states. The woman received illegal remunerations in exchange for these referrals. She was the fifteenth individual to be sentenced in an investigation targeting a combination of inpatient psychiatric hospitals, illegal kickback activities, and patient brokering schemes. The investigation focused on the intricate relationship among hospital associates who pay kickbacks in return for patient referrals to hospitals; patient brokers who profit from the trade in patient referrals; and patient referral sources who accept money from hospitals or patient brokers in exchange for referrals.

- A podiatrist was sentenced to 2 years probation and payment of $16,200 in restitution for violating the antikickback statute. The podiatrist illegally received kickbacks from a DME company owner in return for the referral of patients requiring lymphedema pumps.

- An employee of a diagnostic laboratory was sentenced to 3 years probation and a $4,000 fine for conspiracy to violate the antikickback statute and tax evasion. The man paid kickbacks to a clinic manager in return for laboratory testing referrals. In January 1998, the man waived indictment and pled guilty to conspiracy and tax evasion for his role in the scheme.

- A woman was sentenced for engaging illegal kickback activity. Her sentence included 3 years probation and a $3,000 fine. The sole proprietor of a radiology facility, the woman paid a physician kickbacks in exchange for the referral of patients in need of ultrasound testing.

- A woman was sentenced to 1-year probation and $2,050 in fines for her role in accepting kickbacks as a middle person on behalf of a rheumatologist with a medical practice. The woman received money from a DME supplier for facilitating a kickback arrangement with the rheumatologist. Her sentencing concludes a case involving several doctors and podiatrists who participated in a kickback conspiracy among health care providers in two states.

- An osteopath was sentenced to 3 months in a halfway house, 2 years probation, and a $5,000 fine for filing falsified Medicare and Medicaid claims. The indictment charged the osteopath with accepting kickbacks from a home health care company.

- Three persons were sentenced to prison for their participation in a scheme to defraud Medicare, the Social Security Administration (SSA), the Department of Labor (DOL), and various private insurance companies. One person was ordered to serve 27 months in prison and to pay restitution of $49,400 to insurance companies. She had falsified nursing receipts submitted to the companies for reimbursement. A second person was ordered to serve 24 months and to pay $66,900 to SSA and an insurance company for falsifying her own disability claims to receive reimbursement.

  A third person, a psychologist, was sentenced to 87 months in prison and ordered to pay restitution of $590,600, of which $515,900 went to Medicare and the remainder to DOL and various insurance companies. The psychologist diagnosed people, brought to her by an individual who pled guilty earlier, with post-traumatic stress disorder as a result of auto accidents that never happened. She then billed Medicare, DOL, and various insurance companies for services not performed. Some beneficiaries received money for their part in the scheme.

- A podiatrist was sentenced for mail fraud, making a false statement, and fraud in relation to false Medicare claims after he had been excluded from the program. In 1991, the podiatrist pled guilty and was sentenced in Pennsylvania for defrauding the Medicaid program, and as a result was excluded from Medicare and state health care programs for 8 years. Later, while still on probation, he moved to Florida and applied for and received a Medicare provider number after making false statements on his application. He then billed Medicare, through the practices with which he was associated, for services to beneficiaries in nursing homes, adult living facilities, and outpatient surgery centers as well as at the medical office. He was sentenced to 18 months imprisonment, followed by 3 years supervised release, and ordered to make restitution of $29,739.

- A psychiatrist and two unlicensed psychotherapists were each excluded for 10 years after being convicted of defrauding the Medicaid program. They had devised a scheme where *unlicensed individuals* undertook psychiatric counseling sessions and their clinic billed Medi-Cal as if a psychiatrist had been present throughout the entire session. The loss to the Medi-Cal program as a result of this scheme was in excess of $500,000. [italics added]

- A physician was required to make restitution to Medicare of $190,000 after being convicted for his part in a conspiracy to defraud Medicare in which he received remuneration for referring patients to a psychologist. After his conviction, he was excluded for 10 years.

- The owner of a clinic was convicted of defrauding Medicaid by submitting claims for the services of an unlicensed physician. The court ordered her to pay restitution of $100,000. After being convicted, the clinic owner was excluded for 10 years.

- A mental health rehabilitation provider and her company were each excluded for 10 years. Her exclusion was based on her conviction for defrauding the Medicaid program of $280,000 by billing for services that had to be ordered by a physician, or in some instances, performed under the supervision of a physician when no such order existed or no physician supervision was provided.

- A dentist was found guilty of involuntary manslaughter after giving a patient a fatal overdose of sedatives during gum surgery. After this conviction, the dentist was excluded for 15 years.

- The owner of a medical center was convicted of defrauding insurance companies by submitting fraudulent medical bills and reports to them. He was ordered to pay over $106,000 in restitution to the insurance companies. As a result of this conviction, he was excluded for 10 years from program participation.

- A 10-year exclusion was imposed on the manager of a medical service for his part in a scheme to defraud health insurance companies. He had instructed company staff to fabricate fraudulent medical bills and reports describing medical treatment purportedly rendered to personal injury clients and to submit the claims to the insurance companies. He was ordered to pay restitution of $100,000 to the insurance companies.

- A podiatrist agreed to pay $100,000 to resolve his civil liability for submitting improper Medicare claims. Between 1993 and 1995, the podiatrist billed for whirlpool treatments each time a patient visited his office. He also billed for removal of skin lesions when in fact he was performing noncovered routine foot care. The improper billing resulted in an overpayment of approximately $61,000.

- A physician and acupuncturist were sentenced for conspiracy in fraudulently billing Medicare $1.9 million. The acupuncturist and her former husband, who co-owned six acupuncture clinics, hired the physician and other medical doctors to prescribe physical therapy when the couple had performed non-billable acupuncture. The physician also backdated physical examinations, and had others backdate them, to make them appear to have been done before the couple began treatments. The physician was sentenced to 30 months in prison and ordered to repay $144,390. The acupuncturist, who pled guilty and testified against him, was sentenced to 36 months probation and ordered to pay back $927,000, the actual amount Medicare overpaid. Her former husband is a fugitive and is believed to have fled to Hong Kong.

- The former chief executive officer of a vascular diagnostic testing laboratory was sentenced to 51 months incarceration. Over a 3-year period, the officer used his position to cause submission of Medicare and Medicaid claims for services not performed. He was convicted on 100 counts of false claims, one count of attempting to induce a witness to give false testimony before a grand jury, and one count of giving false testimony himself to the grand jury. He was fined $65,000 and ordered to pay $219,600 in restitution. At the time, he was on parole as a result of a 1985 conviction for Medicare/Medicaid fraud and related drug charges.

- A physician was sentenced to 36 months incarceration and fined $195,000 for billing Medicare, Blue Cross Blue Shield, and a private insurance company for physical therapy services that were not provided. The physician and his office manager also participated in a scheme involving insurance fraud. The office manager claimed injury from a no-contact auto accident, for which the physician submitted 159 false insurance claims. The physician also claimed payment for two sigmoidoscopies performed on the office manager, which she claimed she could not recall. The physician's conviction was the result of the testimony of the office manager, who was dismissed earlier as a defendant.

- A urologist was sentenced to 24 months in prison for submitting false claims to Medicare. He had pled guilty to submitting claims for complex procedures he did not perform. Earlier he agreed to pay $440,000 in damages and penalties, which were paid before the sentencing. The urologist will be excluded from Medicare for 10 years because of aggravating circumstances: he performed invasive procedures such as cystourethroscopies (visual examinations of the bladder and urethra) and cystometrograms (assessments of the bladder's neuromuscular function), which he admitted were not medically necessary. He has surrendered his medical license.

- A chiropractor pled guilty to one count of submitting a false claim to an employee welfare benefit program. The chiropractor also billed Medicare and the Department of Labor for services for patients who missed or canceled their appointments. The plea agreement called for him to pay a total of $102,110 in restitution, fines, and civil monetary penalties. He was immediately sentenced to 3 years probation.

- A psychiatrist was sentenced for conspiracy and mail fraud related to submitting false Medicare and private insurer claims. The psychiatrist was sentenced to 15 months incarceration and 3 years probation, and ordered to pay $85,930 in restitution. He allowed his brother-in-law, who operated an optometry practice, to use his license to charge for tests that were either never performed or medically unnecessary. The brother-in-law was sentenced earlier to 5 months in jail and 5 months home detention, and ordered to pay restitution of $150,000.

- A woman was sentenced to a year and a day in prison and ordered to make restitution of $41,500 she had stolen in Medicare and Medicaid checks. *While employed by a doctor as an office manager,* she submitted claims for a personal friend, although no services were performed. When the checks came in, the two split the proceeds, with the woman taking the larger amount. The friend was sentenced to a year of probation and fined $2,550. [italics added]

- Through its six owners, a company entered into an agreement to pay $85,000 to resolve federal civil false claims liability. The company conducted diagnostic testing, primarily at nursing homes, and filed false Medicare claims for services that were either not performed or not medically necessary. The claims, which resulted in a $46,570 overpayment, were submitted by an employee, who pled guilty separately. The civil agreement with the owners is based on their "reckless disregard" of company and employee activities.

- The former business manager of three physical therapy clinics was sentenced to 1 year probation, ordered to perform 40 hours community service, and fined $100 for Medicare fraud. One of several employees hired by the owner and operator of the clinics, she falsified working hours, wages, and personnel qualifications of unlicensed assistants and aides, which the owner used to claim more therapy hours than were actually provided. The Medicare fiscal intermediary identified $4 million in overpayments and disallowances through cost reports filed by the owner's companies. She was sentenced earlier to 21 months in jail and excluded from Medicare and state health care programs. The business manager's light sentence was the result of her cooperation in the investigation and her testimony against the owner. A civil case is pending against the owner.

- A neurologist was sentenced for his part in a scheme to defraud the Medicare and Medi-Cal programs. He previously pled guilty to four felony counts of mail fraud. The physician submitted claims for nerve conduction studies and upcoded claims for office visits and EMGs. He was sentenced to 6 months home detention and 3 years probation. He was also ordered to pay $118,750 in restitution and perform 3,000 hours of community service.

- With the expansion of exclusion authority under the Health Insurance Portability and Accountability Act of 1996 (HIPAA) to include the sanctioning of individuals controlling previously sanctioned entities, a Maryland doctor was excluded from program participation for 10 years. The doctor was the owner of a methadone clinic in Maryland, which had been convicted for knowingly and willfully making false statements in applications for payment to Medicaid. The clinic paid restitution in the amount of $290,000 based upon an overpayment of $95,000, and was excluded for 10 years.

- The HIPAA established OIG mandatory authority to exclude any individual who has been convicted of a felony relating to controlled substance violations. The HIPAA also expanded the mandatory exclusion authority to exclude any individual convicted of a felony relating to health care fraud.

The following are OIG comments on patient dumping and physician certifications.

Civil Penalties for Patient Dumping. Section 1867 of the Social Security Act (42 U.S.C. 1395dd) provides that when an individual presents to the emergency room for examination or treatment, a hospital which has a Medicare provider agreement is required to provide an appropriate medical screening examination to determine whether that individual has an emergency medical condition. If an individual has such a condition, the hospital must provide, within the capabilities of the staff and facilities available at the hospital, treatment to stabilize the condition, unless a physician certifies that the individual should be transferred because the benefits of medical treatment elsewhere outweigh the risks associated with transfer. If a transfer is ordered, the transferring hospital must arrange for a safe transfer, which includes providing stabilizing treatment to minimize the risks of transfer, making sure the receiving hospital has agreed to accept the transfer and effecting the transfer through qualified personnel and transportation equipment. A hospital is prohibited from delaying provision of examination or treatment for an emergency condition to inquire about an individual's method of payment or insurance status. Further, a participating hospital with specialized capabilities or facilities may not refuse to accept an appropriate transfer of an individual who needs those services if the hospital has the capacity to treat the individual.

The OIG is authorized to impose CMPs of up to $25,000 against small hospitals (less than 100 beds) and up to $50,000 against larger hospitals (100 beds or more) for each instance where the hospital negligently violated any of the section 1867 requirements. In addition, OIG may impose a CMP of up to $50,000 against a participating physician, including an on-call physician, for each negligent violation of any of the section 1867 requirements, and impose a program exclusion in certain cases. Between 10/31/98 and 3/31/99, OIG collected $985,000 in CMPs from 34 hospitals and physicians.

Special Fraud Alert: Physician Certifications. During this reporting period, OIG issued a special fraud alert entitled "Physician Liability for Certifications in the Provision of Medical Equipment and Supplies and Home Health Services." It was published in the Federal Register on January 12, 1999. The fraud alert was issued to educate and inform physicians of the significance of the certifications they make in connection with items and services they order for home health services and DME. Under the Medicare program, physicians prescribing home health care or DME, such as hospital beds, wheelchairs and oxygen delivery systems, must certify that the services are medically necessary and that the beneficiary meets the requirements to qualify for the benefit. This fraud alert is an effort to assist providers in their compliance efforts by explaining in clear language the physicians' responsibilities in making certifications and the legal significance of the certifications.

Endnotes

1. Sometimes physicians and/or their billing staff find out that Medicare will not deny their claims as a noncovered service if they bill another, similar CPT® code or use a certain diagnosis code even though the codes are not descriptive of the services provided or the patient's condition. Often, this occurs without the physician's or supervisor's knowledge and again illustrates the importance of voluntary compliance efforts such as an internal audit of billing practices.

How to Request an Advisory Opinion

The Office of Inspector General (OIG) includes detailed instructions for requesting an advisory opinion at the Web site, http://oig.hhs.gov/fraud/advisoryopinions.html.

In accordance with section 1128D (b) (5) (A) (v) of the Social Security Act and 42 CFR 1008.47 of our regulations, advisory opinions issued by the Office of Inspector General are being made available to the general public through this OIG website. One purpose of the advisory opinion process is to provide meaningful advice on the application of the anti-kickback statute and other OIG sanction statutes in specific factual situations.

Please note, however, that advisory opinions are binding and may legally be relied upon only by the requestor. Since each opinion will apply legal standards to a set of facts involving certain known persons who provide specific statements about key factual issues, no third parties are bound nor may they legally rely on these advisory opinions.

We have redacted specific information regarding the requestor and certain privileged, confidential or financial information associated with the individual or entity, unless otherwise specified by the requestor.

Advisory Opinion Regulations

The OIG Interim Final Rule (62 FR 7350)pdf and Revised Final Rule (63 FR 38311)pdf, addressing the procedural aspects for submitting a request and obtaining a formal advisory opinion from the Office of Inspector General, can be found under the OIG Regulations section of this web site.

[Note: At this time, readers will need to access both the interim final rule and the revised final rule to ascertain the current regulatory text set forth in 42 CFR 1008.]

Information Regarding Preliminary Questions and Supplementary Information for Obtaining OIG Advisory Opinions

Set forth below are the proposed preliminary questions and supplementary information for addressing requests for OIG advisory opinions in accordance with section 1128D of the Social Security Act and 42 CFR 1008.18 of our regulations. A Federal Register notice published on March 21, 1997 (62 FR 13621) specifically solicited public comments on this information collection activity. After receipt and due consideration of public comments, the OIG will submit the proposed preliminary questions to the Office of Management and Budget (OMB) for approval under the Paperwork Reduction Act (44 U.S.C. 2501-2530). We will provide public notice when a formal request is submitted to OMB. The preliminary questions will not be used until approved by OMB.

Recommended Preliminary Questions and Supplementary Information for Addressing Requests for OIG

Advisory Opinions In Accordance With Section 1128D of the Social Security Act and 42 CFR Part 1008. [See below or go to oig.hhs.gov/fraud/docs/advisoryopinions/prequestions.htm]

Preliminary Checklist for Advisory Opinion Requests (revised June 1999): Updated checklist to reflect revised OIG final regulations on the Advisory Opinion Process (63 FR 38311; July 16, 1998) [See below or go to oig.hhs.gov/fraud/docs/advisoryopinions/precheck.htm]

HCFA Advisory Opinion Website

For HCFA Advisory Opinions under the Stark Physician Self-Referral rule, go to www.hcfa.gov/regs/aop/.

Requesting an Advisory Opinion

The OIG Web site http://oig.hhs.gov/fraud/docs/advisoryopinions/prequestions.htm provides the following information:

Recommended Preliminary Questions and Supplementary Information for Addressing Requests for OIG Advisory Opinions in Accordance With Section 1128D of the Social Security Act and 42 CFR Part 1008

I. Introduction

In requesting an advisory opinion from the Office of Inspector General (OIG), you must fully and accurately provide the information required by regulations set forth at 42 CFR part 1008. In addition, you are encouraged, but not required, to respond to the suggested questions set forth below, as appropriate to the subject matter of your request. Providing the information that corresponds to the subject matter of your inquiry for an advisory opinion may expedite the processing of your request by the OIG. The Office of Inspector General reserves the right to modify or add suggested questions at any time.

For the purposes of the questions listed below, we will refer to the factual context of the question as the "arrangement" and use the following definitions. We ask that persons requesting an opinion use the same definitions in any submission.

- **"Referral"** means referral of a patient or the purchasing, leasing, ordering (or arranging for or recommending purchasing, leasing, or ordering) of any good, facility, service or item if any portion of that patient's care or the cost of the good, facility, service or item may be paid in whole or in part by Medicare, Medicaid, or any other Federal health care program.

- **"Fair market value"** means the value that would be assigned to the item or service in question by individuals or entities who have an arms-length relationship and who have no ability to influence referrals of any health care business to each other.

- **"Federal Health Care Program"** means any plan or program that provides health benefits, whether directly or indirectly, through insurance, or otherwise, which is funded directly, in whole or in part, by the United States Government (other than the health insurance program under 5 U.S.C. 89).

- **"Party or Parties"** are all individuals or entities that will or may participate in any way with the arrangement, including indirect ownership interests. This also includes any parties or third-party beneficiaries to contracts, as well as others affected by the arrangement. Generally, anyone who may pay or receive remuneration as a result of the arrangement is a party to the arrangement.

- **"Remuneration"** means anything of value, whether tangible or intangible. For example, a reduction or discount, like a direct payment, is remuneration.

II. Subject Areas

Set forth below are three specific subject areas for which we are providing suggested questions to be answered in advisory opinion requests.

Subject Areas

— If the subject matter of your inquiry concerns —
  1. What constitutes prohibited remuneration within the meaning of section 1128B(b) of the Social Security Act; or
  2. Whether an activity, or proposed activity, constitutes grounds for the imposition of sanctions under section 1128B(b) of the Social Security Act.

Please refer to the suggested questions contained in attachment A.

— If the subject matter of your inquiry concerns —
  1. Whether an arrangement, or proposed arrangement, satisfies the criteria set forth in section 1128B(b)(3) of the Social Security Act for activities which do not result in prohibited remuneration;
  2. Whether an arrangement, or proposed arrangement, satisfies the criteria set forth in 42 CFR 1001.952 for activities which do not result in prohibited remuneration; or

  3. Whether an arrangement, or proposed arrangement, although not satisfying the criteria of 1. or 2. above, is sufficiently similar to activities set forth in section 1128B(b)(3) or 42 CFR 1001.952 that it should not constitute grounds for the imposition of sanctions under section 1128B(b) of the Social Security Act.

Please refer to the suggested questions contained in attachment B.

— If the subject matter of your inquiry concerns —
  1. What constitutes an inducement to reduce or limit services to individuals entitled to benefits under title 18 or 19 of the Social Security Act within the meaning of section 1128A(b) of the Act(1)?

Please refer to the suggested questions contained in attachment C.

Attachment A

1. What parties or potential parties to the arrangement have the ability to influence the referral of health care business to other parties?

2. For each party or potential party who has the ability to influence the referral of such business, describe the reasons for and extent of such ability.

3. What remuneration may or will be paid to or from parties to the arrangement?

   The answer to this question should identify each potential remuneration relationship and for each such relationship:
   (a) Identify the payor and recipient of remuneration for that relationship;
   (b) Explain the nature of the remuneration that will or may be paid through that relationship;
   (c) Set forth the amount of remuneration and explain how the amount of remuneration will be calculated;
   (d) Explain any variation in the amount of remuneration to be paid by or to various parties, the reasons for such variations and how they are calculated;
   (e) For each party that is receiving remuneration, describe the services or other consideration that party is providing for the remuneration; and
   (f) For each recipient of remuneration in the arrangement, does the remuneration received constitute the fair market value for the consideration that

party is providing (as set forth in response to sub-part (e) above)?

4. To the extent health care services or items are provided in accordance with the arrangement, are such items or services covered or reimbursed by any Federal health care program?

5. Please address whether the arrangement may result in any of the following:
   (a) An increase or decrease in access to health care services;
   (b) An increase or decrease in the quality of health care services;
   (c) An increase or decrease in patient freedom of choice among health care providers;
   (d) An increase or decrease in competition among health care providers;
   (e) An increase or decrease in the ability of health care facilities to provide services in medically underserved areas or to medically underserved populations;
   (f) An increase or decrease in the cost to Federal health care programs; or
   (g) The existence or nonexistence of any potential financial benefit to a health care professional or provider which may vary based on his or her decisions of-
       (i) Whether to order a health care item or service; or
       (ii) Whether to arrange for a referral of health care items or services to a particular practitioner or provider.

6. Describe any other business arrangements or transactions among the parties, either in existence or planned.

7. Describe what factors or characteristics of the arrangement will prevent the kinds of abuse addressed by the anti-kickback statute.

8. Provide any other information that the requestor believes is relevant, e.g. a description of the requestor's compliance program, if any.

Attachment B

1. Describe the arrangement in detail.

2. To the extent health care services or items are provided pursuant to the arrangement, are such items or services covered or reimbursed by any Federal health care program?

3. Please address how the arrangement meets or fails to meet each of the elements of the relevant safe harbor at 42 CFR 1001.952 or the relevant subsection of section 1128B(b)(3) of the Social Security Act.

4. Please address whether the subject arrangement may result in any of the following:
   (a) An increase or decrease in access to health care services;
   (b) An increase or decrease in the quality of health care services;
   (c) An increase or decrease in patient freedom of choice among health care providers;
   (d) An increase or decrease in competition among health care providers;
   (e) An increase or decrease in the ability of health care facilities to provide services in medically underserved areas or to medically underserved populations;
   (f) An increase or decrease in the cost to Federal health care programs; or
   (g) The existence or nonexistence of any potential financial benefit to a health care professional or provider which may vary based on his or her decisions of-
       (i) Whether to order a health care item or service; or
       (ii) Whether to arrange for a referral of health care items or services to a particular practitioner or provider.

5. Describe what factors or characteristics of the arrangement will prevent the kinds of abuse addressed by the anti-kickback statute.

6. Describe any other business relationships or transactions among the parties, either in existence or planned.

7. Provide any other information that the requestor believes is relevant, e.g. a description of the requestor's compliance program, if any.

Attachment C

1. How does the hospital calculate the remuneration provided to physicians?

2. Does the hospital make any distinction between physicians in calculating the amounts of remuneration? If yes, describe and explain the distinctions.

3. Does the hospital make any distinctions between patients in determining the amounts of remuneration? If yes, describe and explain the distinctions.

4. What is the relationship, if any, between the amount and type of care provided to a Medicare or Medicaid beneficiary under the direct care of a physician and the amount of payments made to that physician?

5. Do the physicians receiving the payments have direct care responsibilities over Medicare or Medicaid beneficiaries?

6. How many patients are considered when determining the amount of the payment?

7. What is the physician's total income from the treatment of patients at the hospital?

8. What is the amount of payments made to the physician pursuant to the arrangement?

9. Are the payments calculated based on the practices of more than one physician? If so, how many physicians are in the pool used to calculate the incentive payments?

10. What is the period of time over which the amount of the payment is determined?

11. What safeguards does the hospital utilize to detect and deter poor care or underutilization by physicians?

12. Would the remuneration be allowable under the standards at 42 CFR 417.479 if made by an organization rather than a hospital? Explain why or why not.

13. Provide any other information that the requestor believes is relevant, e.g. a description of the requestor's utilization review and/or quality assurance program, patient grievance procedures, review of denials of care.

Footnote:

1. Although the statute refers to section 1128B(b), the reference is apparently intended to be section 1128A(b).

Preliminary Checklist

The OIG's Web site http://oig.hhs.gov/fraud/docs/advisoryopinions/precheck.htm includes the following checklist for submitting a request for an advisory opinion.

Preliminary Checklist for Advisory Opinion Requests

Updated July 1999, this checklist reflects the OIG final regulations published in the *Federal Register* on July 16, 1998 (63 FR 38311). This version of the checklist is not substantially different from the previous versions set forth. The checklist is for informational purposes only and should not be a substitute for reading the regulations on issuance of OIG advisory opinions.

A. Technical Requirements

1. The requestor is a party to the arrangement. (42 CFR 1008.11) _____

2. The request is for an existing arrangement or one which the requestor in good faith plans to undertake.
   (42 CFR 1008.15(a)) _____

3. The requestor has included:
   a. A non-refundable check or money order for $250, payable to the Treasury of the United States. (42 CFR 1008.31(b) and 1008.36(b)(6)) _____
   b. A request for a written estimate of the cost involved in processing the advisory opinion. (Optional) (42 CFR 1008.31(d)(2)) _____
   c. A designated triggering dollar amount. (Optional) (42 CFR 1008.31(d)(3)) _____
   d. An original and two copies. (42 CFR 1008.36(a)) _____
   e. The name and addresses of the requestor and all other actual and potential parties to the extent known to the requestor. (42 CFR 1008.36(b)(1)) _____
   f. The name, title, address, and daytime telephone number of a contact person. (42 CFR 1008.36(b)(2)) _____
   g. Each requesting party's Taxpayer Identification Number. (42 CFR 1008.36(b)(8)) _____
   h. Full and complete information as to the identity of each entity owned or controlled by the individual, and of each person with an ownership or control interest in the entity. (42 CFR 1008.37) _____
   i. If applicable, a statement that some or all of the information or documents provided are trade secrets or are privileged or confidential commercial or financial information and are not subject to disclosure under the Freedom of Information Act (42 CFR 1008.36(b)(4)(v)) _____

B. Describing the Issues and the Arrangement

The request includes:

1. A declaration of the subject category or categories for which the opinion is requested. (42 CFR 1008.36(b)(3)) _____

2. A complete and specific description of all relevant information bearing on the arrangement and on the circumstances of the conduct. (42 CFR 1008.36(b)(4)) _____

3. All relevant background information. (42 CFR 1008.36(b)(4)(i)) _____

4. Complete copies of all operative documents, if applicable, or narrative descriptions of those documents. (42 CFR 1008.36(b)(4)) _____

5. Detailed statements of all collateral or oral understandings (if any). (42 CFR 1008.36(b)(4)(iii)) _____

C. Certifications

1. The request includes a signed certification that all of the information provided is true and correct and constitutes a complete description of the facts regarding which an advisory opinion is sought. (42 CFR 1008.38(a)) _____

2. The certification is signed by-
    a. The requestor if the requestor is an individual. (42 CFR 1008.38(c)(1)) _____

    b. The CEO or comparable officer if the requestor is a corporation. (42 CFR 1008.38(c)(2)) _____
    c. The managing partner if the requestor is a partnership. (42 CFR 1008.38(c)(3)) _____

3. If the request is for a proposed arrangement, it contains a signed certification that the arrangement is one that the requestor in good faith plans to undertake. (42 CFR 1008.38(b)) _____

The Office of Inspector General reserves the right to modify this checklist at any time or to request additional information not specified on this checklist.

Advisory Opinions Issued in 1997, 1998, 1999, 2000, 2001, 2002 (through June 21, 2002)

As of June 21, 2002, http://oig.hhs.gov/fraud/advisoryopinions/opinions.html included the following advisory opinions (the summary sentences are from the Web site):

2002 Advisory Opinions (Through June 21, 2002)

June 21, 2002 Advisory Opinion 02-9—(concerning whether a proposed single-specialty ambulatory surgical center that would be wholly-owned by a physician would violate the administrative authorities related to the anti-kickback statute)

June 19, 2002 Advisory Opinion 02-8—(concerning whether a political subdivision of a State that owns and operates an ambulance service can treat operating revenues received from local taxes as payments of applicable copayments and deductibles due from residents)

June 11, 2002 Advisory Opinion 02-7—(concerning the proposed waiver of coinsurance for portable x-ray services provided to nursing facility residents who are eligible for Medicare and Medicaid, but who do not meet the eligibility requirements for Qualified Medicare beneficiaries)

May 22, 2002 Advisory Opinion 02-6—(concerning whether a proposal to offer a refund program to hospital consumers who purchase the hospital's blood-filtering device for treatment of rheumatoid arthritis would constitute grounds for the imposition of sanctions under the OIG's exclusion and civil money penalty authorities)

May 14, 2002 Advisory Opinion No.02-5—(concerning whether the proposed reorganization of an existing radiation oncology group practice would violate the administrative authorities related to the anti-kickback statute)

April 26, 2002 Advisory Opinion No. 02-4—(concerning a durable medical equipment company's proposal to place its portable oxygen systems onsite at certain local hospitals, clinics, and physician offices for distribution to certain departing patients)

April 4, 2002 Advisory Opinion No. 02-3—(concerning an ambulance restocking program that will satisfy the criteria for a "general replenishing" arrangement within the terms of the recently issued ambulance restocking safe harbor)

April 4, 2002 Advisory Opinion No. 02-2—(concerning an ambulance restocking program that will satisfy the criteria for a "general replenishing" arrangement within the terms of the recently issued ambulance restocking safe harbor)

April 4, 2002 Advisory Opinion No. 02-1—(concerning a non-profit, tax-exempt, charitable corporation funded largely by drug companies that would provide financial assistance to subsidize, in whole or in part, the Part B cost-sharing amounts and Medigap premiums of financially needy Medicare beneficiaries suffering from relatively rare chronic diseases)

2001 Advisory Opinions

November 26, 2001 Advisory Opinion No. 01-21—(concerning a medical center's proposed acquisition of an ownership interest in an operating ambulatory surgical center that is currently owned by a group of gastroenterologists)

November 21, 2001 Advisory Opinion No. 01-20—(concerning a payment arrangement between a Medicare-certified hospice and certain nursing facilities for services provided to residents of such facilities who are eligible both for Medicaid and Medicare hospice benefits ["Dually Eligibles"]. Specifically, for Dually Eligibles, the hospice pays the nursing facilities the full Medicaid nursing facility per diem rate for non-hospice patients, which covers pharmacy services, plus a separate payment for drugs used by Dually Eligibles in connection with their terminal illness. You have asked whether such an arrangement would constitute grounds for the imposition of sanctions under the exclusion authority at section 1128(b)(7) of the Social Security Act [the "Act"] or the civil monetary penalty provision at section 1128A(a)(7) of the Act, as those sections relate to the commission of acts described in section 1128B(b) of the Act.)

November 21, 2001 Advisory Opinion No. 01-19—(concerning a hospital's proposed donation of free office space to an entity that provides free end-of-life services to patients with terminal illnesses. Specifically, whether that donation would constitute grounds for the imposition of sanctions under the exclusion authority at section 1128(b)(7) of the Social Security Act [the "Act"] or the civil monetary penalty provision at section 1128A(a)(7) of the Act, as those sections relate to the commission of acts described in section 1128B(b) of the Act)

November 7, 2001 Advisory Opinion No. 01-18—(concerning an exclusive contract for emergency ambulance services between County A, State B and Medical Center C under which County A has assumed the obligation to pay otherwise uncollected coinsurance amounts on behalf of County A residents. Specifically, whether such an arrangement would constitute grounds for the imposition of sanctions under the exclusion authority at section 1128(b)(7) of the Social Security Act [the "Act"] or the civil monetary penalty provision at section 1128A(a)(7) of the Act, as those sections relate to the commission of acts described in section 1128B(b) of the Act, or under the civil monetary penalties provision for illegal remuneration to beneficiaries at section 1128A(a)(5) of the Act.)

October 17, 2001 Advisory Opinion No. 01-17—(concerning whether an existing ambulatory surgical center ["ASC"] joint venture between a hospital-affiliated entity and an entity owned indirectly by five ophthalmologists, together with the execution of three related ancillary agreements [the "Arrangement"], constitutes grounds for the imposition of sanctions under the exclusion authority at section 1128(b)(7) of the Social Security Act [the "Act"] or the civil monetary penalty provision at section 1128A(a)(7) of the Act, as those sections relate to the commission of acts described in section 1128B(b) of the Act)

October 5, 2001 Advisory Opinion No. 01-16—(concerning a managed care organization's employment of an excluded individual and potential sanctions under section 1320a-7a(a)(6) of the SSA)

September 27, 2001 Advisory Opinion No. 01-15—(concerning a managed care organization's proposal to subsidize the Medicare+Choice premiums and copayments of its members eligible for both Medicare and certain limited Medicaid benefits)

September 4, 2001 Advisory Opinion No. 01-14—(concerning a hospital's policy of waiving out-of-pocket copayments and deductibles for screening services and certain follow-up services that the hospital offers to promote early detection of breast and gynecological cancers)

August 24, 2001 Advisory Opinion No. 01-13—(concerning the "coordination of benefits" provisions of a provider agreement between . . . a health maintenance organization or "HMO", and the skilled nursing facilities in its provider network [the "Nursing Facilities"])

August 24, 2001 Final Notice of Modification of OIG Advisory Opinion No. 98-5—(concerning Advisory Opinion No. 98-5, which was issued on April 17, 1998. In OIG Advisory Opinion No. 98-5, we concluded that the Requestor's contract with a managed care organization [in particular, its coordination of benefits provision, hereafter the "COB provision"] could violate the anti-kickback statute, and we could not conclude that the COB provision posed little or no risk of Federal health care program fraud and abuse.)

July 26, 2001 Advisory Opinion No. 01-12—(concerning an exclusive contract between a city and an ambulance company for the provision of emergency medical services for city residents that includes a requirement that the contracting ambulance company waive out-of pocket Medicare copayments for city residents)

July 26, 2001 Advisory Opinion No. 01-11—(concerning a municipal corporation that owns and operates an ambulance service and that treats the operating revenues received from local taxes as payment of otherwise applicable copayments and deductibles due from the residents)

July 26, 2001 Advisory Opinion No. 01-10—(concerning a political subdivision of a State that owns and operates an ambulance service and that treats the operating revenues received from local taxes as payment of otherwise applicable copayments and deductibles due from the residents)

July 26, 2001 Advisory Opinion No. 01-09—(concerning a proposed grant from a hospital to a community health center to defray the costs of providing services to uninsured patients)

July 10, 2001 Advisory Opinion No. 01-8—(concerns a comprehensive program that a manufacturer of therapeutic mattresses and other support services markets and sells to State-licensed nursing facilities to manage pressure ulcers)

July 3, 2001 Advisory Opinion No. 01-7—(concerning the practice of accepting reimbursement from third-party payers plus certain payments)

May 29, 2001 Advisory Opinion No. 01-6—(concerning "payments by vendors to a group purchasing organization [GPO] owned by entities affiliated with health care providers that purchase items covered by the GPO's vendor contracts")

May 23, 2001 Advisory Opinion No. 01-5—(concerning "a proposed lease of cardiac diagnostic equipment to emergency medical services providers for a nominal charge")

May 10, 2001 Advisory Opinion No. 01-4—(concerning "a proposed arrangement between a hospital and a new physician whom the hospital would like to recruit to practice within its service area")

May 10, 2001 Advisory Opinion No. 01-3—(concerning "whether proposed contracts for discounted services between a Federally-recognized Indian tribe and local hospitals would constitute grounds for the imposition of exclusions under section 1128(b)(7) of the Act or civil money penalties under section 1128A(a)(7) of the Act")

March 27, 2001 Advisory Opinion No. 01-2—(concerning an annual charity golf tournament for which some of its vendors and suppliers pay money as sponsors and tournament participants)

January 18, 2001 Advisory Opinion No. 01-1—(concerning a proposed arrangement in which a hospital will share with a group of cardiac surgeons a percentage of the hospital's cost savings)

2000 Advisory Opinions

December 28, 2000 Advisory Opinion No. 00-11—(regarding approval of a charitable donation from a hospital to a volunteer emergency medical services provider to pay for new equipment and paramedic training)

December 28, 2000 Advisory Opinion No. 00-10—(regarding a program designed by a drug manufacturer to promote an expensive new drug used to prevent certain respiratory infections in pediatric patients)

December 21, 2000 Advisory Opinion No. 00-09—(whether a hospital proposal to provide free restocking of medical supplies and drugs for volunteer emergency medical services would violate the anti-kickback statute)

December 21, 2000 Advisory Opinion No. 00-8—(concerning whether a housing referral for the elderly would be subject to sanctions arising under the anti-kickback statute)

November 24, 2000 Advisory Opinion No. 00-7—(regarding free transportation services that a hospital offers to certain patients who have been referred to the hospital for extended courses of treatment involving)

October 6, 2000 Advisory Opinion No. 00-6—(concerning proposed donation of its ownership interest in a portion of a medical office building to an agency of the State for use by the Medical School)

July 7, 2000 Advisory Opinion No. 00-5—(whether waiving Medicare Part A and Part B copayment and deductible obligations for participants in a clinical study sponsored by the Health Care Financing Administration and the National Heart, Lung, and Blood Institute)

June 27, 2000 Advisory Opinion No. 00-4—(concerning a lifestyle modification program for individuals with chronic disease that uses physicians to monitor and evaluate the program's participants)

April 18, 2000 Advisory Opinion No. 00-3—(concerning an arrangement to provide various services free of charge to patients with terminal illnesses)

April 18, 2000 Advisory Opinion No. 00-2—(about a proposed cost-savings program pursuant to which (the Hospital) would reward its nonphysician employees for submitting cost-savings suggestions)

March 16, 2000 Advisory Opinion No. 00-1—(concerning a consulting firm's contractual payment arrangements for the performance of auditing services to identify hospital undercharges and overcharges associated with private payers)

1999 Advisory Opinions

December 7, 1999 Advisory Opinion No. 99-13—(regarding certain arrangements for discounted pathology services provided to physicians)

December 6, 1999 Advisory Opinion No. 99-12—(a proposed marketing program involving the use of physician practices and health care clinics to distribute coupons redeemable by certain retailers [including grocery stores, pharmacies, and Internet companies] for discounts on items or services that are not reimbursable by any Federal health care program)

November 1, 1999 Advisory Opinion No. 99-11—(concerning an arrangement sponsored by Coalition A [the "Coalition"] to provide psychotherapy services at free or reduced prices using residents from local teaching facilities as clinicians [the "Arrangement"])

November 1, 1999 Advisory Opinion No. 99-10—(concerning a corporate sponsorship program between Drug Company A ["Company A"] and Charity B ["Charity B"] [the "Proposed Arrangement"])

October 7, 1999 Advisory Opinion No. 99-9—(a proposed contractual arrangement between a self-insured employer health plan and a single-specialty managed care organization to provide managed podiatry benefits for the employer's retirees)

July 13, 1999 Advisory Opinion No. 99-8—(whether an arrangement to provide for personal appearances by podiatrists to certain retail stores constitutes grounds for sanctions under the anti-kickback statute)

July 8, 1999 Advisory Opinion No. 99-7—(whether an across-the-board waiver of any out-of-pocket beneficiary copayments for medical services covered by the national Eye Care Project constitutes grounds for the imposition of a sanction under section 1128A[a][5] of the Act)

April 14, 1999 Advisory Opinion No. 99-6—(whether the longstanding policy of a hospital, specializing in pediatric oncology research, of not billing its patients for any amounts associated with their treatment, including copayment amounts)

April 8, 1999 Advisory Opinion No. 99-5—(whether an annual fee imposed by city ordinance on ambulance companies wishing to provide ambulance services in the city [the "Ambulance Fee"] constitutes prohibited remuneration under the anti-kickback statute, section 1128B[b] of the Social Security Act [the "Act"], and, if so, whether the Ambulance Fee assessment constitutes grounds for the imposition of sanctions)

April 8, 1999 Advisory Opinion No. 99-4—(whether a proposed agreement [the "Proposed Agreement"], pursuant to which Hospital District No. 1 ["District One" or the "Requestor"] would locate a medical clinic within the geographic boundaries of Hospital District No. 2 ["District Two"], would constitute grounds for sanctions under the anti-kickback statute, section 1128B[b] of the Social Security Act [the "Act"], the exclusion authority for kickbacks)

March 23, 1999 Advisory Opinion No. 99-3—(whether a proposed pricing arrangement for a package of therapeutic mattresses for SNF patients to be marketed by a company, and certain commissioned agents, would result in prohibited remuneration under the anti-kickback statute)

March 4, 1999 Advisory Opinion No. 99-2—(whether certain arrangements for discounted ambulance services provided to residents of Medicare skilled nursing facilities would result in prohibited remuneration and sanctions under the anti-kickback statute)

January 27, 1999 Advisory Opinion No. 99-1—(whether the Arrangement constitutes prohibited remuneration within the meaning of the anti-kickback statute, section 1128B[b] of the Social Security Act [the "Act"])

1998 Advisory Opinions

March 19, 1998 Advisory Opinion No. 98-1 pdf—(whether a contractual arrangement for distribution and billing services between Company A and Company B [the "Arrangement"] constitutes grounds for sanction under the anti-kickback statute)

April 8, 1998 Advisory Opinion No. 98-2 pdf—(certain pharmaceutical discount pricing arrangements that are limited to arrangements between a manufacturer and wholesalers [the "Proposed Arrangement"] will subject you to sanction under the anti-kickback statute)

April 14, 1998 Advisory Opinion No. 98-3 pdf—(whether a hospital system's provision of an ambulance to a municipal fire department as described in your request)

April 14, 1998 Advisory Opinion No. 98-4 pdf—(whether a proposed management services contract between a medical practice management company and a physician practice, which provides that the management company will be reimbursed for its costs and paid a percentage of net practice revenues)

April 24, 1998 Advisory Opinion No. 98-5 pdf—(which seeks our opinion regarding the "coordination of benefits" ["COB"] provisions of a provider agreement between Nursing Home A [the "Nursing Home"] and a health care plan)

April 24, 1998 Advisory Opinion No. 98-6 pdf—(whether waiving coinsurance obligations for participants in a clinical study sponsored by the Health Care Financing Administration and the National Heart, Lung, and Blood Institute [the "Proposed Arrangement"])

June 11, 1998 Advisory Opinion No. 98-7 pdf—(whether an ambulance restocking and continuing education arrangement [the "Arrangement"] constitutes prohibited remuneration under the anti-kickback statute, section 1128B[b] of the Social Security Act [the "Act"])

July 6, 1998 Advisory Opinion No. 98-8 pdf—(whether Company A ["Company A"], a wholly-owned subsidiary of Company B ["Company B"] [collectively referred to as "Company AB"] would be subject to exclusion from Federal health care programs pursuant to 42 U.S.C. §1320a-7[b])

July 13, 1998 Advisory Opinion No. 98-9—(whether a compensation arrangement for registered nurses and certain other employees pursuant to a collective bargaining agreement with the nurses' union)

September 8, 1998 Advisory Opinion No. 98-10—(whether the payment of a sales commission to an independent manufacturers' representative [the "Arrangement"] constitutes grounds for sanctions under the anti-kickback statute, section 1128B[b] of the Social Security Act [the "Act"])

September 21, 1998 Advisory Opinion No. 98-11—(whether a proposed purchasing arrangement involving a trade association, its nursing home members, and an electrical utility consultant [the "Proposed Arrangement"] constitutes prohibited remuneration under the anti-kickback statute, section 1128B[b] of the Social Security Act [the "Act"])

September 23, 1998 Advisory Opinion No. 98-12—(whether a proposed joint venture among several orthopedic surgeons and anesthesiologists specializing in pain management to establish an ambulatory surgical center, as described in your request letter and supplemental submissions [the "Proposed Arrangement"], would generate prohibited remuneration.)

September 30, 1998 Advisory Opinion No. 98-13—(whether an ambulance restocking program, coordinated through a local emergency medical services council [the "Program"], constitutes prohibited remuneration under the anti-kickback statute, section 1128B[b] of the Social Security Act [the "Act"], and, if so, whether the Program constitutes grounds for the imposition of sanctions under the antikickback statute)

October 28, 1998 Advisory Opinion No. 98-14—(whether an existing pharmaceutical restocking program [the "Drug Program"] and a proposed medical supplies restocking program [the "Supply Program"] [collectively, the "Arrangements"] constitute prohibited remuneration under the anti-kickback statute, section 1128B[b] of the Social Security Act [the "Act"])

November 10, 1998 Advisory Opinion No. 98-15—(whether an arrangement for contracted pharmacy services between University A and Pharmacy Company B to facilitate an outpatient pharmacy program for the University's hemophilia center pursuant to section 340B of the Public Health Service Act [the "Proposed Arrangement"] would constitute grounds for sanctions under the anti-kickback statute)

November 10, 1998 Advisory Opinion No. 98-16—(whether a proposed arrangement under which [name redacted] would assign an employee pharmacist to work in designated hospital transplant centers for the purpose of providing pharmacy-related products and services [the "Proposed Arrangement"] would constitute prohibited remuneration under the anti-kickback statute)

November 13, 1998 Advisory Opinion No. 98-17—(whether donations by Company X ["Company X"] to Organization A ["Organization A"] [an independent, 501(c)(3) charitable organization] for the purpose of funding a program to pay for Supplementary Medical Insurance ["Medicare Part B"] or Medicare Supplementary Health Insurance ["Medigap"] premiums for financially needy Medicare beneficiaries with end-stage renal disease)

December 3, 1998 Advisory Opinion No. 98-18—(whether an ophthalmologist's proposed sublease to an optometrist of certain imaging equipment [the "Sublease"] would meet the criteria of the equipment rental safe harbor, 42 C.F.R. §1001.952[c])

December 21, 1998 Advisory Opinion No. 98-19—(whether an arrangement whereby an independent physician association would acquire an equity interest in a managed care organization would constitute grounds for the imposition of sanctions under the anti-kickback statute, section 1128B[b] of the Social Security Act [the "Act"], the exclusion authority for kickbacks)

1997 Advisory Opinions

June 11, 1997 Advisory Opinion No. 97-1 pdf—(it is permissible for a charitable organization partly funded by kidney dialysis providers to pay Medicare Part B, Medigap and other health insurance premiums for end-stage renal disease patients who are financially needy) Media Advisory

July 28, 1997 Advisory Opinion No. 97-2 pdf—(asks whether a state-funded program that pays for insurance premiums for financially needy Medicare beneficiaries with end-stage renal disease would constitute grounds for the imposition of a civil monetary penalty under Section 231[h] of the Health Insurance Portability and Accountability Act of 1996)

August 22, 1997 Advisory Opinion No. 97-3 pdf—(asks whether Mrs. P's transfer of assets to her nephew, Mr. S, and subsequent application for Medicaid benefits, subjects her to sanction under 42 U.S.C. 1320a-7b[a][6], which prohibits certain dispositions of assets for the purpose of qualifying for Medicaid)

October 2, 1997 Advisory Opinion No. 97-4 pdf—(asks whether declining to pursue collection of copayments from certain patients who have employer-sponsored Medicare complementary coverage constitutes grounds for imposition of sanctions under Section 231[h] of the Health Insurance Portability and Accountability Act ["HIPAA"] [42 U.S.C. §1320a-7a(a)(5)] or under Sections 1128B[b] [the anti-kickback statute] or 1128A[7] [relating to payment of kickbacks] of the Social Security Act [42 U.S.C. §§1320a-7b(b) and 1320a-7(b)(7)]).

October 15, 1997 Advisory Opinion No. 97-5 pdf—(asks whether an outpatient radiology imaging center joint venture owned by a medical group specializing in radiology and a hospital care provider [I] generates prohibited remuneration within the meaning of the anti-kickback statute, Section 1128B of the Social Security Act ["act"]; [ii] constitutes grounds for the imposition of an exclusion under Section 1128[b][7] of the Act [as it applies to kickbacks]; [iii] constitutes grounds for criminal sanctions under Section 1128B[b] of the Act; and/or [iv] satisfies the criteria set out in Section 1128B[b][3] of the Act or associated regulations, 42 C.F.R. §1001.952)

October 20, 1997 Advisory Opinion No. 97-6 pdf—(asks whether a proposed arrangement for restocking ambulance supplies and medications [the "Proposed Arrangement"] would constitute illegal remuneration as defined in the antikickback statute, 42 U.S.C. §1320a-7b[b])

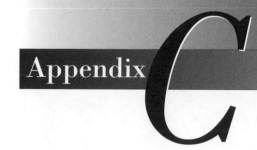

OIG Compliance Program Guidance for Individual and Small Group Physician Practices

This appendix includes the OIG *Compliance Program Guidance for Individual and Small Group Physician Practices* and the press release announcing its publication.

In addition to compliance guidance, the document also discusses some of the areas of fraud and abuse that are of concern to the OIG.

Note: In this revised edition, some Web site addresses provided in the original 9/25/2000 *Federal Register* document have been changed to reflect current government internet locations.

Office of Inspector General
Public Affairs

330 Independence Ave., SW
Washington, DC 20201

NEWS RELEASE

FOR IMMEDIATE RELEASE
Monday, September 25, 2000
Contact: Judy Holtz (202) 619-0260
or Ben St. John (202) 619-1028

Inspector General Issues Voluntary Compliance
Program Guidance for Physician Practices

The Department of Health and Human Services' Office of Inspector General ("OIG")
today issued final guidance to help physicians in individual and small group practices
design voluntary compliance programs.

"The intent of the guidance is to provide a roadmap to develop a voluntary compliance
program that best fits the needs of that individual practice. The guidance itself provides
great flexibility as to how a physician practice could implement compliance efforts in a
manner that fits with the practice's existing operations and resources," Inspector
General June Gibbs Brown said.

The final guidance—Compliance Program Guidance for Individual and Small Group
Physician Practices—is scheduled for publication this week as a Federal Register notice
and is being posted today on the OIG website. Inspector General Brown further com-
mented, "We are encouraging physician practices to adopt the active application of compliance principles in their practice, rather than implement rigid, costly, formal procedures.
Our goal in issuing this final guidance was to show physician practices that compliance
can become a part of the practice culture without the practice having to expend substantial monetary or time resources."

The OIG believes the great majority of physicians are honest and committed to providing
high quality medical care to Medicare beneficiaries.

Under the law, physicians are not subject to civil, administrative or criminal penalties for
innocent errors, or even negligence. The Government's primary enforcement tool, the
civil False Claims Act, covers only offenses that are committed with actual knowledge of
the falsity of the claim, reckless disregard or deliberate ignorance of the truth or falsity of
a claim. The False Claims Act does not cover mistakes, errors or negligence. The OIG is
very mindful of the difference between innocent errors ("erroneous claims") and reckless or intentional conduct ("fraudulent claims").

A voluntary compliance program can help physicians identify both erroneous and fraudulent claims and help ensure that submitted claims are true and accurate. It can also help
the practice by speeding up and optimizing proper payment of claims, minimizing billing
mistakes and avoiding conflicts with the self-referral and anti-kickback statutes.

Unlike other guidance previously issued by the OIG, the final physician guidance does not suggest that physician practices implement all seven standard components of a full scale compliance program. While the seven components provide a solid basis upon which a physician practice can create a compliance program, the OIG acknowledges that full implementation of all components may not be feasible for smaller physician practices. Instead, the guidance emphasizes a step by step approach for those practices to follow in developing and implementing a voluntary compliance program. As a first step, physician practices can begin by identifying risk areas which, based on a practice's specific history with billing problems and other compliance issues, might benefit from closer scrutiny and corrective/educational measures.

The step by step approach is as follows: 1) conducting internal monitoring and auditing through the performance of periodic audits; 2) implementing compliance and practice standards through the development of written standards and procedures; 3) designating a compliance officer or contact(s) to monitor compliance efforts and enforce practice standards; 4) conducting appropriate training and education on practice standards and procedures; 5) responding appropriately to detected violations through the investigation of allegations and the disclosure of incidents to appropriate Government entities; 6) developing open lines of communication, such as discussions at staff meetings regarding erroneous or fraudulent conduct issues and community bulletin boards, to keep practice employees updated regarding compliance activities; and 7) enforcing disciplinary standards through well-publicized guidelines.

The final guidance identifies four specific compliance risk areas for physicians: 1) proper coding and billing; 2) ensuring that services are reasonable and necessary; 3) proper documentation; and 4) avoiding improper inducements, kickbacks and self-referrals. These risk areas reflect areas in which the OIG has focused its investigations and audits related to physician practices.

Recognizing the financial and staffing resource constraints faced by physician practices, the final guidance stresses flexibility in the manner a practice implements voluntary compliance measures. The OIG encourages physician practices to participate in the compliance programs of other providers, such as hospitals or other settings in which the physicians practice. A physician practice's participation in such compliance programs could be a way, at least partly, to augment the practice's own compliance efforts.

The final guidance also provides direction to larger practices in developing compliance programs by recommending that they use both the physician guidance and previously issued guidance, such as the Third-Party Medical Billing Company Compliance Program Guidance or the Clinical Laboratory Compliance Program Guidance, to create a compliance program that meets the needs of the larger practice.

The final guidance includes several appendices outlining additional risk areas about which various physicians expressed interest, as well as information about criminal, civil and administrative statutes related to the Federal health care programs. There is also information about the OIG's provider self-disclosure protocol and Internet resources that may be useful to physician practices.

###

Note: The final physician guidance is available on the Office of Inspector General Web site at http://oig.hhs.gov/authorities/docs/physician.pdf.

OIG Compliance Program Guidance for Individual and Small Group Physician Practices

The compliance program guidance below is available at the OIG Web site, http://oig.hhs.gov.

The Office of Inspector General
Compliance Program Guidance for Individual and
Small Group Physician Practices

September 2000

Table Of Contents

Office of Inspector General's Compliance Program Guidance for Individual and Small Group Physician Practices

I. Introduction

This compliance program guidance is intended to assist individual and small group physician practices ("physician practices")[1] in developing a voluntary compliance program that promotes adherence to statutes and regulations applicable to the Federal health care programs ("Federal health care program requirements"). The goal of voluntary compliance programs is to provide a tool to strengthen the efforts of health care providers to prevent and reduce improper conduct. These programs can also benefit physician practices[2] by helping to streamline business operations.

Many physicians have expressed an interest in better protecting their practices from the potential for erroneous or fraudulent conduct through the implementation of voluntary compliance programs. The Office of Inspector General (OIG) believes that the great majority of physicians are honest and share our goal of protecting the integrity of Medicare and other Federal health care programs. To that

end, all health care providers have a duty to ensure that the claims submitted to Federal health care programs are true and accurate. The development of voluntary compliance programs and the active application of compliance principles in physician practices will go a long way toward achieving this goal.

Through this document, the OIG provides its views on the fundamental components of physician practice compliance programs, as well as the principles that a physician practice might consider when developing and implementing a voluntary compliance program. While this document presents basic procedural and structural guidance for designing a voluntary compliance program, it is not in and of itself a compliance program. Indeed, as recognized by the OIG and the health care industry, there is no "one size fits all" compliance program, especially for physician practices. Rather, it is a set of guidelines that physician practices can consider if they choose to develop and implement a compliance program.

As with the OIG's previous guidance,[3] these guidelines are not mandatory. Nor do they represent an all-inclusive document containing all components of a compliance program. Other OIG outreach efforts, as well as other Federal agency efforts to promote compliance,[4] can also be used in developing a compliance program. However, as explained later, if a physician practice adopts a voluntary and active compliance program, it may well lead to benefits for the physician practice.

A. Scope of the Voluntary Compliance Program Guidance

This guidance focuses on voluntary compliance measures related to claims submitted to the Federal health care programs. Issues related to private payor claims may also be covered by a compliance plan if the physician practice so desires.

The guidance is also limited in scope by focusing on the development of voluntary compliance programs for individual and small group physician practices. The difference between a small practice and a large practice cannot be determined by stating a particular number of physicians. Instead, our intent in narrowing the guidance to the small practices subset was to provide guidance to those physician practices whose financial or staffing resources would not allow them to implement a full scale, institutionally structured compliance program as set forth in the Third Party Medical Billing Guidance or other previously released OIG guidance. A compliance program can be an important tool for physician practices of all sizes and does not have to be costly, resource-intensive or time-intensive.

B. Benefits of a Voluntary Compliance Program

The OIG acknowledges that patient care is, and should be, the first priority of a physician practice. However, a practice's focus on patient care can be enhanced by the adoption of a voluntary compliance program. For example, the increased accuracy of documentation that may result from a compliance program will actually assist in enhancing patient care. The OIG believes that physician practices can realize numerous other benefits by implementing a compliance program. A well-designed compliance program can:

- speed and optimize proper payment of claims;

- minimize billing mistakes;

- reduce the chances that an audit will be conducted by HCFA or the OIG; and

- avoid conflicts with the self-referral and anti-kickback statutes.

The incorporation of compliance measures into a physician practice should not be at the expense of patient care, but instead should augment the ability of the physician practice to provide quality patient care.

Voluntary compliance programs also provide benefits by not only helping to prevent erroneous or fraudulent claims, but also by showing that the physician practice is making additional good faith efforts to submit claims appropriately. Physicians should view compliance programs as analogous to practicing preventive medicine for their practice. Practices that embrace the active application of compliance principles in their practice culture and put efforts towards compliance on a continued basis can help to prevent problems from occurring in the future.

A compliance program also sends an important message to a physician practice's employees that while the practice recognizes that mistakes will occur, employees have an affirmative, ethical duty to come forward and report erroneous or fraudulent conduct, so that it may be corrected.

C. Application of Voluntary Compliance Program Guidance

The applicability of these recommendations will depend on the circumstances and resources of the particular physician practice. Each physician practice can undertake reasonable steps to implement compliance measures, depending on the size and resources of that practice. Physician practices can rely, at least in part, upon standard protocols and current practice procedures to develop an appropriate compliance program for that practice. In fact, many physician practices already have established the framework of a compliance program without referring to it as such.

D. The Difference Between "Erroneous" and "Fraudulent" Claims To Federal Health Programs

There appear to be significant misunderstandings within the physician community regarding the critical differences between what the government views as innocent "erroneous" claims on the one hand and "fraudulent" (intentionally or recklessly false) health care claims on the other. Some physicians feel that Federal law enforcement agencies have maligned medical professionals, in part, by a perceived focus on innocent billing errors. These physicians are under the impression that innocent billing errors can subject them to civil penalties, or even jail. These impressions are mistaken.

To address these concerns, the OIG would like to emphasize the following points. First, the OIG does not disparage physicians, other medical professionals or medical enterprises. In our view, the great majority of physicians are working ethically to render high quality medical care and to submit proper claims.

Second, under the law, physicians are not subject to criminal, civil or administrative penalties for innocent errors, or even negligence. The Government's primary enforcement tool, the civil False Claims Act, covers only offenses that are committed with actual knowledge of the falsity of the claim, reckless disregard, or deliberate ignorance of the falsity of the claim.[5] The False Claims Act does not encompass mistakes, errors, or negligence. The Civil Monetary Penalties Law, an administrative remedy, similar in scope and effect to the False Claims Act, has exactly the same standard of proof.[6] The OIG is very mindful of the difference between innocent errors ("erroneous claims") on one hand, and reckless or intentional conduct ("fraudulent claims") on the other. For criminal penalties, the standard is even higher—criminal intent to defraud must be proved beyond a reasonable doubt.

Third, even ethical physicians (and their staffs) make billing mistakes and errors through inadvertence or negligence. When physicians discover that their billing errors, honest mistakes, or negligence result in erroneous claims, the physician practice should return the funds erroneously claimed, but without penalties. In other words, absent a violation of a civil, criminal or administrative law, erroneous claims result only in the return of funds claimed in error.

Fourth, innocent billing errors are a significant drain on the Federal health care programs. All parties (physicians, providers, carriers, fiscal intermediaries, Government agencies, and beneficiaries) need to work cooperatively to reduce the overall error rate.

Finally, it is reasonable for physicians (and other providers) to ask: what duty do they owe the Federal health care programs" The answer is that all health care providers have a duty to reasonably ensure that the claims submitted to Medicare and other Federal health care programs are true and accurate. The OIG continues to engage the provider community in an extensive, good faith effort to work cooperatively on voluntary compliance to minimize errors and to prevent potential penalties for improper billings before they occur. We encourage all physicians and other providers to join in this effort.

II. Developing a Voluntary Compliance Program

A. The Seven Basic Components of a Voluntary Compliance Program

The OIG believes that a basic framework for any voluntary compliance program begins with a review of the seven basic components of an effective compliance program. A review of these components provides physician practices with an overview of the scope of a fully developed and implemented compliance program. The following list of components, as set forth in previous OIG compliance program guidances, can form the basis of a voluntary compliance program for a physician practice:

- conducting internal monitoring and auditing through the performance of periodic audits;

- implementing compliance and practice standards through the development of written standards and procedures;

- designating a compliance officer or contact(s) to monitor compliance efforts and enforce practice standards;

- conducting appropriate training and education on practice standards and procedures;

- responding appropriately to detected violations through the investigation of allegations and the disclosure of incidents to appropriate Government entities;

- developing open lines of communication, such as (1) discussions at staff meetings regarding how to avoid erroneous or fraudulent conduct and (2) community bulletin boards, to keep practice employees updated regarding compliance activities; and

- enforcing disciplinary standards through well-publicized guidelines.

These seven components provide a solid basis upon which a physician practice can create a compliance program. The OIG acknowledges that full implementation of all components may not be feasible for all physician practices. Some physician practices may never fully implement all of the components. However, as a first step, physician practices can begin by adopting only those components which, based on a practice's specific history with billing problems and other compliance issues, are most likely to provide an identifiable benefit.

The extent of implementation will depend on the size and resources of the practice. Smaller physician practices may incorporate each of the components in a manner that best suits the practice. By contrast, larger physician practices often have the means to incorporate the components in a more systematic manner. For example, larger physician practices can use both this guidance and the Third-Party Medical Billing Compliance Program Guidance, which provides a more detailed compliance program structure, to create a compliance program unique to the practice.

The OIG recognizes that physician practices need to find the best way to achieve compliance for their given circumstances. Specifically, the OIG encourages physician practices to participate in other provider's compliance programs, such as the compliance programs of the hospitals or other settings in which the physicians practice. Physician Practice Management companies also may serve as a source of compliance program guidance. A physician practice's participation in such compliance programs could be a way, at least partly, to augment the practice's own compliance efforts.

The opportunities for collaborative compliance efforts could include participating in training and education programs or using another entity's policies and procedures as a template from which the physician practice creates its own version. The OIG encourages this type of collaborative effort, where the content is appropriate to the setting involved (i.e., the training is relevant to physician practices as well as the sponsoring provider), because it provides a means to promote the desired objective without imposing excessive burdens on the practice or requiring physicians to undertake duplicative action. However, to prevent possible anti-kickback or self-referral issues, the OIG recommends that physicians consider limiting their participation in a sponsoring provider's compliance program to the areas of training and education or policies and procedures.

The key to avoiding possible conflicts is to ensure that the entity providing compliance services to a physician practice (its referral source) is not perceived as nor is it operating the practice compliance program at no charge. For example, if the sponsoring entity conducted claims review for the physician practice as part of a compliance program or provided compliance oversight without charging the practice fair market value for those services, the anti-kickback and Stark self-referral laws would be implicated. The payment of fair market value by referral sources for compliance services will generally address these concerns.

B. Steps for Implementing a Voluntary Compliance Program

As previously discussed, implementing a voluntary compliance program can be a multi-tiered process. Initial development of the compliance program can be focused on practice risk areas that have been problematic for the practice such as coding and billing. Within this area, the practice should examine its claims denial history or claims that have resulted in repeated overpayments, and identify and correct the most frequent sources of those denials or overpayments. A review of claim denials will help the practice scrutinize a significant risk area and improve its cash flow by submitting correct claims that will be paid the first time they are submitted. As this example illustrates, a compliance program for a physician practice often makes sound business sense.

The following is a suggested order of the steps a practice could take to begin the development of a compliance program. The steps outlined below articulate all seven components of a compliance program and there are numerous suggestions for implementation within each component. Physician practices should keep in mind, as stated earlier, that it is up to the practice to determine the manner in which and the extent to which the practice chooses to implement these voluntary measures.

Step One: Auditing and Monitoring

An ongoing evaluation process is important to a successful compliance program. This ongoing evaluation includes not only whether the physician practice's standards and procedures are in fact current and accurate, but also whether the compliance program is working, i.e., whether individuals are properly carrying out their responsibilities and claims are submitted appropriately. Therefore, an audit is an excellent way for a physician practice to ascertain what, if any, problem areas exist and focus on the risk areas that are associated with those problems. There are two types of reviews that can be performed as part of this evaluation: (1) a standards and procedures review; and (2) a claims submission audit.

1. Standards and procedures

It is recommended that an individual(s) in the physician practice be charged with the responsibility of periodically reviewing the practice's standards and procedures to determine if they are current and complete. If the standards and procedures are found to be ineffective or outdated, they should be updated to reflect changes in

Government regulations or compendiums generally relied upon by physicians and insurers (i.e., changes in Current Procedural Terminology (CPT) and ICD-9-CM codes).

2. Claims Submission Audit

In addition to the standards and procedures themselves, it is advisable that bills and medical records be reviewed for compliance with applicable coding, billing and documentation requirements. The individuals from the physician practice involved in these self-audits would ideally include the person in charge of billing (if the practice has such a person) and a medically trained person (e.g., registered nurse or preferably a physician (physicians can rotate in this position)). Each physician practice needs to decide for itself whether to review claims retrospectively or concurrently with the claims submission. In the Third-Party Medical Billing Compliance Program Guidance, the OIG recommended that a baseline, or "snapshot," be used to enable a practice to judge over time its progress in reducing or eliminating potential areas of vulnerability. This practice, known as "benchmarking," allows a practice to chart its compliance efforts by showing a reduction or increase in the number of claims paid and denied. The practice's self-audits can be used to determine whether:

- bills are accurately coded and accurately reflect the services provided (as documented in the medical records);

- documentation is being completed correctly;

- services or items provided are reasonable and necessary; and

- any incentives for unnecessary services exist.

A baseline audit examines the claim development and submission process, from patient intake through claim submission and payment, and identifies elements within this process that may contribute to non-compliance or that may need to be the focus for improving execution.[7] This audit will establish a consistent methodology for selecting and examining records, and this methodology will then serve as a basis for future audits.

There are many ways to conduct a baseline audit. The OIG recommends that claims/services that were submitted and paid during the initial three months after implementation of the education and training program be examined, so as to give the physician practice a benchmark against which to measure future compliance effectiveness.

Following the baseline audit, a general recommendation is that periodic audits be conducted at least once each

year to ensure that the compliance program is being followed. Optimally, a randomly selected number of medical records could be reviewed to ensure that the coding was performed accurately. Although there is no set formula to how many medical records should be reviewed, a basic guide is five or more medical records per Federal payor (i.e., Medicare, Medicaid), or five to ten medical records per physician. The OIG realizes that physician practices receive reimbursement from a number of different payors, and we would encourage a physician practice's auditing/monitoring process to consist of a review of claims from all Federal payors from which the practice receives reimbursement. Of course, the larger the sample size, the larger the comfort level the physician practice will have about the results. However, the OIG is aware that this may be burdensome for some physician practices, so, at a minimum, we would encourage the physician practice to conduct a review of claims that have been reimbursed by Federal health care programs.

If problems are identified, the physician practice will need to determine whether a focused review should be conducted on a more frequent basis. When audit results reveal areas needing additional information or education of employees and physicians, the physician practice will need to analyze whether these areas should be incorporated into the training and educational system.

There are many ways to identify the claims/services from which to draw the random sample of claims to be audited. One methodology is to choose a random sample of claims/services from either all of the claims/services a physician has received reimbursement for or all claims/services from a particular payor. Another method is to identify risk areas or potential billing vulnerabilities. The codes associated with these risk areas may become the universe of claims/services from which to select the sample. The OIG recommends that the physician practice evaluate claims/services selected to determine if the codes billed and reimbursed were accurately ordered, performed, and reasonable and necessary for the treatment of the patient.

One of the most important components of a successful compliance audit protocol is an appropriate response when the physician practice identifies a problem. This action should be taken as soon as possible after the date the problem is identified. The specific action a physician practice takes should depend on the circumstances of the situation. In some cases, the response can be as straight forward as generating a repayment with appropriate explanation to Medicare or the appropriate payor from which the overpayment was received. In others, the physician practice may want to consult with a coding/billing expert to determine the next best course of action. There is no boilerplate solution to how to handle problems that are identified.

It is a good business practice to create a system to address how physician practices will respond to and report potential problems. In addition, preserving information relating to identification of the problem is as important as preserving information that tracks the physician practice's reaction to, and solution for, the issue.

Step Two: Establish Practice Standards and Procedures
After the internal audit identifies the practice's risk areas, the next step is to develop a method for dealing with those risk areas through the practice's standards and procedures. Written standards and procedures are a central component of any compliance program. Those standards and procedures help to reduce the prospect of erroneous claims and fraudulent activity by identifying risk areas for the practice and establishing tighter internal controls to counter those risks, while also helping to identify any aberrant billing practices. Many physician practices already have something similar to this called "practice standards" that include practice policy statements regarding patient care, personnel matters and practice standards and procedures on complying with Federal and State law.

The OIG believes that written standards and procedures can be helpful to all physician practices, regardless of size and capability. If a lack of resources to develop such standards and procedures is genuinely an issue, the OIG recommends that a physician practice focus first on those risk areas most likely to arise in its particular practice.[8] Additionally, if the physician practice works with a physician practice management company (PPMC), independent practice association (IPA), physician-hospital organization, management services organization (MSO) or third-party billing company, the practice can incorporate the compliance standards and procedures of those entities, if appropriate, into its own standards and procedures. Many physician practices have found that the adoption of a third party's compliance standards and procedures, as appropriate, has many benefits and the result is a consistent set of standards and procedures for a community of physicians as well as having just one entity that can then monitor and refine the process as needed. This sharing of compliance responsibilities assists physician practices in rural areas that do not have the staff to perform these functions, but do belong to a group that does have the resources. Physician practices using another entity's compliance materials will need to tailor those materials to the physician practice where they will be applied.

Physician practices that do not have standards or procedures in place can develop them by: (1) developing a written standards and procedures manual; and (2) updating clinical forms periodically to make sure they facilitate and encourage clear and complete documentation of patient care. A practice's standards could also identify the clinical protocol(s), pathway(s), and other treatment guidelines followed by the practice.

Creating a resource manual from publicly available information may be a cost-effective approach for developing additional standards and procedures. For example, the practice can develop a "binder" that contains the practice's written standards and procedures, relevant HCFA directives and carrier bulletins, and summaries of informative OIG documents (e.g., Special Fraud Alerts, Advisory Opinions, inspection and audit reports).[9] If the practice chooses to adopt this idea, the binder should be updated as appropriate and located in a readily accessible location.

If updates to the standards and procedures are necessary, those updates should be communicated to employees to keep them informed regarding the practice's operations. New employees can be made aware of the standards and procedures when hired and can be trained on their contents as part of their orientation to the practice. The OIG recommends that the communication of updates and training of new employees occur as soon as possible after either the issuance of a new update or the hiring of a new employee.

1. Specific Risk Areas
The OIG recognizes that many physician practices may not have in place standards and procedures to prevent erroneous or fraudulent conduct in their practices. In order to develop standards and procedures, the physician practice may consider what types of fraud and abuse related topics need to be addressed based on its specific needs. One of the most important things in making that determination is a listing of risk areas where the practice may be vulnerable.

To assist physician practices in performing this initial assessment, the OIG has developed a list of four potential risk areas affecting physician practices. These risk areas include: (a) coding and billing; (b) reasonable and necessary services; (c) documentation; and (d) improper inducements, kickbacks and self-referrals. This list of risk areas is not exhaustive, or all-encompassing. Rather, it should be viewed as a starting point for an internal review of potential vulnerabilities within the physician practice.[10] The objective of such an assessment is to ensure that key personnel in the physician practice are aware of these major risk areas and that steps are taken to minimize, to the extent possible, the types of problems identified. While there are many ways to accomplish this objective, clear written standards and procedures that are communicated to all employees are important to ensure the effectiveness of a compliance program. Specifically, the following are discussions of risk areas for physician practices:[11]

a. Coding and Billing

A major part of any physician practice's compliance program is the identification of risk areas associated with coding and billing. The following risk areas associated with billing have been among the most frequent subjects of investigations and audits by the OIG:

- billing for items or services not rendered or not provided as claimed;[12]

- submitting claims for equipment, medical supplies and services that are not reasonable and necessary;[13]

- double billing resulting in duplicate payment;[14]

- billing for non-covered services as if covered;[15]

- knowing misuse of provider identification numbers, which results in improper billing;[16]

- unbundling (billing for each component of the service instead of billing or using an all-inclusive code);[17]

- failure to properly use coding modifiers;[18]

- clustering;[19] and

- upcoding the level of service provided.[20]

The physician practice written standards and procedures concerning proper coding reflect the current reimbursement principles set forth in applicable statutes, regulations[21] and Federal, State or private payor health care program requirements and should be developed in tandem with coding and billing standards used in the physician practice. Furthermore, written standards and procedures should ensure that coding and billing are based on medical record documentation. Particular attention should be paid to issues of appropriate diagnosis codes and individual Medicare Part B claims (including documentation guidelines for evaluation and management services).[22] A physician practice can also institute a policy that the coder and/or physician review all rejected claims pertaining to diagnosis and procedure codes. This step can facilitate a reduction in similar errors.

b. Reasonable and Necessary Services

A practice's compliance program may provide guidance that claims are to be submitted only for services that the physician practice finds to be reasonable and necessary in the particular case. The OIG recognizes that physicians should be able to order any tests, including screening tests, they believe are appropriate for the treatment of their patients. However, a physician practice should be aware that Medicare will only pay for services that meet the Medicare definition of reasonable and necessary.[23]

Medicare (and many insurance plans) may deny payment for a service that is not reasonable and necessary according to the Medicare reimbursement rules. Thus, when a physician provides services to a Medicare beneficiary, he or she should only bill those services that meet the Medicare standard of being reasonable and necessary for the diagnosis and treatment of a patient. A physician practice can bill in order to receive a denial for services, but only if the denial is needed for reimbursement from the secondary payor. Upon request, the physician practice should be able to provide documentation, such as a patient's medical records and physician's orders, to support the appropriateness of a service that the physician has provided.

c. Documentation

Timely, accurate and complete documentation is important to clinical patient care. This same documentation serves as a second function when a bill is submitted for payment, namely, as verification that the bill is accurate as submitted. Therefore, one of the most important physician practice compliance issues is the appropriate documentation of diagnosis and treatment. Physician documentation is necessary to determine the appropriate medical treatment for the patient and is the basis for coding and billing determinations. Thorough and accurate documentation also helps to ensure accurate recording and timely transmission of information.

i. Medical Record Documentation
    In addition to facilitating high quality patient care, a properly documented medical record verifies and documents precisely what services were actually provided. The medical record may be used to validate: (a) the site of the service; (b) the appropriateness of the services provided; (c) the accuracy of the billing; and (d) the identity of the care giver (service provider). Examples of internal documentation guidelines a practice might use to ensure accurate medical record documentation include the following:[24]
    - The medical record is complete and legible;
    - The documentation of each patient encounter includes the reason for the encounter; any relevant history; physical examination findings; prior diagnostic test results; assessment,

clinical impression, or diagnosis; plan of care; and date and legible identity of the observer;

- If not documented, the rationale for ordering diagnostic and other ancillary services can be easily inferred by an independent reviewer or third party who has appropriate medical training;
- CPT and ICD-9-CM codes used for claims submission are supported by documentation and the medical record; and
- Appropriate health risk factors are identified. The patient's progress, his or her response to, and any changes in, treatment, and any revision in diagnosis is documented.

The CPT and ICD-9-CM codes reported on the health insurance claims form should be supported by documentation in the medical record and the medical chart should contain all necessary information. Additionally, HCFA and the local carriers should be able to determine the person who provided the services. These issues can be the root of investigations of inappropriate or erroneous conduct, and have been identified by HCFA and the OIG as a leading cause of improper payments.

One method for improving quality in documentation is for a physician practice to compare the practice's claim denial rate to the rates of other practices in the same specialty to the extent that the practice can obtain that information from the carrier. Physician coding and diagnosis distribution can be compared for each physician within the same specialty to identify variances.

ii. HCFA 1500 Form
Another documentation area for physician practices to monitor closely is the proper completion of the HCFA 1500 form. The following practices will help ensure that the form has been properly completed:

- link the diagnosis code with the reason for the visit or service;
- use modifiers appropriately;
- provide Medicare with all information about a beneficiary's other insurance coverage under the Medicare Secondary Payor (MSP) policy, if the practice is aware of a beneficiary's additional coverage.

d. Improper Inducements, Kickbacks and Self-Referrals
A physician practice would be well advised to have standards and procedures that encourage compliance with the anti kickback statute[25] and the physician self-referral

law.[26] Remuneration for referrals is illegal because it can distort medical decision-making, cause overutilization of services or supplies, increase costs to Federal health care programs, and result in unfair competition by shutting out competitors who are unwilling to pay for referrals. Remuneration for referrals can also affect the quality of patient care by encouraging physicians to order services or supplies based on profit rather than the patients' best medical interests.[27]

In particular, arrangements with hospitals, hospices, nursing facilities, home health agencies, durable medical equipment suppliers, pharmaceutical manufacturers and vendors are areas of potential concern. In general the anti-kickback statute prohibits knowingly and willfully giving or receiving anything of value to induce referrals of Federal health care program business. It is generally recommended that all business arrangements wherein physician practices refer business to, or order services or items from, an outside entity should be on a fair market value basis.[28] Whenever a physician practice intends to enter into a business arrangement that involves making referrals, the arrangement should be reviewed by legal counsel familiar with the anti-kickback statute and physician self-referral statute.

In addition to developing standards and procedures to address arrangements with other health care providers and suppliers, physician practices should also consider implementing measures to avoid offering inappropriate inducements to patients.[29] Examples of such inducements include routinely waiving coinsurance or deductible amounts without a good faith determination that the patient is in financial need or failing to make reasonable efforts to collect the cost-sharing amount.[30]

Possible risk factors relating to this risk area that could be addressed in the practice's standards and procedures include:

- financial arrangements with outside entities to whom the practice may refer Federal health care program business;[31]

- joint ventures with entities supplying goods or services to the physician practice or its patients;[32]

- consulting contracts or medical directorships;

- office and equipment leases with entities to which the physician refers; and

- soliciting, accepting or offering any gift or gratuity of more than nominal value to or from those who may benefit from a physician practice's referral of Federal health care program business.[33]

In order to keep current with this area of the law, a physician practice may obtain copies, available on the OIG web site or in hard copy from the OIG, of all relevant OIG Special Fraud Alerts and Advisory Opinions that address the application of the anti-kickback and physician self-referral laws to ensure that the standards and procedures reflect current positions and opinions.

2. Retention of Records

In light of the documentation requirements faced by physician practices, it would be to the practice's benefit if its standards and procedures contained a section on the retention of compliance, business and medical records. These records primarily include documents relating to patient care and the practice's business activities. A physician practice's designated compliance contact could keep an updated binder or record of these documents, including information relating to compliance activities. The primary compliance documents that a practice would want to retain are those that relate to educational activities, internal investigations and internal audit results. We suggest that particular attention should be paid to documenting investigations of potential violations uncovered by the compliance program and the resulting remedial action. Although there is no requirement that the practice retain its compliance records, having all the relevant documentation relating to the practice's compliance efforts or handling of a particular problem can benefit the practice should it ever be questioned regarding those activities.

Physician practices that implement a compliance program might also want to provide for the development and implementation of a records retention system. This system would establish standards and procedures regarding the creation, distribution, retention, and destruction of documents. If the practice decides to design a record system, privacy concerns and Federal or State regulatory requirements should be taken into consideration.[34]

While conducting its compliance activities, as well as its daily operations, a physician practice would be well advised, to the extent it is possible, to document its efforts to comply with applicable Federal health care program requirements. For example, if a physician practice requests advice from a Government agency (including a Medicare carrier) charged with administering a Federal health care program, it is to the benefit of the practice to document and retain a record of the request and any written or oral response (or nonresponse). This step is extremely important if the practice intends to rely on that

response to guide it in future decisions, actions, or claim reimbursement requests or appeals.

In short, it is in the best interest of all physician practices, regardless of size, to have procedures to create and retain appropriate documentation. The following record retention guidelines are suggested:

- The length of time that a practice's records are to be retained can be specified in the physician practice's standards and procedures (Federal and State statutes should be consulted for specific time frames, if applicable);

- Medical records (if in the possession of the physician practice) need to be secured against loss, destruction, unauthorized access, unauthorized reproduction, corruption, or damage; and

- Standards and procedures can stipulate the disposition of medical records in the event the practice is sold or closed.

Step Three: Designation of a Compliance Officer/Contact(s)

After the audits have been completed and the risk areas identified, ideally one member of the physician practice staff needs to accept the responsibility of developing a corrective action plan, if necessary, and oversee the practice's adherence to that plan. This person can either be in charge of all compliance activities for the practice or play a limited role merely to resolve the current issue. In a formalized institutional compliance program there is a compliance officer who is responsible for overseeing the implementation and day-to-day operations of the compliance program. However, the resource constraints of physician practices make it so that it is often impossible to designate one person to be in charge of compliance functions.

It is acceptable for a physician practice to designate more than one employee with compliance monitoring responsibility. In lieu of having a designated compliance officer, the physician practice could instead describe in its standards and procedures the compliance functions for which designated employees, known as "compliance contacts," would be responsible. For example, one employee could be responsible for preparing written standards and procedures, while another could be responsible for conducting or arranging for periodic audits and ensuring that billing questions are answered. Therefore, the compliance-related responsibilities of the designated person or persons may be only a portion of his or her duties.

Another possibility is that one individual could serve as compliance officer for more than one entity. In situations where staffing limitations mandate that the practice cannot afford to designate a person(s) to oversee compliance activities, the practice could outsource all or part of the functions of a compliance officer to a third party, such as a consultant, PPMC, MSO, IPA or third-party billing company. However, if this role is outsourced, it is beneficial for the compliance officer to have sufficient interaction with the physician practice to be able to effectively understand the inner workings of the practice. For example, consultants that are not in close geographic proximity to a practice may not be effective compliance officers for the practice.

One suggestion for how to maintain continual interaction is for the practice to designate someone to serve as a liaison with the outsourced compliance officer. This would help ensure a strong tie between the compliance officer and the practice's daily operations. Outsourced compliance officers, who spend most of their time off-site, have certain limitations that a physician practice should consider before making such a critical decision. These limitations can include lack of understanding as to the inner workings of the practice, accessibility and possible conflicts of interest when one compliance officer is serving several practices.

If the physician practice decides to designate a particular person(s) to oversee all compliance activities, not just those in conjunction with the audit-related issue, the following is a list of suggested duties that the practice may want to assign to that person(s):

- overseeing and monitoring the implementation of the compliance program;

- establishing methods, such as periodic audits, to improve the practice's efficiency and quality of services, and to reduce the practice's vulnerability to fraud and abuse;

- periodically revising the compliance program in light of changes in the needs of the practice or changes in the law and in the standards and procedures of Government and private payor health plans;

- developing, coordinating and participating in a training program that focuses on the components of the compliance program, and seeks to ensure that training materials are appropriate;

- ensuring that the HHS-OIG's List of Excluded Individuals and Entities, and the General Services Administration's (GSA's) List of Parties Debarred from

Federal Programs have been checked with respect to all employees, medical staff and independent contractors;[35] and

- investigating any report or allegation concerning possible unethical or improper business practices, and monitoring subsequent corrective action and/or compliance.

Each physician practice needs to assess its own practice situation and determine what best suits that practice in terms of compliance oversight.

Step Four: Conducting Appropriate Training and Education

Education is an important part of any compliance program and is the logical next step after problems have been identified and the practice has designated a person to oversee educational training. Ideally, education programs will be tailored to the physician practice's needs, specialty and size and will include both compliance and specific training.

There are three basic steps for setting up educational objectives:

- determining who needs training (both in coding and billing and in compliance);

- determining the type of training that best suits the practice's needs (e.g., seminars, in-service training, self-study or other programs); and

- determining when and how often education is needed and how much each person should receive.

Training may be accomplished through a variety of means, including in-person training sessions (i.e., either on site or at outside seminars), distribution of newsletters,[36] or even a readily accessible office bulletin board. Regardless of the training modality used, a physician practice should ensure that the necessary education is communicated effectively and that the practice's employees come away from the training with a better understanding of the issues covered.

1. Compliance Training

Under the direction of the designated compliance officer/contact, both initial and recurrent training in compliance is advisable, both with respect to the compliance program itself and applicable statutes and regulations. Suggestions for items to include in compliance training are: the operation and importance of the compliance program; the consequences of violating the standards and procedures set forth in the program; and the role of each employee in the operation of the compliance program.

There are two goals a practice should strive for when conducting compliance training: (1) all employees will receive training on how to perform their jobs in compliance with the standards of the practice and any applicable regulations; and (2) each employee will understand that compliance is a condition of continued employment. Compliance training focuses on explaining why the practice is developing and establishing a compliance program. The training should emphasize that following the standards and procedures will not get a practice employee in trouble, but violating the standards and procedures may subject the employee to disciplinary measures. It is advisable that new employees be trained on the compliance program as soon as possible after their start date and employees should receive refresher training on an annual basis or as appropriate.

2. Coding and Billing Training
Coding and billing training on the Federal health care program requirements may be necessary for certain members of the physician practice staff depending on their respective responsibilities. The OIG understands that most physician practices do not employ a professional coder and that the physician is often primarily responsible for all coding and billing. However, it is in the practice's best interest to ensure that individuals who are directly involved with billing, coding or other aspects of the Federal health care programs receive extensive education specific to that individual's responsibilities. Some examples of items that could be covered in coding and billing training include:

- coding requirements;

- claim development and submission processes;

- signing a form for a physician without the physician's authorization;

- proper documentation of services rendered;

- proper billing standards and procedures and submission of accurate bills for services or items rendered to Federal health care program beneficiaries; and

- the legal sanctions for submitting deliberately false or reckless billings.

3. Format of the Training Program
Training may be conducted either in-house or by an outside source.[37] Training at outside seminars, instead of internal programs and in-service sessions, may be an effective way to achieve the practice's training goals. In fact, many community colleges offer certificate or associate degree programs in billing and coding, and professional associations provide various kinds of continuing education and certification programs. Many carriers also offer billing training.

The physician practice may work with its third-party billing company, if one is used, to ensure that documentation is of a level that is adequate for the billing company to submit accurate claims on behalf of the physician practice. If it is not, these problem areas should also be covered in the training. In addition to the billing training, it is advisable for physician practices to maintain updated ICD-9, HCPCS and CPT manuals (in addition to the carrier bulletins construing those sources) and make them available to all employees involved in the billing process. Physician practices can also provide a source of continuous updates on current billing standards and procedures by making publications or Government documents that describe current billing policies available to its employees.[38]

Physician practices do not have to provide separate education and training programs for the compliance and coding and billing training. All in-service training and continuing education can integrate compliance issues, as well as other core values adopted by the practice, such as quality improvement and improved patient service, into their curriculum.

4. Continuing Education on Compliance Issues
There is no set formula for determining how often training sessions should occur. The OIG recommends that there be at least an annual training program for all individuals involved in the coding and billing aspects of the practice. Ideally, new billing and coding employees will be trained as soon as possible after assuming their duties and will work under an experienced employee until their training has been completed.

Step Five: Responding to Detected Offenses and Developing Corrective Action Initiatives
When a practice determines it has detected a possible violation, the next step is to develop a corrective action plan and determine how to respond to the problem. Violations of a physician practice's compliance program, significant failures to comply with applicable Federal or State law, and other types of misconduct threaten a practice's status as a reliable, honest, and trustworthy provider of health care. Consequently, upon receipt of reports or reasonable indications of suspected noncompliance, it is important that the compliance contact or other practice employee look into the allegations to determine whether a significant violation of applicable law or the requirements of the compliance program has

indeed occurred, and, if so, take decisive steps to correct the problem.[40] As appropriate, such steps may involve a corrective action plan,[41] the return of any overpayments, a report to the Government,[42] and/or a referral to law enforcement authorities.

One suggestion is that the practice, in developing its compliance program, develop its own set of monitors and warning indicators. These might include: significant changes in the number and/or types of claim rejections and/or reductions; correspondence from the carriers and insurers challenging the medical necessity or validity of claims; illogical patterns or unusual changes in the pattern of CPT-4, HCPCS or ICD-9 code utilization; and high volumes of unusual charge or payment adjustment transactions. If any of these warning indicators become apparent, then it is recommended that the practice follow up on the issues. Subsequently, as appropriate, the compliance procedures of the practice may need to be changed to prevent the problem from recurring.

For potential criminal violations, a physician practice would be well advised in its compliance program procedures to include steps for prompt referral or disclosure to an appropriate Government authority or law enforcement agency. In regard to overpayment issues, it is advised that the physician practice take appropriate corrective action, including prompt identification and repayment of any overpayment to the affected payor.

It is also recommended that the compliance program provide for a full internal assessment of all reports of detected violations. If the physician practice ignores reports of possible fraudulent activity, it is undermining the very purpose it hoped to achieve by implementing a compliance program.

It is advised that the compliance program standards and procedures include provisions to ensure that a violation is not compounded once discovered. In instances involving individual misconduct, the standards and procedures might also advise as to whether the individuals involved in the violation either be retrained, disciplined, or, if appropriate, terminated. The physician practice may also prevent the compounding of the violation by conducting a review of all confirmed violations, and, if appropriate, self-reporting the violations to the applicable authority.

The physician practice may consider the fact that if a violation occurred and was not detected, its compliance program may require modification. Physician practices that detect violations could analyze the situation to determine whether a flaw in their compliance program failed to anticipate the detected problem, or whether the compliance program's procedures failed to prevent the violation. In any event, it is prudent, even absent the detection of any violations, for physician practices to periodically review and modify their compliance programs.

Step Six: Developing Open Lines of Communication

In order to prevent problems from occurring and to have a frank discussion of why the problem happened in the first place, physician practices need to have open lines of communication. Especially in a smaller practice, an open line of communication is an integral part of implementing a compliance program. Guidance previously issued by the OIG has encouraged the use of several forms of communication between the compliance officer/committee and provider personnel, many of which focus on formal processes and are more costly to implement (e.g., hotlines and e-mail). However, the OIG recognizes that the nature of some physician practices is not as conducive to implementing these types of measures. The nature of a small physician practice dictates that such communication and information exchanges need to be conducted through a less formalized process than that which has been envisioned by prior OIG guidance.

In the small physician practice setting, the communication element may be met by implementing a clear "open door" policy between the physicians and compliance personnel and practice employees. This policy can be implemented in conjunction with less formal communication techniques, such as conspicuous notices posted in common areas and/or the development and placement of a compliance bulletin board where everyone in the practice can receive up-to-date compliance information.[43]

A compliance program's system for meaningful and open communication can include the following:

- the requirement that employees report conduct that a reasonable person would, in good faith, believe to be erroneous or fraudulent;

- the creation of a user-friendly process (such as an anonymous drop box for larger practices) for effectively reporting erroneous or fraudulent conduct;

- provisions in the standards and procedures that state that a failure to report erroneous or fraudulent conduct is a violation of the compliance program;

- the development of a simple and readily accessible procedure to process reports of erroneous or fraudulent conduct;

- if a billing company is used, communication to and from the billing company's compliance officer/contact and other responsible staff to coordinate billing and compliance activities of the practice and the billing company, respectively. Communication can include, as appropriate, lists of reported or identified concerns, initiation and the results of internal assessments, training needs, regulatory changes, and other operational and compliance matters;

- the utilization of a process that maintains the anonymity of the persons involved in the reported possible erroneous or fraudulent conduct and the person reporting the concern; and

- provisions in the standards and procedures that there will be no retribution for reporting conduct that a reasonable person acting in good faith would have believed to be erroneous or fraudulent.

The OIG recognizes that protecting anonymity may not be feasible for small physician practices. However, the OIG believes all practice employees, when seeking answers to questions or reporting potential instances of erroneous or fraudulent conduct, should know to whom to turn for assistance in these matters and should be able to do so without fear of retribution. While the physician practice may strive to maintain the anonymity of an employee's identity, it also needs to make clear that there may be a point at which the individual's identity may become known or may have to be revealed in certain instances.

Step Seven: Enforcing Disciplinary Standards Through Well-Publicized Guidelines

Finally, the last step that a physician practice may wish to take is to incorporate measures into its practice to ensure that practice employees understand the consequences if they behave in a non-compliant manner. An effective physician practice compliance program includes procedures for enforcing and disciplining individuals who violate the practice's compliance or other practice standards. Enforcement and disciplinary provisions are necessary to add credibility and integrity to a compliance program. The OIG recommends that a physician practice's enforcement and disciplinary mechanisms ensure that violations of the practice's compliance policies will result in consistent and appropriate sanctions, including the

possibility of termination, against the offending individual. At the same time, it is advisable that the practice's enforcement and disciplinary procedures be flexible enough to account for mitigating or aggravating circumstances. The procedures might also stipulate that individuals who fail to detect or report violations of the compliance program may also be subject to discipline. Disciplinary actions could include: warnings (oral); reprimands (written); probation; demotion; temporary suspension; termination; restitution of damages; and referral for criminal prosecution. Inclusion of disciplinary guidelines in in-house training and procedure manuals is sufficient to meet the "well publicized" standard of this element.

It is suggested that any communication resulting in the finding of non-compliant conduct be documented in the compliance files by including the date of incident, name of the reporting party, name of the person responsible for taking action, and the follow-up action taken. Another suggestion is for physician practices to conduct checks to make sure all current and potential practice employees are not listed on the OIG or GSA lists of individuals excluded from participation in Federal health care or Government procurement programs.[44]

C. Assessing A Voluntary Compliance Program
A practice's commitment to compliance can best be assessed by the active application of compliance principles in the day-to-day operations of the practice. Compliance programs are not just written standards and procedures that sit on a shelf in the main office of a practice, but are an everyday part of the practice operations. It is by integrating the compliance program into the practice culture that the practice can best achieve maximum benefit from its compliance program.

III. Conclusion

Just as immunizations are given to patients to prevent them from becoming ill, physician practices may view the implementation of a voluntary compliance program as comparable to a form of preventive medicine for the practice. This voluntary compliance program guidance is intended to assist physician practices in developing and implementing internal controls and procedures that promote adherence to Federal health care program requirements.

As stated earlier, physician compliance programs do not need to be time or resource intensive and can be developed in a manner that best reflects the nature of each individual practice. Many of the recommendations set forth in this document are ones that many physician practices already have in place and are simply good business practices that can be adhered to with a reasonable amount of effort. By implementing an effective compliance program, appropriate for its size and resources, and making compliance principles an active part of the practice culture, a physician practice can help prevent and reduce erroneous or fraudulent conduct in its practice. These efforts can also streamline and improve the business operations within the practice and therefore help to innoculate it against future problems.

Endnotes

[1]   For the purpose of this guidance, the term "physician" is defined as: (1) a doctor of medicine or osteopathy; (2) a doctor of dental surgery or of dental medicine; (3) a podiatrist; (4) an optometrist; or (5) a chiropractor, all of whom must be appropriately licensed by the State. 42 U.S.C. 1395x(r).

[2]   Much of this guidance can also apply to other independent practitioners, such as psychologists, physical therapists, speech language pathologists, and occupational therapists.

[3]   Currently, the OIG has issued compliance program guidance for the following eight industry sectors: hospitals, clinical laboratories, home health agencies, durable medical equipment suppliers, third-party medical billing companies, hospices, Medicare+Choice organizations offering coordinated care plans, and nursing facilities. The guidance listed here and referenced in this document is available on the OIG web site at oig.hhs.gov in the Electronic Reading Room or by calling the OIG Public Affairs office at (202) 619-1343.

[4]   The OIG has issued Advisory Opinions responding to specific inquiries concerning the application of the OIG's authorities, in particular, the anti-kickback statute, and Special Fraud Alerts setting forth activities that raise legal and enforcement issues. These documents, as well as reports from the OIG's Office of Audit Services and Office of Evaluation and Inspections can be obtained via the Internet address or phone number provided in Footnote 3. Physician practices can also review the Health Care Financing Administration (HCFA) web site on the Internet at cms.hhs.gov, for up-to-date regulations, manuals, and program memoranda related to the Medicare and Medicaid programs.

[5]   31 U.S.C. 3729.

[6]   42 U.S.C. 1320a-7a.

[7]   *See* Appendix D.II. referencing the Provider Self-Disclosure Protocol for information on how to conduct a baseline audit.

[8]   Physician practices with laboratories or arrangements with third-party billing companies can also check the risk areas included in the OIG compliance program guidance for those industries.

[9]   The OIG and HCFA are working to compile a list of basic documents issued by both entities that could be included in such a binder. We expect to complete this list later this fall, and will post it on the OIG and HCFA web sites as well as publicize this list to physician organizations and representatives (information on how to contact the OIG is contained in Footnote 3; HCFA information can be obtained at www.hcfa.gov/medlearn or by calling 1-800-MEDICARE).

[10]   Physician practices seeking additional guidance on potential risk areas can review the OIG's Work Plan to identify vulnerabilities and risk areas on which the OIG will focus in the future. In addition, physician practices can also review the OIG's semiannual reports, which identify program vulnerabilities and risk areas that the OIG has targeted during the preceding six months. All of these documents are available on the OIG's webpage at oig.hhs.gov.

[11]   Appendix A of this document lists additional risk areas that a physician practice may want to review and incorporate into their practice standards and procedures.

[12]   For example, Dr. X, an ophthalmologist, billed for laser surgery he did not perform. As one element of proof, he did not even have laser equipment or access to such equipment at the place of service designated on the claim form where he performed the surgery.

[13]   Billing for services, supplies and equipment that are not reasonable and necessary involves seeking reimbursement for a service that is not warranted by a patient's documented medical condition. See 42 U.S.C. 1395i(a)(1)(A) ("no payment may be made under part A or part B [of Medicare] for any expenses incurred for items or services which . . . are not reasonable and necessary for the diagnosis or treatment of illness or injury or to improve the functioning of the malformed body member"). *See also* Appendix A for further discussion on this topic.

[14]   Double billing occurs when a physician bills for the same item or service more than once or another party billed the Federal health care program for an item or service also billed by the physician. Although duplicate billing can occur due to simple error, the knowing submission of duplicate claims—which is sometimes evidenced by systematic or repeated double billing—can create liability under criminal, civil, and/or administrative law.

[15]   For example, Dr. Y bills Medicare using a covered office visit code when the actual service was a non-covered annual physical. Physician practices should remember that "necessary" does not always constitute "covered" and that this example is a misrepresentation of services to the Federal health care programs.

[16]   An example of this is when the practice bills for a service performed by Dr. B, who has not yet been issued a Medicare provider number, using Dr. A's Medicare provider number. Physician practices need to bill using the correct Medicare provider number,

even if that means delaying billing until the physician receives his/her provider number.

17   Unbundling is the practice of a physician billing for multiple components of a service that must be included in a single fee. For example, if dressings and instruments are included in a fee for a minor procedure, the provider may not also bill separately for the dressings and instruments.

18   A modifier, as defined by the CPT-4 manual, provides the means by which a physician practice can indicate a service or procedure that has been performed has been altered by some specific circumstance, but not changed in its definition or code. Assuming the modifier is used correctly and appropriately, this specificity provides the justification for payment for those services. For correct use of modifiers, the physician practice should reference the appropriate sections of the *Medicare Provider Manual. See Medicare Carrier Manual* § 4630. For general information on the correct use of modifiers, a physician practice can consult the National Correct Coding Initiative (NCCI). *See* Appendix F for information on how to download the NCCI edits. The NCCI coding edits are updated on a quarterly basis and are used to process claims and determine payments to physicians.

19   This is the practice of coding/charging one or two middle levels of service codes exclusively, under the philosophy that some will be higher, some lower, and the charges will average out over an extended period (in reality, this overcharges some patients while undercharging others).

20   Upcoding is billing for a more expensive service than the one actually performed. For example, Dr. X intentionally bills at a higher evaluation and management (E&M) code than what he actually renders to the patient.

21   The official coding guidelines are promulgated by HCFA, the National Center for Health Statistics, the American Hospital Association, the American Medical Association and the American Health Information Management Association. *See* International Classification of Diseases, 9th Revision, Clinical Modification (ICD-9 CM)(and its successors); 1998 Health Care Financing Administration Common Procedure Coding System (HCPCS) (and its successors); and Physicians' CPT. In addition, there are specialized coding systems for specific segments of the health care industry. Among these are ADA (for dental procedures), DSM IV (psychiatric health benefits) and DMERCs (for durable medical equipment, prosthetics, orthotics and supplies).

22   The failure of a physician practice to: (i) document items and services rendered; and (ii) properly submit the corresponding claims for reimbursement is a major area of potential erroneous or fraudulent conduct involving Federal health care programs. The OIG has undertaken numerous audits, investigations, inspections and national enforcement initiatives in these areas.

23   " . . . for the diagnosis or treatment of illness or injury or to improve the functioning of a malformed body member." 42 U.S.C. 1395y(a)(1)(A).

24   *For additional information on proper documentation, physician practices should also reference the Documentation Guidelines for Evaluation and Management Services*, published by HCFA. Currently, physicians may document based on the 1995 or 1997 E&M Guidelines, whichever is most advantageous to the physician. A new set of draft guidelines were announced in June 2000, and are undergoing pilot testing and revision, but are not in current use.

25   The anti-kickback statute provides criminal penalties for individuals and entities that knowingly offer, pay, solicit, or receive bribes or kickbacks or other remuneration in order to induce business reimbursable by Federal health care programs. See 42 U.S.C. 1320a-7b(b). Civil penalties, exclusion from participation in the Federal health care programs, and civil False Claims Act liability may also result from a violation of the prohibition. *See* 42 U.S.C. 1320a-7a(a)(5), 42 U.S.C. 1320a-7(b)(7), and 31 U.S.C. 3729-3733.

26   The physician self-referral law, 42 U.S.C. 1395nn (also known as the "Stark law"), prohibits a physician from making a referral to an entity with which the physician or any member of the physician's immediate family has a financial relationship if the referral is for the furnishing of designated health services, unless the financial relationship fits into an exception set forth in the statute or implementing regulations.

27   *See* Appendix B for additional information on the anti-kickback statute.

28   The OIG's definition of "fair market value" excludes any value attributable to referrals of Federal program business or the ability to influence the flow of such business. See 42 U.S.C. 1395nn(h)(3). Adhering to the rule of keeping business arrangements at fair market value is not a guarantee of legality, but is a highly useful general rule.

29   See 42 U.S.C. 1320a-7a(a)(5).

30   In the OIG Special Fraud Alert "Routine Waiver of Part B Co-payments/ Deductibles" (May 1991), the OIG describes several reasons why routine waivers of these cost-sharing amounts pose concerns. The Alert sets forth the circumstances under which it may be appropriate to waive these amounts. *See also* 42 U.S.C. 1320a-7a(a)(5).

[31] All physician contracts and agreements with parties in a position to influence Federal health care program business or to whom the doctor is in such a position to influence should be reviewed to avoid violation of the anti-kickback, self-referral, and other relevant Federal and State laws. The OIG has published safe harbors that define practices not subject to the anti-kickback statute, because such arrangements would be unlikely to result in fraud or abuse. Failure to comply with a safe harbor provision does not make an arrangement per se illegal. Rather, the safe harbors set forth specific conditions that, if fully met, would assure the entities involved of not being prosecuted or sanctioned for the arrangement qualifying for the safe harbor. One such safe harbor applies to personal services contracts. *See* 42 CFR 1001.952(d).

[32] *See* OIG Special Fraud Alert "Joint Venture Arrangements" (August 1989) available on the OIG web site at oig.hhs.gov. *See also* OIG Advisory Opinion 97-5.

[33] Physician practices should establish clear standards and procedures governing gift-giving because such exchanges may be viewed as inducements to influence business decisions.

[34] There are various Federal regulations governing the privacy of patient records and the retention of certain types of patient records. Many states also have record retention statutes. Practices should check with their state medical society and/or affiliated professional association for assistance in ascertaining these requirements for their particular specialty and location.

[35] The HHS-OIG "List of Excluded Individuals/Entities" provides information to health care providers, patients, and others regarding individuals and entities that are excluded from participation in Federal health care programs. This report, in both an on-line searchable and downloadable database, can be located on the Internet at oig.hhs.gov. The OIG sanction information is readily available to users in two formats on over 15,000 individuals and entities currently excluded from program participation through action taken by the OIG. The on-line searchable database allows users to obtain information regarding excluded individuals and entities sorted by: (1) the legal bases for exclusions; (2) the types of individuals and entities excluded by the OIG; and (3) the States where excluded individuals reside or entities do business. In addition, the General Services Administration maintains a monthly listing of debarred contractors.

[36] HCFA also offers free online training for general fraud and abuse issues at http://www.hcfa.gov/medlearn. See Appendix F for additional information.

[37] As noted earlier in this guidance, another way for physician practices to receive training is for the physicians and/or the employees of the practice to attend training programs offered by outside entities, such as a hospital, a local medical society or a carrier. This sort of collaborative effort is an excellent way for the practice to meet the desired training objective without having to expend the resources to develop and implement in-house training.

[38] Some publications, such as OIG's Special Fraud Alerts, audit and inspection reports, and Advisory Opinions are readily available from the OIG and can provide a basis for educational courses and programs for physician practice employees. See Appendix F for a partial listing of these documents. *See* Footnote 3 for information on how to obtain copies of these documents.

[39] Currently, the OIG is monitoring a significant number of corporate integrity agreements that require many of these training elements. The OIG usually requires a minimum of one hour annually for basic training in compliance areas. Additional training may be necessary for specialty fields such as claims development and billing.

[40] Instances of noncompliance must be determined on a case-by-case basis. The existence or amount of a monetary loss to a health care program is not solely determinative of whether the conduct should be investigated and reported to governmental authorities. In fact, there may be instances where there is no readily identifiable monetary loss to a health care provider, but corrective actions are still necessary to protect the integrity of the applicable program and its beneficiaries, e.g., where services required by a plan of care are not provided.

[41] The physician practice may seek advice from its legal counsel to determine the extent of the practice's liability and to plan the appropriate course of action.

[42] The OIG has established a Provider Self-Disclosure Protocol that encourages providers to voluntarily report suspected fraud. The concept of voluntary self-disclosure is premised on a recognition that the Government alone cannot protect the integrity of the Medicare and other Federal health care programs. Health care providers must be willing to police themselves, correct underlying problems, and work with the Government to resolve these matters. The Provider Self-Disclosure Protocol can be located on the OIG's web site at: oig.hhs.gov. *See* Appendix D for further information on the Provider Self-Disclosure Protocol.

[43] In addition to whatever other method of communication is being utilized, the OIG recommends that physician practices post the HHS-OIG Hotline telephone number (1-800-HHS-TIPS) in a prominent area.

[44] *See* Footnote 35 for information on how to access these lists.

Appendix A: Additional Risk Areas

Appendix A describes additional risk areas that a physician practice may wish to address during the development of its compliance program. If any of the following risk areas are applicable to the practice, the practice may want to consider addressing the risk areas by incorporating them into the practice's written standards and procedures manual and addressing them in its training program.

I. Reasonable and Necessary Services

A. Local Medical Review Policy

An area of concern for physicians relating to determinations of reasonable and necessary services is the variation in local medical review policies (LMRPs) among carriers. Physicians are supposed to bill the Federal health care programs only for items and services that are reasonable and necessary. However, in order to determine whether an item or service is reasonable and necessary under Medicare guidelines, the physician must apply the appropriate LMRP.[1]

With the exception of claims that are properly coded and submitted to Medicare solely for the purpose of obtaining a written denial, physician practices are to bill the Federal health programs only for items and services that are covered. In order to determine if an item or service is covered for Medicare, a physician practice must be knowledgeable of the LMRPs applicable to its practice's jurisdiction. The practice may contact its carrier to request a copy of the pertinent LMRPs, and once the practice receives the copies, they can be incorporated into the practice's written standards and procedures manual. When the LMRP indicates that an item or service may not be covered by Medicare, the physician practice is responsible to convey this information to the patient so that the patient can make an informed decision concerning the health care services he/she may want to receive. Physician practices convey this information through Advance Beneficiary Notices (ABNs).

B. Advance Beneficiary Notices

Physicians are required to provide ABNs before they provide services that they know or believe Medicare does not consider reasonable and necessary. (The one exception to this requirement is for services that are performed pursuant to EMTALA requirements as described in section II.A). A properly executed ABN acknowledges that coverage is uncertain or yet to be determined, and stipulates that the patient promises to pay the bill if

Medicare does not. Patients who are not notified before they receive such services are not responsible for payment. The ABN must be sufficient to put the patient on notice of the reasons why the physician believes that the payment may be denied. The objective is to give the patient sufficient information to allow an informed choice as to whether to pay for the service.

Accordingly, each ABN should:

1. be in writing;

2. identify the specific service that may be denied (procedure name and CPT/HCPC code is recommended);

3. state the specific reason why the physician believes that service may be denied; and

4. be signed by the patient acknowledging that the required information was provided and that the patient assumes responsibility to pay for the service.

The *Medicare Carrier's Manual*[2] provides that an ABN will not be acceptable if: (1) the patient is asked to sign a blank ABN form; or (2) the ABN is used routinely without regard to a particularized need. The routine use of ABNs is generally prohibited because the ABN must state the specific reason the physician anticipates that the specific service will not be covered.

A common risk area associated with ABNs is in regard to diagnostic tests or services. There are three steps that a physician practice can take to help ensure it is in compliance with the regulations concerning ABNs for diagnostic tests or services:

1. determine which tests are not covered under national coverage rules;

2. determine which tests are not covered under local coverage rules such as LMRPs (contact the practice's carrier to see if a listing has been assembled); and

3. determine which tests are only covered for certain diagnoses.

The OIG is aware that the use of ABNs is an area where physician practices experience numerous difficulties. Practices can help to reduce problems in this area by educating their physicians and office staff on the correct use of ABNs, obtaining guidance from the carrier regarding their interpretation of whether an ABN is necessary where the service is not covered, developing a standard form for all diagnostic tests (most carriers have a developed model), and developing a process for handling patients who refuse to sign ABNs.

C. Physician Liability for Certifications in the Provision of Medical Equipment and Supplies and Home Health Services

In January 1999, the OIG issued a Special Fraud Alert on this topic, which is available on the OIG web site at oig.hhs.gov/fraud/fraudalerts.html. The following is a summary of the Special Fraud Alert.

The OIG issued the Special Fraud Alert to reiterate to physicians the legal and programmatic significance of physician certifications made in connection with the ordering of certain items and services for Medicare patients. In light of information obtained through OIG provider audits, the OIG deemed it necessary to remind physicians that they may be subject to criminal, civil and administrative penalties for signing a certification when they know that the information is false or for signing a certification with reckless disregard as to the truth of the information. (See Appendix B and Appendix C for more detailed information on the applicable statutes).

Medicare has conditioned payment for many items and services on a certification signed by a physician attesting that the physician has reviewed the patient's condition and has determined that an item or service is reasonable and necessary. Because Medicare primarily relies on the professional judgment of the treating physician to determine the reasonable and necessary nature of a given service or supply, it is important that physicians provide complete and accurate information on any certifications they sign. Physician certification is obtained through a variety of forms, including prescriptions, orders, and Certificates of Medical Necessity (CMNs). Two areas where physician certification as to whether an item or service is reasonable and necessary is essential and which are vulnerable to abuse are: (1) home health services; and (2) durable medical equipment. By signing a CMN, the physician represents that:

1. he or she is the patient's treating physician and that the information regarding the physician's address and unique physician identification number (UPIN) is correct;

2. the entire CMN, including the sections filled out by the supplier, was completed prior to the physician's signature; and

3. the information in section B relating to whether the item or service is reasonable and necessary is true, accurate, and complete to the best of the physician's knowledge.

Activities such as signing blank CMNs, signing a CMN without seeing the patient to verify the item or service is reasonable and necessary, and signing a CMN for a service that the physician knows is not reasonable and necessary are activities that can lead to criminal, civil and administrative penalties.

Ultimately, it is advised that physicians carefully review any form of certification (order, prescription or CMN) before signing it to verify that the information contained in the certification is both complete and accurate.

D. Billing for Non-covered Services as if Covered

In some instances, we are aware that physician practices submit claims for services in order to receive a denial from the carrier, thereby enabling the patient to submit the denied claim for payment to a secondary payer.

A common question relating to this risk area is: If the medical services provided are not covered under Medicare, but the secondary or supplemental insurer requires a Medicare rejection in order to cover the services, then would the original submission of the claim to Medicare be considered fraudulent? Under the applicable regulations, the OIG would not consider such submissions to be fraudulent. For example, the denial may be necessary to establish patient liability protections as stated in section 1879 of the Social Security Act (the Act) (codified at 42 U.S.C. 1395pp). As stated, Medicare denials may also be required so that the patient can seek payment from a secondary insurer. In instances where a claim is being submitted to Medicare for this purpose, the physician should indicate on the claim submission that the claim is being submitted for the purpose of receiving a denial, in order to bill a secondary insurance carrier. This step should assist carriers and prevent inadvertent payments to which the physician is not entitled.

In some instances, however, the carrier pays the claim even though the service is non-covered, and even though the physician did not intend for payment to be made. When this occurs,
the physician has a responsibility to refund the amount paid and indicate that the service is not covered.

II. Physician Relationships with Hospitals

A. The Physician Role in EMTALA

The Emergency Medical Treatment and Active Labor Act (EMTALA), 42 U.S.C. 1395dd, is an area that has been receiving increasing scrutiny. The statute is intended to ensure that all patients who come to the emergency department of a hospital receive care, regardless of their insurance or ability to pay. Both hospitals and physicians need to work together to ensure compliance with the provisions of this law.

The statute imposes three fundamental requirements upon hospitals that participate in the Medicare program with regard to patients requesting emergency care. First, the hospital must conduct an appropriate medical screening examination to determine if an emergency medical condition exists.[3] Second, if the hospital determines that an emergency medical condition exists, it must either provide the treatment necessary to stabilize the emergency medical condition or comply with the statute's requirements to effect a proper transfer of a patient whose condition has not been stabilized.[4] A hospital is considered to have met this second requirement if an individual refuses the hospital's offer of additional examination or treatment, or refuses to consent to a transfer, after having been informed of the risks and benefits.[5]

If an individual's emergency medical condition has not been stabilized, the statute's third requirement is activated. A hospital may not transfer an individual with an unstable emergency medical condition unless: (1) the individual or his or her representative makes a written request for transfer to another medical facility after being informed of the risk of transfer and the transferring hospital's obligation under the statute to provide additional examination or treatment; (2) a physician has signed a certification summarizing the medical risks and benefits of a transfer and certifying that, based up on the information available at the time of transfer, the medical benefits reasonably expected from the transfer outweigh the increased risks; or (3) if a physician is not physically present when the transfer decision is made, a qualified medical person signs the certification after the physician, in consultation with the qualified medical person, has made the determination that the benefits of transfer outweigh the increased risks. The physician must later countersign the certification.[6]

Physician and/or hospital misconduct may result in violations of the statute.[7] One area of particular concern is physician on-call responsibilities. Physician practices whose members serve as on-call emergency room physicians with hospitals are advised to familiarize themselves with the hospital's policies regarding on-call physicians. This can be done by reviewing the medical staff bylaws or policies and procedures of the hospital that must define the responsibility of on-call physicians to respond to, examine, and treat patients with emergency medical conditions. Physicians should also be aware of the requirement that, when medically indicated, on-call physicians must generally come to the hospital to examine the patient. The exception to this requirement is that a patient may be sent to see the on-call physician at a hospital-owned contiguous or on-campus facility to conduct or complete the medical screening examination as long as:

1. all persons with the same medical condition are moved to this location;

2. there is a bona fide medical reason to move the patient; and

3. qualified medical personnel accompany the patient.

B. Teaching Physicians

Special regulations apply to teaching physicians' billings. Regulations provide that services provided by teaching physicians in teaching settings are generally payable under the physician fee schedule only if the services are personally furnished by a physician who is not a resident or the services are furnished by a resident in the presence of a teaching physician.[8]

Unless a service falls under a specified exception, such as the Primary Care Exception,[9] the teaching physician must be present during the key portion of any service or procedure for which payment is sought.[10] Physicians should ensure the following with respect to services provided in the teaching physician setting:[11]

• only services actually provided are billed;

• every physician who provides or supervises the provision of services to a patient is responsible for the correct documentation of the services that were rendered;

• every physician is responsible for assuring that in cases where the physician provides evaluation and management (E&M) services, a patient's medical record includes appropriate documentation of the applicable key components of the E&M services provided or supervised by the physician (e.g., patient history, physician examination, and medical decision making), as well as documentation to adequately reflect the procedure or portion of the services provided by the physician; and

• unless specifically excepted by regulation, every physician must document his or her presence during the key portion of any service or procedure for which payment is sought.

C. Gainsharing Arrangements and Civil Monetary Penalties for Hospital Payments to Physicians to Reduce or Limit Services to Beneficiaries

In July 1999, the OIG issued a Special Fraud Alert on this topic, which is available on the OIG web site at oig.hhs.gov/fraud/fraudalerts.html. The following is a summary of the Special Fraud Alert.

The term "gainsharing" typically refers to an arrangement in which a hospital gives a physician a percentage share of any reduction in the hospital's costs for patient care attributable in part to the physician's efforts. The civil monetary penalty (CMP) that applies to gainsharing arrangements is set forth in 42 U.S.C. 1320a-7a(b)(1). This section prohibits any hospital or critical access hospital from knowingly making a payment directly or indirectly to a physician as an inducement to reduce or limit services to Medicare or Medicaid beneficiaries under a physician's care.

It is the OIG's position that the Civil Monetary Penalties Law clearly prohibits any gainsharing arrangements that involve payments by, or on behalf of, a hospital to physicians with clinical care responsibilities to induce a reduction or limitation of services to Medicare or Medicaid beneficiaries. However, hospitals and physicians are not prohibited from working together to reduce unnecessary hospital costs through other arrangements. For example, hospitals and physicians may enter into personal services contracts where hospitals pay physicians based on a fixed fee at fair market value for services rendered to reduce costs rather than a fee based on a share of cost savings.

D. Physician Incentive Arrangements

The OIG has identified potentially illegal practices involving the offering of incentives by entities in an effort to recruit and retain physicians. The OIG is concerned that the intent behind offering incentives to physicians may not be to recruit physicians, but instead the offer is intended as a kickback to obtain and increase patient referrals from physicians. These recruitment incentive arrangements are implicated by the Anti-Kickback Statute because they can constitute remuneration offered to induce, or in return for, the referral of business paid for by Medicare or Medicaid.

Some examples of questionable incentive arrangements are:

- provision of free or significantly discounted billing, nursing, or other staff services.

- payment of the cost of a physician's travel and expenses for conferences.

- payment for a physician's services that require few, if any, substantive duties by the physician.

- guarantees that if the physician's income fails to reach a predetermined level, the entity will supplement the remainder up to a certain amount.

III. Physician Billing Practices

A. Third-Party Billing Services

Physicians should remember that they remain responsible to the Medicare program for bills sent in the physician's name or containing the physician's signature, even if the physician had no actual knowledge of a billing impropriety. The attestation on the HCFA 1500 form, i.e., the physician's signature line, states that the physician's services were billed properly. In other words, it is no defense for the physician if the physician's billing service improperly bills Medicare.

One of the most common risk areas involving billing services deals with physician practices contracting with billing services on a percentage basis. Although percentage based billing arrangements are not illegal per se, the Office of Inspector General has a longstanding concern that such arrangements may increase the risk of intentional upcoding and similar abusive billing practices.[12]

A physician may contract with a billing service on a percentage basis. However, the billing service can not directly receive the payment of Medicare funds into a bank account that it solely controls. Under 42 U.S.C. 1395u(b)(6), Medicare payments can only be made to either the beneficiary or a party (such as a physician) that furnished the services and accepted assignment of the beneficiary's claim. A billing service that contracts on a percentage basis does not qualify as a party that furnished services to a beneficiary, thus a billing service cannot directly receive payment of Medicare funds. According to the Medicare Carriers Manual § 3060(A), a payment is considered to be made directly to the billing service if the service can convert the payment to its own use and control without the payment first passing through the control of the physician. For example, the billing service should not bill the claims under its own name or tax identification number. The billing service should bill claims under the physician's name and tax identification number. Nor should a billing service receive the payment of Medicare funds directly into a bank account over which the billing service maintains sole control. The Medicare payments should instead be deposited into a bank account over which the provider has signature control.

Physician practices should review the third-party medical billing guidance for additional information on third-party billing companies and the compliance risk areas associated with billing companies.

B. Billing Practices by Non-Participating Physicians
Even though nonparticipating physicians do not accept payment directly from the Medicare program, there are a number of laws that apply to the billing of Medicare beneficiaries by non-participating physicians.

Limiting Charges
42 U.S.C. 1395w-4(g) prohibits a nonparticipating physician from knowingly and willfully billing or collecting on a repeated basis an actual charge for a service that is in excess of the Medicare limiting charge. For example, a nonparticipating physician may not bill a Medicare beneficiary $50 for an office visit when the Medicare limiting charge for the visit is $25. Additionally, there are numerous provisions that prohibit nonparticipating physicians from knowingly and willfully charging patients in excess of the statutory charge limitations for certain specified procedures, such as cataract surgery, mammography screening and coronary artery bypass surgery. Failure to comply with these sections can result in a fine of up to $10,000 per violation or exclusion from participation in Federal health care programs for up to five years.

Refund of Excess Charges
42 U.S.C. 1395w-4(g) mandates that if a nonparticipating physician collects an actual charge for a service that is in excess of the limiting charge, the physician must refund the amount collected above the limiting charge to the individual within 30 days notice of the violation. For example, if a physician collected $50 from a Medicare beneficiary for an office visit, but the limiting charge for the visit was $25, the physician must refund $25 to the beneficiary, which is the difference between the amount collected ($50) and the limiting charge ($25). Failure to comply with this requirement may result in a fine of up to $10,000 per violation or exclusion from participation in Federal health care programs for up to five years.

42 U.S.C. 1395u(l)(A)(iii) mandates that a nonparticipating physician must refund payments received from a Medicare beneficiary if it is later determined by a Peer Review Organization or a Medicare carrier that the services were not reasonable and necessary. Failure to comply with this requirement may result in a fine of up to $10,000 per violation or exclusion from participation in Federal health care programs for up to five years.

C. Professional Courtesy
The term "professional courtesy" is used to describe a number of analytically different practices. The traditional definition is the practice by a physician of waiving all or a part of the fee for services provided to the physician's office staff, other physicians, and/or their families. In recent times, "professional courtesy" has also come to mean the waiver of coinsurance obligations or other out-of-pocket expenses for physicians or their families (i.e., "insurance only" billing), and similar payment arrangements by hospitals or other institutions for services provided to their medical staffs or employees. While only the first of these practices is truly "professional courtesy," in the interests of clarity and completeness, we will address all three.

In general, whether a professional courtesy arrangement runs afoul of the fraud and abuse laws is determined by two factors: (i) how the recipients of the professional courtesy are selected; and (ii) how the professional courtesy is extended. If recipients are selected in a manner that directly or indirectly takes into account their ability to affect past or future referrals, the anti-kickback statute—which prohibits giving anything of value to generate Federal health care program business—may be implicated. If the professional courtesy is extended through a waiver of copayment obligations (i.e., "insurance only" billing), other statutes may be implicated, including the prohibition of inducements to beneficiaries, section 1128A(a)(5) of the Act (codified at 42 U.S.C. 1320a-7a(a)(5)). Claims submitted as a result of either practice may also implicate the civil False Claims Act.

The following are general observations about professional courtesy arrangements for physician practices to consider:

- A physician's regular and consistent practice of extending professional courtesy by waiving the entire fee for services rendered to a group of persons (including employees, physicians, and/or their family members) may not implicate any of the OIG's fraud and abuse authorities so long as membership in the group receiving the courtesy is determined in a manner that does not take into account directly or indirectly any group member's ability to refer to, or otherwise generate Federal health care program business for, the physician.

- A physician's regular and consistent practice of extending professional courtesy by waiving otherwise applicable copayments for services rendered to a group of persons (including employees, physicians, and/or their family members), would not implicate the anti-kickback statute so long as membership in the group is determined in a manner that does not take into account directly or indirectly any group member's ability to refer to, or otherwise generate Federal health care program business for, the physician.

- Any waiver of copayment practice, including that described in the preceding bullet, does implicate section 1128A(a)(5) of the Act if the patient for whom the copayment is waived is a Federal health care program beneficiary who is not financially needy.

The legality of particular professional courtesy arrangements will turn on the specific facts presented, and, with respect to the anti-kickback statute, on the specific intent of the parties. A physician practice may wish to consult with an attorney if it is uncertain about its professional courtesy arrangements.

IV. Other Risk Areas

A. Rental of Space in Physician Offices by Persons or Entities to which Physicians Refer

In February 2000, the OIG issued a Special Fraud Alert on this topic, which is available on the OIG web site at **oig.hhs.gov/fraud/fraudalerts.html**. The following is a summary of the Special Fraud Alert.

Among various relationships between physicians and labs, hospitals, home health agencies, etc., the OIG has identified potentially illegal practices involving the rental of space in a physician's office by suppliers that provide items or services to patients who are referred or sent to the supplier by the physician-landlord. An example of a suspect arrangement is the rental of physician office space by a durable medical equipment (DME) supplier in a position to benefit from referrals of the physician's patients. The OIG is concerned that in such arrangements the rental payments may be disguised kickbacks to the physician-landlord to induce referrals.

Space Rental Safe Harbor to the Anti-Kickback Statute

To avoid potentially violating the anti-kickback statute, the OIG recommends that rental agreements comply with all of the following criteria for the space rental safe harbor:

- The agreement is set out in writing and signed by the parties.

- The agreement covers all of the space rented by the parties for the term of the agreement and specifies the space covered by the agreement.

- If the agreement is intended to provide the lessee with access to the space for periodic intervals of time rather than on a full-time basis for the term of the rental agreement, the rental agreement specifies exactly the schedule of such intervals, the precise length of each interval, and the exact rent for each interval.

- The term of the rental agreement is for not less than one year.

- The aggregate rental charge is set in advance, is consistent with fair market value, and is not determined in a manner that takes into account the volume or value of any referrals or business otherwise generated between the parties for which payment may be made in whole or in part under Medicare or a State health care program.

- The aggregate space rented does not exceed that which is reasonably necessary to accomplish the commercially reasonable business purpose of the rental.

B. Unlawful Advertising

42 U.S.C. 1320b-10 makes it unlawful for any person to advertise using the names, abbreviations, symbols, or emblems of the Social Security Administration, Health Care Financing Administration, Department of Health and Human Services, Medicare, Medicaid or any combination or variation of such words, abbreviations, symbols or emblems in a manner that such person knows or should know would convey the false impression that the advertised item is endorsed by the named entities. For instance, a physician may not place an ad in the newspaper that reads "Dr. X is a cardiologist approved by both the Medicare and Medicaid programs." A violation of this section may result in a penalty of up to $5,000 ($25,000 in the case of a broadcast or telecast) for each violation.

Endnotes

[1]   HCFA has recently developed a web site which, when completed by the end of the year 2000, will contain the LMRPs for each of the contractors across the country. The web site can be accessed at http://www.lmrp.net.

[2]   The relevant manual provisions are located at MCM, Part III, §§ 7300 and 7320. This section of the manual also includes the carrier's recommended form of an ABN.

[3]   See 42 U.S.C. 1395dd(a).

[4]   See 42 U.S.C. 1395dd(b)(1).

[5]   See 42 U.S.C. 1395dd(b)(2) and (3).

[6]   See 42 U.S.C. 1395dd(c)(1)(A).

[7]   Hospitals and physicians, including on-call physicians, who violate the statute may face penalties that include civil fines of up to $50,000 (or not more than $25,000 in the case of a hospital with less than 100 beds) per violation, and physicians may be excluded from participation in the Federal health care programs.

[8]   42 CFR 415.150 through 415.190.

[9]   42 CFR 415.174

[10]   *Id.*

[11]   This section is not intended to be and is not a complete reference for teaching physicians. It is strongly recommended that those physicians who practice in a teaching setting consult their respective hospitals for more guidance.

[12]   This concern is noted in Advisory Opinion No. 98-4 and also the Office of Inspector General Compliance Program Guidance for Third-Party Medical Billing Companies. Both are available on the OIG web site at oig.hhs.gov.

Appendix B: Criminal Statutes

This Appendix contains a description of criminal statutes related to fraud and abuse in the context of health care. The Appendix is not intended to be a compilation of all Federal statutes related to health care fraud and abuse. It is merely a summary of some of the more frequently cited Federal statutes.

I. Health Care Fraud (18 U.S.C. 1347)

Description of Unlawful Conduct

It is a crime to knowingly and willfully execute (or attempt to execute) a scheme to defraud any health care benefit program, or to obtain money or property from a health care benefit program through false representations. Note that this law applies not only to Federal health care programs, but to most other types of health care benefit programs as well.

Penalty for Unlawful Conduct

The penalty may include the imposition of fines, imprisonment of up to 10 years, or both. If the violation results in serious bodily injury, the prison term may be increased to a maximum of 20 years. If the violation results in death, the prison term may be expanded to include any number of years, or life imprisonment.

Examples

1. Dr. X, a chiropractor, intentionally billed Medicare for physical therapy and chiropractic treatments that he never actually rendered for the purpose of fraudulently obtaining Medicare payments.

2. Dr. X, a psychiatrist, billed Medicare, Medicaid, TRI-CARE, and private insurers for psychiatric services that were provided by his nurses rather than himself.

II. Theft or Embezzlement in Connection with Health Care (18 U.S.C. 669)

Description of Unlawful Conduct

It is a crime to knowingly and willfully embezzle, steal or intentionally misapply any of the assets of a health care benefit program. Note that this law applies not only to Federal health care programs, but to most other types of health care benefit programs as well.

Penalty for Unlawful Conduct

The penalty may include the imposition of a fine, imprisonment of up to 10 years, or both. If the value of the asset is $100 or less, the penalty is a fine, imprisonment of up to a year, or both.

Example

An office manager for Dr. X knowingly embezzles money from the bank account for Dr. X's practice. The bank account includes reimbursement received from the Medicare program; thus, intentional embezzlement of funds from this account is a violation of the law.

III. False Statements Relating to Health Care Matters (18 U.S.C. 1035)

Description of Unlawful Conduct

It is a crime to knowingly and willfully falsify or conceal a material fact, or make any materially false statement or use any materially false writing or document in connection with the delivery of or payment for health care benefits, items or services. Note that this law applies not only to Federal health care programs, but to most other types of health care benefit programs as well.

Penalty for Unlawful Conduct

The penalty may include the imposition of a fine, imprisonment of up to five years, or both.

Example

Dr. X certified on a claim form that he performed laser surgery on a Medicare beneficiary when he knew that the surgery was not actually performed on the patient.

IV. Obstruction of Criminal Investigations of Health Care Offenses (18 U.S.C. 1518)

Description of Unlawful Conduct

It is a crime to willfully prevent, obstruct, mislead, delay or attempt to prevent, obstruct, mislead, or delay the communication of records relating to a Federal health care offense to a criminal investigator. Note that this law applies not only to Federal health care programs, but to most other types of health care benefit programs as well.

Penalty for Unlawful Conduct

The penalty may include the imposition of a fine, imprisonment of up to five years, or both.

Examples

1. Dr. X instructs his employees to tell OIG investigators that Dr. X personally performs all treatments when, in fact, medical technicians do the majority of the treatment and Dr. X is rarely present in the office.

2. Dr. X was under investigation by the FBI for reported fraudulent billings. Dr. X altered patient records in an attempt to cover up the improprieties.

V. Mail and Wire Fraud
(18 U.S.C. 1341 and 1343)

Description of Unlawful Conduct

It is a crime to use the mail, private courier, or wire service to conduct a scheme to defraud another of money or property. The term "wire services" includes the use of a telephone, fax machine or computer. Each use of a mail or wire service to further fraudulent activities is considered a separate crime. For instance, each fraudulent claim that is submitted electronically to a carrier would be considered a separate violation of the law.

Penalty for Unlawful Conduct

The penalty may include the imposition of a fine, imprisonment of up to five years, or both.

Examples

1. Dr. X knowingly and repeatedly submits electronic claims to the Medicare carrier for office visits that he did not actually provide to Medicare beneficiaries with the intent to obtain payments from Medicare for services he never performed.

2. Dr. X, a neurologist, knowingly submitted claims for tests that were not reasonable and necessary and intentionally upcoded office visits and electromyograms to Medicare.

VI. Criminal Penalties for Acts Involving Federal Health Care Programs
(42 U.S.C. 1320a-7b)

Description of Unlawful Conduct

False Statement and Representations
It is a crime to knowingly and willfully:

1. make, or cause to be made, false statements or representations in applying for benefits or payments under all Federal health care programs;

2. make, or cause to be made, any false statement or representation for use in determining rights to such benefit or payment;

3. conceal any event affecting an individual's initial or continued right to receive a benefit or payment with the intent to fraudulently receive the benefit or payment either in an amount or quantity greater than that which is due or authorized;

4. convert a benefit or payment to a use other than for the use and benefit of the person for whom it was intended;

5. present, or cause to be presented, a claim for a physician's service when the service was not furnished by a licensed physician;

6. for a fee, counsel an individual to dispose of assets in order to become eligible for medical assistance under a State health program, if disposing of the assets results in the imposition of an ineligibility period for the individual.

Anti-Kickback Statute
It is a crime to knowingly and willfully solicit, receive, offer, or pay remuneration of any kind (e.g., money, goods, services):

- for the referral of an individual to another for the purpose of supplying items or services that are covered by a Federal health care program; or

- for purchasing, leasing, ordering, or arranging for any good, facility, service, or item that is covered by a Federal health care program.

There are a number of limited exceptions to the law, also known as "safe harbors," which provide immunity from criminal prosecution and which are described in greater detail in the statute and related regulations (found at 42 CFR 1001.952 and oig.hhs.gov/fraud/safeharborregulations.html. Current safe harbors include:

- investment interests;

- space rental;

- equipment rental;

- personal services and management contracts;

- sale of practice;

- referral services;

- warranties;

- discounts;

- employment relationships;

- waiver of Part A co-insurance and deductible amounts;

- group purchasing organizations;

- increased coverage or reduced cost sharing under a risk-basis or prepaid plan; and

- charge reduction agreements with health plans.

Penalty for Unlawful Conduct

The penalty may include the imposition of a fine of up to $25,000, imprisonment of up to five years, or both. In addition, the provider can be excluded from participation in Federal health care programs. The regulations defining the aggravating and mitigating circumstances that must be reviewed by the OIG in making an exclusion determination are set forth in 42 CFR part 1001.

Examples

1. Dr. X accepted payments to sign Certificates of Medical Necessity for durable medical equipment for patients she never examined.

2. Home Health Agency disguises referral fees as salaries by paying referring physician Dr. X for services Dr. X never rendered to the Medicare beneficiaries or by paying Dr. X a sum in excess of fair market value for the services he rendered to the Medicare beneficiaries.

Appendix C: Civil and Administrative Statutes

This Appendix contains a description of civil and administrative statutes related to fraud and abuse in the context of health care. The Appendix is not intended to be a compilation of all federal statutes related to health care fraud and abuse. It is merely a summary of some of the more frequently cited Federal statutes.

I. The False Claims Act (31 U.S.C. 3729-3733)

Description of Unlawful Conduct

This is the law most often used to bring a case against a health care provider for the submission of false claims to a Federal health care program. The False Claims Act prohibits knowingly presenting (or causing to be presented) to the Federal Government a false or fraudulent claim for payment or approval. Additionally, it prohibits knowingly making or using (or causing to be made or used) a false record or statement to get a false or fraudulent claim paid or approved by the Federal Government or it agents, like a carrier, other claims processor, or State Medicaid program.

Definitions

False Claim—A "false claim" is a claim for payment for services or supplies that were not provided specifically as presented or for which the provider is otherwise not entitled to payment. Examples of false claims for services or supplies that were not provided specifically as presented include, but are not limited to:

- a claim for a service or supply that was never provided.

- a claim indicating the service was provided for some diagnosis code other than the true diagnosis code in order to obtain reimbursement for the service (which would not be covered if the true diagnosis code were submitted).

- a claim indicating a higher level of service than was actually provided.

- a claim for a service that the provider knows is not reasonable and necessary.

- a claim for services provided by an unlicensed individual.

Knowingly—To "knowingly" present a false or fraudulent claim means that the provider: (1) has actual knowledge that the information on the claim is false; (2) acts in deliberate ignorance of the truth or falsity of the information on the claim; or (3) acts in reckless disregard of the truth or falsity of the information on the claim. It is important to note the provider does not have to deliberately intend to defraud the Federal Government in order to be found liable under this Act. The provider need only "knowingly" present a false or fraudulent claim in the manner described above.

Deliberate Ignorance—To act in "deliberate ignorance" means that the provider has deliberately chosen to ignore the truth or falsity of the information on a claim submitted for payment, even though the provider knows, or has notice, that information may be false. An example of a provider who submits a false claim with deliberate ignorance would be a physician who ignores provider update bulletins and thus does not inform his/her staff of changes in the Medicare billing guidelines or update his/her billing system in accordance with changes to the Medicare billing practices. When claims for non-reimbursable services are submitted as a result, the False Claims Act has been violated.

Reckless Disregard—To act in "reckless disregard" means that the provider pays no regard to whether the information on a claim submitted for payment is true or false. An example of a provider who submits a false claim with reckless disregard would be a physician who assigns the billing function to an untrained office person without inquiring whether the employee has the requisite knowledge and training to accurately file such claims.

Penalty for Unlawful Conduct

The penalty for violating the False Claims Act is a minimum of $5,500 up to a maximum of $11,000 for each false claim submitted. In addition to the penalty, a provider could be found liable for damages of up to three times the amount unlawfully claimed.

Examples

1. A physician submitted claims to Medicare and Medicaid representing that he had personally performed certain services when, in reality, the services were performed by a nonphysician and they were not reimbursable under the Federal health care programs.

2. Dr. X intentionally upcoded office visits and angioplasty consultations that were submitted for pay-

ment to Medicare.

3. Dr. X, a podiatrist, knowingly submitted claims to the Medicare and Medicaid programs for non-routine surgical procedures when he actually performed routine, non-covered services such as the cutting and trimming of toenails and the removal of corns and calluses.

II. Civil Monetary Penalties Law (42 U.S.C. 1320a-7a)

Description of Unlawful Conduct

The Civil Monetary Penalties Law (CMPL) is a comprehensive statute that covers an array of fraudulent and abusive activities and is very similar to the False Claims Act. For instance, the CMPL prohibits a health care provider from presenting, or causing to be presented, claims for services that the provider "knows or should know" were:

- not provided as indicated by the coding on the claim;

- not medically necessary;

- furnished by a person who is not licensed as a physician (or who was not properly supervised by a licensed physician);

- furnished by a licensed physician who obtained his or her license through misrepresentation of a material fact (such as cheating on a licensing exam);

- furnished by a physician who was not certified in the medical specialty that he or she claimed to be certified in; or

- furnished by a physician who was excluded from participation in the Federal health care program to which the claim was submitted.

  Additionally, the CMPL contains various other prohibitions, including:

- offering remuneration to a Medicare or Medicaid beneficiary that the person knows or should know is likely to influence the beneficiary to obtain items or services billed to Medicare or Medicaid from a particular provider;

- employing or contracting with an individual or entity that the person knows or should know is excluded from participation in a Federal health care program.

The term "should know" means that a provider: (1) acted in deliberate ignorance of the truth or falsity of the information; or (2) acted in reckless disregard of the truth or falsity of the information. The Federal Government does not have to show that a provider specifically intended to defraud a Federal health care program in order to prove a provider violated the statute.

Penalty for Unlawful Conduct

Violation of the CMPL may result in a penalty of up to $10,000 per item or service and up to three times the amount unlawfully claimed. In addition, the provider may be excluded from participation in Federal health care programs. The regulations defining the aggravating and mitigating circumstances that must be reviewed by the OIG in making an exclusion determination are set forth in 42 CFR part 1001.

Examples

1. Dr. X paid Medicare and Medicaid beneficiaries $20 each time they visited him to receive services and have tests performed that were not preventive care services and tests.

2. Dr. X hired Physician Assistant P to provide services to Medicare and Medicaid beneficiaries without conducting a background check on P. Had Dr. X performed a background check by reviewing the HHS-OIG List of Excluded Individuals/Entities, Dr. X would have discovered that he should not hire P because P is excluded from participation in Federal health care programs for a period of five years.

3. Dr. X and his oximetry company billed Medicare for pulse oximetry that they knew they did not perform and services that had been intentionally upcoded.

III. Limitations on Certain Physician Referrals ("Stark Laws") (42 U.S.C. 1395nn)

Description of Unlawful Conduct

Physicians (and immediate family members) who have an ownership, investment or compensation relationship with an entity providing "designated health services" are prohibited from referring patients for these services where payment may be made by a Federal health care program unless a statutory or regulatory exception applies. An entity providing a designated health service is prohibited from billing for the provision of a service that was provided based on a prohibited referral. Designated health services include: clinical laboratory services; physical therapy services; occupational therapy services; radiology services, including magnetic resonance imaging, axial tomography scans, and ultrasound services; radiation therapy services and supplies; durable medical equipment and supplies; parenteral and enteral nutrients, equipment and supplies; prosthetics, orthotics, prosthetic devices and supplies; home health services; outpatient prescription drugs; and inpatient and outpatient hospital services.

New regulations clarifying the exceptions to the Stark Laws are expected to be issued by HCFA shortly. Current exceptions articulated within the Stark Laws include the following, provided all conditions of each exception as set forth in the statute and regulations are satisfied.

Exceptions for Ownership or Compensation Arrangements

- physician's services;

- in-office ancillary services; and

- prepaid plans.

Exceptions for Ownership or Investment in Publicly Traded Securities and Mutual Funds

- ownership of investment securities which may be purchased on terms generally available to the public;

- ownership of shares in a regulated investment company as defined by Federal law, if such company had, at the end of the company's most recent fiscal year, or on average, during the previous three fiscal years, total assets exceeding $75,000,000;

- hospital in Puerto Rico;

- rural provider; and

- hospital ownership (whole hospital exception).

Exceptions Relating to Other Compensation Arrangements

- rental of office space and rental of equipment;

- bona fide employment relationship;

- personal service arrangement;

- remuneration unrelated to the provision of designated health services;

- physician recruitment;

- isolated transactions;

- certain group practice arrangements with a hospital (pre-1989); and

- payments by a physician for items and services

Penalty for Unlawful Conduct

Violations of the statute subject the billing entity to denial of payment for the designated health services, refund of amounts collected from improperly submitted claims, and a civil monetary penalty of up to $15,000 for each improper claim submitted. Physicians who violate the statute may also be subject to additional fines per prohibited referral. In addition, providers that enter into an arrangement that they know or should know circumvents the referral restriction law may be subject to a civil monetary penalty of up to $100,000 per arrangement.

Examples

1. Dr. A worked in a medical clinic located in a major city. She also owned a free standing laboratory located in a major city. Dr. A referred all orders for laboratory tests on her patients to the laboratory she owned.

2. Dr. X agreed to serve as the Medical Director of Home Health Agency, HHA, for which he was paid a sum substantially above the fair market value for his services. In return, Dr. X routinely referred his Medicare and Medicaid patients to HHA for home health services.

3. Dr. Y received a monthly stipend of $500 from a local hospital to assist him in meeting practice expenses. Dr. Y performed no specific service for the stipend and had no obligation to repay the hospital. Dr. Y referred patients to the hospital for in-patient surgery.

IV. Exclusion of Certain Individuals and Entities From Participation in Medicare and other Federal Health Care Programs (42 U.S.C. 1320a-7)

Mandatory Exclusion

Individuals or entities convicted of the following conduct must be excluded from participation in Medicare and Medicaid for a minimum of five years:

1. a criminal offense related to the delivery of an item or service under Medicare or Medicaid;

2. a conviction under Federal or State law of a criminal offense relating to the neglect or abuse of a patient;

3. a conviction under Federal or State law of a felony relating to fraud, theft, embezzlement, breach of fiduciary responsibility or other financial misconduct against a health care program financed by any Federal, State, or local government agency;

4. a conviction under Federal or State law of a felony relating to the unlawful manufacture, distribution, prescription, or dispensing of a controlled substance.

If there is one prior conviction, the exclusion will be for ten years. If there are two prior convictions, the exclusion will be permanent.

Permissive Exclusion

Individuals or entities convicted of the following offenses, may be excluded from participation in Federal health care programs for a minimum of three years:

1) a criminal offense related to the delivery of an item or service under Medicare or Medicaid;

2) a misdemeanor related to fraud, theft, embezzlement, breach of fiduciary responsibility or other financial misconduct against a health care program financed by any Federal, State, or local government agency;

3) interference with, or obstruction of, any investigation into certain criminal offenses;

4) a misdemeanor related to the unlawful manufacture, distribution, prescription or dispensing of a controlled substance;

5) exclusion or suspension under a Federal or State health care program;

6) submission of claims for excessive charges, unnecessary services or services that were of a quality that fails to meet professionally recognized standards of health care;

7) violating the Civil Monetary Penalties Law or the statute entitled "Criminal Penalties for Acts Involving Federal Health Care Programs;"

8) ownership or control of an entity by a sanctioned individual or immediate family member (spouse, natural or adoptive parent, child, sibling, stepparent, stepchild, stepbrother or stepsister, in-laws, grandparent and grandchild);

9) failure to disclose information required by law;

10) failure to supply claims payment information; and

11) defaulting on health education loan or scholarship obligations.

The above list of offenses is not all inclusive. Additional grounds for permissive exclusion are detailed in the statute.

Examples

1. Nurse R was excluded based on a conviction involving obtaining dangerous drugs by forgery. She also altered prescriptions that were given for her own health problems before she presented them to the pharmacist to be filled.

2. Practice T was excluded due to its affiliation with its excluded owner. The practice owner, excluded from participation in the Federal health care programs for soliciting and receiving illegal kickbacks, was still participating in the day-to-day operations of the practice after his exclusion was effective.

Appendix D: OIG-HHS Contact Information

I. OIG Hotline Number

One method for providers to report potential fraud, waste, and abuse problems is to contact the OIG Hotline number. All HHS and contractor employees have a responsibility to assist in combating fraud, waste and abuse in all departmental programs. As such, providers are encouraged to report matters involving fraud, waste and mismanagement in any departmental program to the OIG. The OIG maintains a hotline that offers a confidential means for reporting these matters.

Contacting the OIG Hotline

By Phone:	1-800-HHS-TIPS (1-800-447-8477)
By E-Mail:	HHSTips@oig.hhs.gov
By Mail:	Office of Inspector General
	Department of Health and Human
	Services
	Attn: HOTLINE
	330 Independence Ave., S.W.
	Washington, D.C. 20201

When contacting the Hotline, please provide the following information to the best of your ability:

- Type of Complaint:
  Medicare Part A
  Medicare Part B
  Indian Health Service
  TRICARE
  Other (please specify)

- HHS Department or program being affected by your allegation of fraud, waste, abuse/mismanagement:

- Health Care Financing Administration (HCFA)
  Indian Health Service
  Other (please specify)

Please provide the following information. (However, if you would like your referral to be submitted anonymously, please indicate such in your correspondence or phone call.)

Your Name
Your Street Address
Your City/County
Your State
Your Zip Code
Your email Address

- Subject/Person/Business/Department that allegation is against.
  Name of Subject
  Title of Subject
  Subject's Street Address
  Subject's City/County
  Subject's State
  Subject's Zip Code

Please provide a brief summary of your allegation and the relevant facts.

II. Provider Self-Disclosure Protocol

The recommended method for a provider to contact the OIG regarding potential fraud or abuse issues that may exist in the provider's own organization is through the use of the Provider Self-Disclosure Protocol. This program encourages providers to voluntarily disclose irregularities in their dealings with Federal health care programs. While voluntary disclosure under the protocol does not guarantee a provider protection from civil, criminal, or administrative actions, the fact that a provider voluntarily disclosed possible wrongdoing is a mitigating factor in OIG's recommendations to prosecuting agencies. Although other agencies may not have formal policies offering immunity or mitigation for self-disclosure, they typically view self-disclosure favorably for the self-disclosing entity. Self-reporting offers providers the opportunity to minimize the potential cost and disruption of a full-scale audit and investigation, to negotiate a fair monetary settlement, and to avoid an OIG permissive exclusion preventing the provider from doing business with Federal health care programs. In addition, if the provider is obligated to enter into an Integrity Agreement (IA) as part of the resolution of a voluntary disclosure, there are three benefits the provider might receive as a result of self-reporting:

- If the provider has an effective compliance program and agrees to maintain its compliance program as part of the False Claims Act settlement, the OIG may not even require an IA;

- In cases where the provider's own audits detected the disclosed problem, the OIG may consider alternatives to the IA's auditing provisions. The provider may be able to perform some or all of its billing audits through internal auditing methods rather than be required to retain an independent review organization to perform the billing review; and

- Self-disclosing can help to demonstrate a provider's trustworthiness to the OIG and may result in the OIG determining that it can sufficiently safeguard the Federal health care programs through an IA without the exclusion remedy for a material breach, which is typically included in an IA.

Specific instructions on how a physician practice can submit a voluntary disclosure under the Provider Self-Disclosure Protocol can be found on the OIG's internet site at oig.hhs.gov or in the Federal Register at 63 FR 58399 (1998). A physician practice may, however, wish to consult with an attorney prior to submitting a disclosure to the OIG.

The Provider Self-Disclosure Protocol can also be a useful tool for baseline audits. The protocol details the OIG's views on the appropriate elements of an effective investigative and audit plan for providers. Physician practices can use the self-disclosure protocol as a model for conducting audits and self-assessments.

In relying on the protocol for audit design and sample selection, a physician practice should pay close attention to the sections on self-assessment and sample selection. These two sections provide valuable guidance regarding how these two functions should be performed.

The self-assessment section of the protocol contains information that can be applied to audit design. Self-assessment is an internal financial assessment to determine the monetary impact of the matter. The approach of a review can include reviewing either all claims affected or a statistically valid sample of the claims.

Sample selection must include several elements. These elements are drawn from the government sampling program known as RAT-STATS.[1] All of these elements are set forth in more detail in the Provider Self-Disclosure Protocol, but the elements are (1) sampling unit, (2) sampling frame, (3) probe, (4) sample size, (5) random numbers, (6) sample design and (7) missing sample items. All of these sampling items should be clearly documented by the physician practice and compiled in the format set forth in the Provider Self-Disclosure Protocol. Use of the format set forth in the Provider Self-Disclosure Protocol will help physician practices to ensure that the elements of their internal audits are in conformance with OIG standards.

Endnote

[1]　Available through the OIG web site at oig.hhs.gov.

Appendix E: Carrier Contact Information

Medicare

A complete list of contact information (address, phone number, email address) for Medicare Part A Fiscal Intermediaries, Medicare Part B Carriers, Regional Home Health Intermediaries, and Durable Medical Equipment Regional Carriers can be found on the HCFA web site at www.hcfa.gov/medicare/incardir.htm.

Medicaid

Contact information (address, phone number, email address) for each State Medicaid carrier can be found on the HCFA web site at www.hcfa.gov/medicaid/mcontact.htm. In addition to a list of Medicaid carriers, the web site includes contact information for each State survey agency and the HCFA Regional Offices.

Contact information for each State Medicaid Fraud Control Unit can be found on the OIG web site at oig.hhs.gov.

Appendix F: Internet Resources

Office of Inspector General-U.S. Department of Health and Human Services

oig.hhs.gov

This web site includes a variety of information relating to Federal health care programs, including the following:

    Advisory Opinions
    Anti-kickback Information
    Compliance Program Guidance
    Corporate Integrity Agreements
    Fraud Alerts
    Links to web pages for the:
    Office of Audit Services (OAS)
    Office of Evaluation and Inspections (OEI)
    Office of Investigations (OI)
    OIG List of Excluded Individuals/Entities
    OIG News
    OIG Regulations
    OIG Semi-Annual Report
    OIG Workplan

Health Care Financing Administration

www.hcfa.gov

This web site includes information on a wide array of topics, including the following:

Medicare
    National Correct Coding Initiative
    Intermediary-Carrier Directory
    Payment
    Program Manuals
    Program Transmittals & Memorandum
    Provider Billing/HCFA Forms
    Statistics and Data

Medicaid
    HCFA Regional Offices
    Letters to State Medicaid Directors
    Medicaid Hotline Numbers
    Policy & Program Information
    State Medicaid Contacts
    State Medicaid Manual
    State Survey Agencies
    Statistics and Data

HCFA Medicare Training

www.hcfa.gov/medlearn

This site provides computer-based training on the following topics:

    HCFA 1500 Form
    Fraud & Abuse
    ICD-9-CM Diagnosis Coding
    Adult Immunization
    Medicare Secondary Payer (MSP)
    Women's Health
    Front Office Management
    Introduction to the World of Medicare
    Home Health Agency
    HCFA 1450 (UB92)

Government Printing Office

www.access.gpo.gov

This site provides access to Federal statutes and regulations pertaining to Federal health care programs.

The U.S. House of Representatives Internet Library

uscode.house.gov/usc.htm

This site provides access to the United States Code, which contains laws pertaining to Federal health care programs.

Index